IN VITRO FERTILISATION IN THE 1990s

In Vitro Fertilisation in the 1990s

Towards a medical, social and ethical evaluation

Edited by
ELISABETH HILDT
DIETMAR MIETH

Ashgate
Aldershot • Brookfield USA • Singapore • Sydney

Published by
Ashgate Publishing Limited
Gower House
Croft Road
Aldershot
Hants GU11 3HR
England

Ashgate Publishing Company
Old Post Road
Brookfield
Vermont 05036
USA

British Library Cataloguing in Publication Data
In vitro fertilisation in the 1990s : towards a medical,
social and ethical evaluation
1. Fertilization in vitro, Human 2. Fertilization in vitro,
Human - Moral and ethical aspects
I. Hildt, Elisabeth II. Mieth, Dietmar
176

Library of Congress Catalog Card Number: 97-76952

ISBN 1 85972 685 2

Printed in Great Britain by The Ipswich Book Company, Suffolk.

Contents

List of contributors

Deryck Beyleveld is Professor of Jurisprudence at the University of Sheffield and Founding Director of the Sheffield Institute of Biotechnological Law and Ethics (SIBLE).

Dieter Birnbacher is Professor of Philosophy at the University of Düsseldorf.

Alberto Bondolfi has a PhD in Theology. His research focusses on biomedical ethics and he is the President of the Swiss Society for Biomedical Ethics.

Aldo Campana is Head of the Department of Obstetrics and Gynaecology of the University Hospital Geneva.

Ian D. Cooke is Professor of Obstetrics and Gynaecology, Jessop Hospital for Women at the University of Sheffield.

Robert G. Edwards is Emeritus Professor of Human Reproduction at the University of Cambridge and Chief Editor of the journal *Human Reproduction.*

Eve-Marie Engels holds the Chair for Ethics in the Life Sciences in the Department of Biology at the University of Tübingen.

Yvon Englert is Head of the Fertility Clinic of the Erasmus Hospital at the Free University of Brussels.

Ulrich Göhring is a gynaecologist at the Gynaecological Hospital in Bielefeld-Rosenhöhe.

Sigrid Graumann is a scholar of the post-graduate college 'Ethics in the Sciences and Humanities' in the Center for Ethics in the Sciences and Humanities at the University of Tübingen.

Hille Haker is Research Assistant for Theological Ethics in Catholic Theology at the University of Tübingen.

Elisabeth Hildt is Scientific Coordinator of the *European Network for Biomedical Ethics* at the Center for Ethics in the Sciences and Humanities of the University of Tübingen.

Jürgen Horst is Chairman of the Department of Human Genetics at the University of Münster.

Carmen Kaminsky is Research Assistant in Philosophy of the University of Düsseldorf.

Hans-Georg Koch is a researcher at the Max Planck Institute (MPI) for Foreign and International Criminal Law in Freiburg i.Br., responsible for development and direction of MPI's 'Law and Medicine' Department.

Lene Koch is Senior Research Fellow at the University of Copenhagen, Institute of Social Medicine.

Lorna Leaston studied Socio-legal Studies. She is writing a PhD thesis on Gewirthian theory at the Sheffield Institute of Biotechnological Law and Ethics.

Walter Lesch is an ethicist at the Interdisciplinary Institute for Ethics and Human Rights at the University of Fribourg.

Brian A. Lieberman is Professor of Gynaecology at the Manchester Fertility Services.

Paulus Liening studied Philosophy and Social Sciences. He is writing a PhD thesis on distributive justice and resource allocation in health care systems.

Calum MacKellar teaches Biological Chemistry in Edinburgh. In addition, he is part-time Editor of the European Journal of Genetics in Society.

Deirdre Madden is Lecturer in Law at the University College Cork, where she specialises in medical law, and is completing a PhD thesis on reproductive technologies.

Barbara Maier is a gynaecologist working in Salzburg at the 'Salzburger Frauenklinik' and teaches medical ethics at Vienna University.

Ulrike Mau is a clinical geneticist in the Department of Anthropology and Human Genetics at the University of Tübingen.

Anne McLaren is Principal Research Associate at the Wellcome Trust/Cancer Research Campaign Institute of Cancer and Developmental Biology.

Dieter Meschede is Research Assistant at the Institute of Human Genetics at the University of Münster.

Dietmar Mieth is Professor of Theological Ethics at Tübingen, leader of the research project *European Network for Biomedical Ethics* and speaker of the Interdisciplinary Center for Ethics in the Sciences and Humanities.

Hansjakob Müller is Professor of Human Genetics and Head of the Department of Medical Genetics of the University Children's Hospital Basel and of the Laboratory of Human Genetics of the Basel University Clinics.

Stefan Müller is Scientific Coordinator of the Research Centre on Biotechnology and Law in Lüneburg.

Stella Reiter-Theil is Research Coordinator at the Centre for Ethics and Law in Medicine, University Hospital Freiburg i. Br.

Lone Schmidt is Assistant Professor at the Institute of Public Health, Department of Health Services Research, University of Copenhagen.

Paul Schotsmans is Professor of Medical Ethics and Director of the Centre for Biomedical Ethics and Law at the School of Medicine, K.U. Leuven.

Egbert Schroten is Professor for Christian Ethics at Utrecht University and Director of the University Centre for Bioethics and Health Law.

Klaus Steigleder is a researcher at the Institute for Philosophy of the University of Stuttgart. His research interests include the foundation and application of ethics.

Monika Stuhlinger studied Theology and Medicine in Tübingen. She is completing a PhD thesis on medical ethics.

Agneta Sutton is Managing Research Fellow of the Centre for Bioethics and Public Policy in London and Managing Editor of the journal *Ethics in Medicine*.

Phil Taylor is chairman of CHILD, a British infertility support group. His wife Kathie Taylor delivered twins after IVF-treatment.

Hans-Rudolf Tinneberg is Professor of Gynaecology at the Gynaecological Hospital in Bielefeld-Rosenhöhe.

Paul J.M. van Tongeren is Professor for Philosophical Ethics at the Catholic University of Nijmegen and Chairman of the Center for Ethics of the Catholic University of Nijmegen (CEKUN).

Günter Virt is Director of the Institute for Ethics in Medicine, Vienna.

Dilys Walker is Clinical Director of the Department of Obstetrics and Gynaecology of the University Hospital Geneva.

Guido de Wert is a Senior Research Fellow at the Institute for Bioethics, Maastricht, and Associate Professor in Medical Ethics at the Erasmus University Rotterdam.

Urban Wiesing is visiting lecturer for medical ethics at the University of Tübingen.

Farhan Yazdani is hospital surgeon in Annecy and member of the Institute Droit et Ethique de la Santé, Lyon.

Hub A.G. Zwart is Scientific Director of the Center for Ethics of the Catholic University of Nijmegen (CEKUN).

Preface

In vitro fertilisation (IVF) was developed as a technology to remedy infertility. Defective functioning of a woman's Fallopian tubes was considered the classical indication. Soon, however, IVF came into use for other fertility malfunctions. In spite of its widespread use, there are still many difficulties linked to this technology. Evaluations of IVF success rates vary greatly; they range from reports of increasing success rates to doubts over any significant success when compared to the occurrence of spontaneous pregnancies. The psychological consequences of IVF for women have been a source of intense controversy. Psychosocial aspects of infertility also have to be considered here. Important ethical questions are related to the status of human embryos and the way in which human embryos are handled in reproductive medicine. In addition, there is a need for consideration of the technological realities behind the wish to have a child.

The extension of diagnostic possibilities to IVF could modify the conditions of access to IVF-programmes and thus fundamentally change the therapy. Whereas IVF previously was restricted to infertility treatment, now in connection with preimplantation diagnosis it may be utilised for the detection and avoidance of hereditary handicaps by selection.

This volume is a collection of the lectures delivered at the symposium 'IVF in the 90s – Methods, Contexts, Consequences' which took place from 16 to 19 January 1997 in Stuttgart, Germany. The symposium was organised by the *European Network for Biomedical Ethics*, a concerted action funded by the European Commission within Biomed 2. The *European Network for Biomedical Ethics* works on ethical problems of IVF with particular regard to its connection with genetic diagnosis and therapy.

The contributions to this book cover different fields of research such as medicine, human genetics, philosophy, theology, social sciences and law. In order to bring out the different points of view and to work towards an interdisciplinary evaluation, each subject area consists of texts written by researchers working in different disciplines, thereby accessing their respective professional backgrounds.

Thus, this book has a thoroughly interdisciplinary character. It may serve as a survey of the great number of aspects offered by IVF to the various disciplines and presents the relevant differences and the ways of reaching agreement. In particular, the differences in the social acceptance and moral assessment of the new reproductive technologies are clarified, as well as the different legal regulations in the various European countries. Of special interest are issues related to infertility, adequate indications for IVF, aspects directly pertaining to IVF treatment, questions surrounding supernumerary embryos, the connections between IVF and preimplantation diagnosis, as well as issues related to the increasing technicalisation of reproduction.

Acknowledgement

This book is a collection of the lectures delivered at the symposium 'IVF in the 90s – Methods, Contexts, Consequences', which was organised by the *European Network for Biomedical Ethics*.

Without the help of many people, the symposium could not have been carried out and this book could not have been prepared. We are especially indebted to Christof Mandry and Katja Ruppel for their intensive and invaluable assistance with various aspects of the *European Network for Biomedical Ethics*, ranging from help in the organisation of the symposium to assistance in the editorial work on this book. We would like to heartily thank Marcus Düwell for his continuous support in the planning and organisation of the network and the symposium, for helpful ideas, advice, and fascinating discussions. We thank Paul Barber and Michael McGettigan for help with proofreading and Albrecht Nestle and Elisabeth Kurfeß for help with the editorial work on this book. We would also like to thank the Center for Ethics in the Sciences and Humanities, University of Tübingen, for technical support, especially Astrid Lutz, Martin Reinke and Simone Sauter. We thank Sigrid Graumann, Hille Haker and Johannes Kraaibeek for advice in the preparation of the network, and Michael von Doering for organisational help.

We are grateful to the European Commission for the generous funding of the *European Network for Biomedical Ethics*, the symposium 'IVF in the 90s – Methods, Contexts, Consequences', and the publication of its results.

List of abbreviations

ART	Assisted reproductive technology
Art.	Article
BMI	Body mass index
CCNE	Comité Consultatif National d'Ethique
CDC	Center for Disease Control
CECOS	Centers for the Study and Conservation of Human Oocytes and Sperm
CF	Cystic fibrosis
CHILD	National infertility support group
CVS	Chorionic villus sampling
DAZ	Deleted in azoospermia
DI	Donor insemination
DNA	Deoxyribonucleic acid
ECHR	European Convention on Human Rights
ESchG	Embryo Protection Law (Embryonenschutzgesetz)
ET	Embryo transfer
EU	European Union
FF	Franc Français
FISH	Fluorescence in situ hybridisation
FIVNAT	French National Association for IVF
FSH	Follicle-stimulating hormone
GCR	Generic conditions of rights
GF	Generic features of agency
GIFT	Gamete intra Fallopian transfer
GLGT	Germline gene therapy
GMC	General Medical Council
GnRH	Gonadotrophin releasing hormone

GP	General practitioner
HCG	Human chorionic gonadotrophin
HFEA	Human Fertilisation and Embryology Authority
HFE Act	Human Fertilisation and Embryology Act
HIV	Human immunodeficiency virus
HMG	Human menopausal gonadotrophin
hr	hours
ICSI	Intracytoplasmic sperm injection
IUI	Intra uterine insemination
IVF	In vitro fertilisation
KNMG	Royal Dutch Society of Medicine
LH	Luteinising hormone
LHRH	Luteinising hormone releasing hormone
MESA	Microsurgical sperm aspiration
MFPR	Multifetal pregnancy reduction
OHSS	Ovarian hyperstimulation syndrome
PCBs	Polychlorinated biphenols
PCDD	Polychlorinated dibenzo-dioxin
PCDFs	Polychlorinated dibenzo-furans
PCP	Pentachlorophenol
PCR	Polymerase chain reaction
PESA	Percutaneous epididymal sperm aspiration
PGC	Principle of generic consistency
PID	Preimplantation diagnosis
PND	Prenatal diagnosis
PRINS	Primed in situ synthesis
TCDD	Tetrachlorodibenzodioxin
TESE	Testicular sperm extraction
TOP	Termination of pregnancy
UK	United Kingdom
UNESCO	United Nations Educational, Scientific, and Cultural Organisation
US	United States
WHO	World Health Organisation
ZIFT	Zygote intra Fallopian transfer

Part One
INTRODUCTION

1 Introduction and development of IVF and its ethical regulation

Robert G. Edwards

Human reproduction in its various forms has always attracted intense ethical attention. Sexuality in its various forms, prostitution, contraception, abortion and sperm donation by intercourse or by artificial insemination have dominated debate over many centuries. In vitro fertilisation (IVF) is a newcomer to this scene, yet it raises many equally important issues. My intention in this paper is to describe the origins of IVF and other forms of assisted human conception and the reasons why the early pioneers began these studies. I will then discuss the ethical role of doctors and scientists in the IVF clinic, and finally consider some modern aspects of the current methods of regulation of assisted human conception, especially the problems of legislation. Currently, ethical responsibility is shared between practising IVF clinics and regulatory agencies which interpret legislation and are responsible to a Minister of State. After welcoming the move to legislation a decade ago, I now have reservations about law as a primary regulator of the many complex personal and clinical situations in assisted human conception.

Scientific and clinical origins of human IVF

IVF has had diverse origins. Much of the initial work carried out on animals was concerned with pure and applied endocrine, embryological and genetic methods, which took almost 50 years to come to fruition. The first investigator contributing to the development of IVF is generally recognised as Heape (1890) who transferred genetically-marked embryos from a female rabbit to the reproductive tract of a recipient, and obtained offspring from the transferred embryos. This study was strictly concerned with embryo transfer, yet it also included a brief period of embryo culture in vitro. The first attempts to culture mammalian embryos through their cleavage stages in vitro were made by Lewis and Gregory (1933), Lewis and Hartman (1933), and Hammond (1949). Embryos of several species were cultured by these investigators through several cell cycles in vitro, using simple culture media. An improved understanding of tissue culture media (Paul 1961) accelerated these studies on embryo culture and led to the first colonies of mammalian (rabbit) embryonic stem cells in vitro (Cole et al. 1966). Meanwhile, Pincus and Saunders (1939) had carried out initial investigations on the maturation of rabbit and human ova in vitro. They aspirated resting (dictyate) oocytes from ovarian follicles and matured them in vitro to metaphase-2, to produce 'ripe' oocytes ready for fertilisation. They concluded that maturation required 12 hours, a mistaken conclusion that misled later investigators who tried to fertilise human oocytes in vitro by adding spermatozoa to oocytes that had been cultured for 12 hours; no fertilisation was recorded in these studies (Menkin and Rock 1968, Shettles 1955, Hayashi 1963). This situation period has been reviewed in detail elsewhere (Edwards and Brody 1995).

Rapidly increasing knowledge on the pituitary gland and hypothalamus in the second quarter of this century resulted in methods of endocrinologically stimulating many follicles in the ovary. These studies led in turn to methods of superovulating immature mice using pregnant mares' serum as an follicle-stimulating hormone (FSH) preparation and human chorionic gonadotrophin (HCG) to induce oestrus and ovulation. The embryos developed normally in foster mothers (Gates and Beatty 1954). Ovarian stimulation was applied to adult mice – the first time in any adult mammal – and also induced timed oestrus and ovulation of many oocytes - often approaching 50 or 100 ('superovulation') (Fowler and Edwards 1957). Oocyte maturation and ovulation were exactly timed, many eggs were fertilised in vivo, and most of them cleaved, implanted and developed to birth (Fowler and Edwards 1957). Many mice had very large numbers of fetuses at full term, multiple births, and rates of fetal mortality in utero and at delivery were very high (Edwards and Fowler 1959).

Between 1950-1970, studies on fertilisation in vitro in animals led to the concept of capacitation of spermatozoa before fertilisation (Austin 1969, Chang 1969). Unfortunately, a widespread belief that spermatozoa became capacitated only in the uterus or oviduct led to immense problems in achieving fertilisation in vitro in mammals except in hamsters, where epididymal spermatozoa were simply mixed with ripe oocytes (Yanagimachi and Chang 1964). Methods of embryo culture were improving, especially with rabbit embryos, but those of mice, hamster, rat, farm animals still displayed blocks in development at different stages, and it was literally impossible to obtain late cleavage embryos in any of these species (see Edwards and Brody 1995).

In the 1960s, the first modern application of assisted human conception involved the use of pituitary extracts and hormone preparations to stimulate ovulation in some amenorrhoeic patients. The first studies were carried out by Gemzell (1967), using pituitary extracts for stimulation and HCG to induce ovulation. Multiple ovulation and births occurred just as in mice. Lunenfeld and Donini (1969) introduced the use of human menopausal gonadotrophins (HMG) for ovarian stimulation, and identified forms of hyperstimulation, multiple pregnancies and the standard use of HMG and HCG for inducing ovulation as a routine treatment in amenorrhoeic women. Clomiphene was also introduced some years later, and proved to be an effective and mild ovarian stimulant (Greenblatt et al. 1961). The induction of superovulation in amenorrhoeic women raised considerable ethical qualms, concerned at first with the establishment of many multiple births, some of a very high order. Recently, it has been discovered that the use of pituitary extracts to stimulate follicle growth in these women infected many of them with Jacob Creutzfeld disease. Many died from this condition several years after treatment.

Innovations in surgery in the early and mid-20th century, an increasing tempo of research on laparoscopy (Palmer 1946, Fragenheim 1964) led to the first attempts at endoscopy to examine the abdominal cavity. Laparoscopy were greatly refined and made safe by the application of cold light sources, and became a routine treatment in gynaecology as shown by Steptoe (1968). By now, laparoscopy (and keyhole surgery) is used in virtually every gynaecological operating theatre, and keyhole surgery in many other forms of surgery.

IVF itself has been practised widely only in the last quarter of the twentieth century, as the necessary hormone preparations, knowledge of oocyte maturation, fertilisation and embryonic growth in vitro, and new surgical methods, combined to facilitate its introduction. My own purposes in introducing IVF were to alleviate various clinical conditions and open new approaches to gaining fundamental knowledge on human conception, as listed in table 1. In fact, the alleviation of infertility has so far been its major application, although analyses of the origin of chromosomal disorders and the preimplantation diagnosis of genetic disease are making excellent progress. IVF raised many new ethical issues such as the status of the embryo in vitro, typing embryos and the possibilities of interference with gametes or embryos. The growth of early embryos in vitro also challenged the nature of parenthood by opening possibilities of oocyte and embryo donation, and of surrogate parenting of a transferred embryo.

Table 1. Original purposes of the introduction of IVF

- Gain fundamental knowledge on human conception
- Investigate the ethics of human conception involved in studies on IVF, contraception, gamete donation, embryo research, etc
- Attempt to alleviate infertility
- Understand and improve methods of contraception
- Identify the causes of human chromosomal disorders
- Design methods for diagnosing and avoiding genetic disease before implantation
- Produce human stem cells in vitro for analyses on differentiation and transplantation

The introduction of modern IVF

By 1955, the necessary techniques to introduce human IVF had been clarified, and new research programmes were essential to bring the method into clinical practice. Fundamental knowledge was needed on the processes of human follicle growth, oocyte maturation, ovulation, the origin of chromosomal anomalies such as trisomy, and fertilisation and embryo growth before and after implantation. Besides leading to the introduction of IVF, each of these studies would raise complex ethical situations, which would have to be debated and assessed.

The first target was to time oocyte maturation in vitro. This knowledge would help to avert the need for studies on patients during these initial investigative stages. Studies in animals had revealed that the duration of maturation in vitro was equal to the interval between an ovulatory injection of HCG and the beginning of follicle rupture at ovulation (Edwards 1965a). Modern IVF actually began when detailed analyses on the maturation of human oocytes in vitro revealed that 37 hours were needed for oocyte ripening to metaphase-2 (Edwards 1965a,b). This discovery enabled some of the studies outlined in table 1 to be carried out, namely the cause of chromosomal anomalies in oocytes, and the use of mature oocytes to study fertilisation in vitro.

Initial attempts at fertilisation in vitro using human oocytes matured in vitro, and at achieving human sperm capacitation by placing them in intrauterine chambers for several hours, were apparently unsuccessful (Edwards et al. 1966, Edwards et al. 1968). A closer analysis of the exact conditions of culture resulted in the first definite evidence of human fertilisation in vitro (Edwards et al. 1969). This was a major step towards clinical work. Related animal studies established the first embryonic stem cells in vitro, using rabbits (Cole et al. 1966), the first successful genetic diagnosis of a mammalian embryo using excised trophectoderm cells from rabbit blastocysts to sex the embryos

(Edwards and Gardner 1968, Gardner and Edwards 1968), and new concepts on the causes of chromosomal anomalies (Henderson and Edwards 1968).

Knowledge on the timing of human maturation in vitro predicted the timing of ovulation in women at 37 hr post-HCG. The optimal time to collect ripe human oocytes from follicles in vivo would therefore be at 35-36 hr, i.e. shortly before ovulation occurred. Maturation in vivo was essential to obtain normal embryonic growth, because Chang (1969) had shown how rabbit oocytes matured in vitro would fail to develop normally unless their initial maturation was triggered within the follicle.

Clinical IVF began in Oldham and Cambridge using modern methods of laparoscopy to time human ovulation and to aspirate ripe oocytes from their follicles (Steptoe and Edwards 1970). The predicted timing of ovulation was 37 hours post-HCG and follicular growth was directly observed laparoscopically at this time. After the use of ovarian stimulation using HMG and HCG, several oocytes were aspirated from each patient at 36 hr post-HCG. Fertilisation and embryonic growth in vitro were accomplished very quickly (Edwards et al. 1970, Steptoe et al. 1971). Embryonic growth appeared to be normal.

The ethical issues were closely studied from the early years of IVF. I had been stimulated by ethical discussions between Professor Conrad Waddington and theologians on the ethics of genetic research, during lectures on the clinical practice of sperm donation, and when working with Professor Alan Parkes of the importance and ethics of contraception and fertility regulation. The first paper on the ethics of IVF in modern society was published in Nature by Edwards and Sharpe (1971), and later a detailed analysis was made of the ethics and law of human conception (Edwards 1974). These papers covered the same ground as the Warnock Report many years later. Ethical issues were constantly debated by Steptoe and I, including the significance of IVF and the need for fertilisation in vitro to alleviate various forms of infertility, the ethics of asking patients to help with research when they had little chance of benefit, how long to grow embryos in vitro, and the possibilities of alleviating infertility and genetic disease. The misuse of IVF, cloning, other forms of embryonic manipulation, surrogacy and egg donation were discussed constantly.

Early ethical objections to IVF stemmed from several sources, including theologians, politicians and some scientists and doctors, some of whom believed that conception was virtually sacred (table 2). Watson, the Nobel Laureate, believed that many children would be born abnormal. Accusations were made by Kass that IVF cured nothing because the wife remained infertile, even if she delivered a child, after the IVF process was completed. We were charged with misleading the infertile with false promises of babies, or hiding data on various experimental procedures in our laboratories. None of these arguments deterred us. All of our work was published openly, often in well-read journals such as Nature and Lancet. Throughout these years, we were fortified by the close collaboration in ethical matters between Steptoe, Jean Purdy and I, i.e. doctor, nurse and scientist. This helped us to maintain a strong discipline in our work, in clinical and ethical matters. This form of close collaboration has persisted in many IVF clinics today, and it still offers the same advantages.

Table 2. Original objections to the introduction of human IVF

- Fertilising human eggs in vitro was unethical
- The human embryo had full rights from fertilisation
- Embryo research should be prohibited
- Announcements about IVF were misleading the infertile with false promises
- Many babies would be born abnormal
- Embryos would be cryopreserved for centuries
- The first step to cloning
- Misuse of IVF such as its use by white supremacists to increase their population by transferring embryos to black women

The replacement of embryos into infertile mothers began in 1972. After various tribulations concerned with establishing a correct luteal phase, short-lived pregnancies were identified in the early 1970s, and an ectopic pregnancy developed to 10 weeks in 1976 (Steptoe and Edwards 1976). Changes in hormone treatments seemed to be one cause of the low success of embryo transfer, so a switch was made to using the natural cycle and adding clomiphene or bromocryptine to the stimulation regimen. Using the natural cycle, three births occurred in 1978 and 1979 (Steptoe and Edwards 1978). Throughout these years, studies on human embryology and IVF had far outstripped comparable work on animals. Capacitation had now been found to occur in vitro in literally all animal species, just as in humans, but embryos of many animal species could still not be grown to blastocysts in vitro.

The pace of development accelerated in 1980. Bourn Hall and new clinics opened world-wide. Many babies were delivered, clomiphene was added to various forms of ovarian stimulation, the luteinising hormone releasing hormone (LHRH) agonists were introduced in the late 1980s, and recombinant gonadotrophins in the 1990s. Detailed follow-up studies revealed that IVF babies had virtually the same degree of anomalies as those conceived in vivo. Clinical problems were investigated including ovarian hyperstimulation, poor ovarian responses to stimulation, low rates of fertilisation in vitro especially in male infertility, multiple pregnancy and multiple births. Maternal and fetal morbidity and mortality were also generally within the same levels as after natural conception, with the exception of the risks imposed by the high frequency of multiple pregnancies and births, still a major clinical problem of human IVF. The diagnosis of genetic disease in human preimplantation embryos was introduced in 1986, the injection of a single spermatozoon into an oocyte (intracytoplasmic sperm injection – ICSI) in 1993, and currently we await the commercial production of LHRH antagonists to simplify current forms of ovarian stimulation.

Taking clinical and ethical decisions in the IVF clinic

The major interest of this meeting lies in the current ethical situation of assisted human conception. In this part of my lecture, I will describe three recent advances in assisted conception and their ethical consequences, stressing how scientists and doctors (professionals) are taking complex ethical decisions during the course of their daily work.

Ovarian stimulation today: time for a change?

Procedures of ovarian stimulation have steadily become more complex since 1980. HMG and HCG are effective in inducing ovulation but unexpected or attenuated luteinising hormone (LH) surges can induce premature ovulation and abnormal forms of luteinisation. Consequently, during the mid-1970s, clomiphene or bromocryptine were added to control short luteal phases or high prolactin levels respectively. Later, in the 1980s, the LHRH agonists were added to stimulation protocols in order to control LH and avoid unwanted LH surges and spontaneous ovulations. Luteal phase support with HCG, oestrogens and progesterone or progestagens was essential. Contraceptive steroids were added to this regimen, to give a better control over the menstrual cycle. The resulting dampening-down of the cycle extended the resulting period of induced amenorrhoea and introduced prolonged treatment with LHRH agonists for days on end. The patient was then 'programmed' by starting HMG as she entered a stimulation cycle on a pre-set day before admission to the IVF clinic. The doctor could therefore plan his workload. Amounts of hormones started to rise, to stimulate more and more follicles and obtain more and more oocytes. Such forms of superovulation – sometimes involving the use of dozens of ampoules of HMG and in the collection of 50 or more oocytes – were expensive, prolonged and not fully understood.

Objections arose within the profession to this ever-increasing stimulation of the ovaries (Edwards et al. 1996). Strong forms of stimulation may be necessary if several embryos are needed, e.g. to provide sufficient for the preimplantation diagnosis of inherited disease. For routine fertility treatment, however, five or fewer oocytes are probably maximal because IVF has become more successful with the introduction of ICSI and more standard culture media. There is no need for large numbers of oocytes in attempts to alleviate infertility. Simpler procedures, using brief and small doses of ovarian stimulants or even modifications of the natural cycle are needed today. Repeated calls are now made by many IVF professionals for such simplified treatments, for briefer regimens, sharp reductions in doses, and questioning existing methods of programming. Costs of treatment must be reduced, and unexpected consequences of high doses of hormones should be identified. Perhaps the imminent introduction of the LHRH antagonists and recombinant gonadotrophins will allow these targets to be reached quickly.

It is worth noting that this stress on proper patient care and well-being, and the criticism of the use of massive doses of hormones, is far more important ethically than some of the situations brought under legislative control in Parliamentary Acts. The health and treatment of patients is a fundamental matter for any State, and massive overstimulation of the ovaries could affect more and more people as IVF expands into new countries and new fields of clinical care. In this example, it is important to note that the proper conditions to achieve an acceptable form of treatment are being established by debates within the IVF profession and not by legislation.

The success of ICSI and its genetic implications

The development of ICSI has raised quite different ethical issues, mostly genetic. This technique is so successful that virtually every man can now achieve fertilisation in vitro. It has changed the treatment of male infertility dramatically, since embryos can be established even if only 10-20 spermatozoa can be recovered from the entire male tract. Highly anomalous spermatozoa can be used to achieve normal fertilisation, and those recovered from epididymis or testis are also highly efficient. Even precursor cells called spermatids can be used to achieve fertilisation. The success of ICSI has sharply reduced the demand for donor insemination.

I wish first to comment on the very high standards of investigation, both clinical and ethical, that established this situation. Detailed follow-up studies show how the children have the same frequencies of morbidity and mortality as arises after natural concpetion. Every attempt has also been made to transmit the method world-wide, so that infertile men virtually everywhere have benefitted. The largest remaining problem is that a skilled IVF team is needed, so the procedures are expensive and so not available to the poor. This problem is, of course, not unique to ICSI, and it behoves investigators to find less expensive substitutes. Good professional care also identified unusual genetic situations when ICSI was applied to men with very severe infertility. Some of the causative genes can be transmitted to offspring, including genes responsible for defects in the vas deferens and which are partially homologous to cystic fibrosis. Some embryos inherit unusual numbers of sex chromosomes. And, most unusually, severe infertility in some men is caused by de novo microdeletions in autosomes or sex chromosomes which impair the normal formation and functions of the testis. Deletion genetics has become a hot topic, within and outside the world of infertility, with many studies on the sites and frequencies of different deletions, their specific effects on the testis and other organs, and their evolutionary significance.

Embryo growth in vitro and the low rates of implantation

My last example concerns the low implantation rates of human embryos, and its related ethical issues affecting patient care. Implantation rates per transferred embryo have not been significantly improved since the Oldham days. Fundamental and applied studies are needed to improve this situation. There is a need to clarify the nature of primary and secondary differentiation, the metabolic needs of human embryos, why so many embryos are chromosomally anomalous, and improve oocyte and embryo cryopreservation. Better culture media and new forms of tissue culture, e.g. the use of co-cultures of endometrial cells, may soon be available (Menezo et al. 1992, Simon 1997). The low rate of implantation remains the largest clinical problem of IVF, since several IVF cycles are needed to establish a pregnancy. It seems that low implantation rates are not due to IVF itself, because the same problems arise in vivo, where only 20 per cent of natural cycles result in pregnancy in couples attempting to conceive. IVF will remain expensive until implantation rates are doubled or trebled.

The search for improved forms of culture raises several ethical issues. Some culture media contain bovine products such as albumin or serum, despite the dangers of transmitting bovine spongioform encephalitis. Animal viruses may also be transmitted. Some clinics still use media containing these products; others use serum, or cell lines, derived from human donors, but this procedure also has an unquantified risk of cross-infection. The debate stresses the need for highly defined, fully-tested media specifically designed to sustain each stage of embryo growth. Many embryos are needed for this research, yet legislators have opposed research on embryos in their own countries. They condemn their citizens to inadequate media and repeated IVF cycles, using methods based on research carried out in patients in other countries. Perfidy indeed! The need for more research also raises the question of establishing embryos for research, which is legal in the UK, but in few other countries. And surely the conception of future citizens must be achieved in the best possible conditions, a duty which is not by banning fundamental research on our own species.

Cryopreservation of embryos also raises ethical issues. Many clinics cryostore all embryos for immediate replacement into the mother. Other clinics do not have such a programme, and instead they use such embryos for research. Their stance raises major questions about the right of a patient to her embryos.

In good clinics, thawed embryos are 80 per cent as effective as fresh embryos in establishing pregnancy, so patients have two or more attempts at embryo replacement after a single oocyte collection. Cumulative pregnancy rates after several transfers can be very high, so the reason why a clinic has no cryopreservation must be explained in detail during patient counselling, which must be a somewhat difficult task.

One explanation offered against cryopreservation is that it involves dangers to the fetus. The overwhelming majority of scientists and doctors do not accept this premise. Indeed all the available data points in the opposite direction, and there is an absence of induced anomalies after long-term cryostorage of mouse embryos over 25 years. A report from Paris (Dulioust et al. 1994) that frozen/thawed embryos of inbred strains developed anomalies in the jaw has been criticised (Testart 1997). It is essential to stress that this work has been strongly criticised elsewhere, and probably has no relevance to human studies. It is also essential to avoid loose talk of anomalies, since it can raise immense concern among parents with children arising from frozen-thawed embryos.

Studies on embryos at implantation could also improve the success of IVF. I will describe two examples. During implantation, small progesterone-sensitive uterine structures called pinopods appear between days 19-21 of the menstrual cycle (Psychoyos 1993). They are believed to be essential since they may extract fluid from the uterine cavity. The embryo is then pressed tightly against the uterine epithelium, and bridging molecules can then join the embryo with the uterine epithelium. Attachment may be facilitated by integrins, a class of cytokines, expressed on pinopods and elsewhere in the uterus and on embryos (Lessey 1997). Embryos may send messages to the uterus, to initiate or sustain these processes, and one such message may be interleukin-1β (Simon 1997).

My second example concerns the optimal time to transfer an embryo to its mother. This may be the blastocyst stage (5-6 days). Growth to this stage may be improved by applying methods such as co-culture, drilling holes in the outer shell of embryo to facilitate its escape ready for hatching, or by improving available media. The production of interleukin-1β by blastocysts may provide a marker to measure embryo viability and so enable the best embryos to be chosen for transfer.

The low rate of human implantation (lower than any other mammal so far investigated) creates a need to transfer several embryos during each cycle. Some clinics elect to replace 4 or more embryos. This ensures high pregnancy rates, since each embryo adds its increment, but it also risks many multiple pregnancies. The high frequency of twins and triplets is a major cause of the high rates of maternal and fetal morbidity after IVF, and an expensive item for the health service. Premature babies must be closely monitored for several weeks. Debates in fertility societies over several years have stressed the urgency to revert to a maximum of two or even one replaced embryos, and to cryopreserve the remainder. Each clinic decides for itself how many embryos to transfer. Perhaps one reason for transferring four or more is to ensure a high place on league ladders of success or a high flow of highly-paying patients. This essential decision to minimise the number of embryos replaced has apparently been omitted from many legislations.

When several embryos are transferred, or several eggs are ovulated after ovulation induction in amenorrhoeic women, the resulting high-order multiple pregnancies can be 'reduced' to twins or singletons mid-way through gestation. Usually, one or both fetuses survive and do not display the full panoply of undersized premature babies. Nevertheless, a strong feeling exists against transferring so many embryos and destroying the excess later in pregnancy. The fetus is reduced to the status of a disposable article, and the IVF procedure becomes a travesty. Yet reduction is still done in some countries. Legislation here would be complex and disputed, perhaps involving modifications existing Abortion Acts, and it would have to interfere with a woman's right to choose what to do with her body. The ethical situation is perhaps best left to professional organisations.

Some investigators believe that more embryos can be transferred safely to patients over the age of 40 or 42. At these ages, fewer embryos implant and multiple pregnancies are reported to be infrequent. This topic is another matter for considerable discussion. Likewise, establishing pregnancies after the menopause has led to differences of opinion among professionals. Postmenopausal women must be given oocytes and hormone support, since their ovaries are non-functional, although the human uterus functions long after the menopause.

Ethics of IVF and its regulation today

I will conclude this paper by comparing the benefits of professional versus legislative control over the practice and ethics of IVF.

It is clearly impossible to legislate for all aspects of IVF. Some legislation is needed, and even welcome. The State obviously has an interest in any procedures that threaten the health or well-being of its citizens, or demotes its authority. Conditions demanded by the State can be regulated in law, performed by organisation responsible to a Secretary of State, delegated to professional organisation such as a General Medical Council (GMC), or left to individuals practising in the clinic. I prefer the GMC. They are highly knowledgeable of the facts and procedures of IVF and other medical procedures. They have the immense advantage of practising medical ethics, as opposed to the imposition of law by politicians, administrators and lawyers. Ethics is not necessarily prohibitive; it is more constructive and responsive to a given situation, and medical ethics is practised by professionals who see and counsel patients every day, and know in detail the intricacies of their field. Law is practised by people who never (or hardly ever) see patients, and who can easily be misled about new advances in science and medicine. Lawyers are expensive, lawsuits very expensive, and appeals courts immensely expensive, another reason for avoiding them if possible. Law is negative ('thou shalt not'), dominated by the wording of individual clauses, difficult to change, and risks the appointment of domineering administrators.

As I have shown above, decisions by professionals involve major matters of care and health of mother, father and child. Decisions left to them are sometimes of far greater ethical significance than those included in legislation. They also act within a framework of a GMC, and a corresponding General Scientific Council to regulate the ethics of laboratory practice is urgently needed. For doctors, the authority of the GMC is perhaps a more powerful deterrent than legal sanctions laid down by various Parliaments.

Is law, and especially the letter of the law, the best way to deal with the ethics of IVF? It is essential to understand that most ethical furores are short-lived. What bothers one generation is of no relevance to the next. How many of the initial objections to human IVF (table 1) are valid today? Cloning is perhaps the only one, witnessed by recent reactions to the birth of Dolly. Nevertheless, even the totally negative situation to cloning may be changing, since it was not banned outright by the 1997 US President's Commission, but merely been put back for 5 years for further consideration. Some doctors believe that patients could be helped by cloning blastomeres of 4-cell embryos to increase the number of embryos available for transfer in weakly-responsive patients. The effect of this procedure would be to produce four identical quadruplets. Of course, cloning from embryonic nuclei is a very different ethical proposition from cloning from adult nuclei. The short-term impact of new ethical situations was also shown when the British Human Fertilisation and Embryology Authority (HFEA) called for a public vote on the use of human fetal ovaries for grafting into amenorrhoeic patients. The result was a resounding 'No', as to be expected from a society inflamed by newspaper headlines. Perhaps the problem of consent, and the right of a child conceived by donation to know something of its parents, may prevent for ever the use of fetal ovarian tissue. To reach a balanced decision, however, means that debate must occur when furores have subsided and rational consideration can be given.

Lawyers and administrators are not the right people to make ethical decisions about IVF or other medical topics. We do not want armies of lawyers threatening and even deciding ethical issues, as in the USA. Yet this situation is creeping into my country, unwittingly encouraged by the need for the HFEA to adhere rigidly to the letter of the law. Recently, this organisation banned a British widow from using the spermatozoa of her dead husband. He had not consented to the collection of his spermatozoa for the insemination of his wife since he was apparently unconscious when his spermatozoa were collected. The letter of the law was imposed on this hapless widow who merely desired to have children by her deeply-loved dead husband. It seems that a marriage licence or love is of no importance when faced by the bureaucracy of the HFEA.

It would surely have been preferable to refer this case to the GMC, where a reprimand (hopefully a gentle one) could be administered to the surgeon who collected the spermatozoa without formal consent. The sample could then have been used to inseminate the widow. Instead, the widow was forced to move from court to court, and finally to the final Appeals Court (House of Lords) to try to obtain her husband's spermatozoa. Even more bizarre, the House of Lords ruled that she could take the spermatozoa out of the UK for her insemination, but it could not be done within the UK. In other words, if she could find a foreign clinic that would perform the deed, she could then come back to the UK to have a child that was originally banned from creation by the HFEA and various courts. This is ethical absurdity. Apart from impugning the ethical standards of an unknown foreign country, it could produce a child conceived out of UK law who will be an English citizen at birth. And the widow has had to spend thousands of pounds in lawsuits, and find a foreign clinic, to produce a child when it could well have been conceived in Sheffield.

A second case involved the destruction of many cryopreserved frozen embryos. A five-year period of embryo cryostorage was written into the Parliamentary Act which established the HFEA. As the 5-year period approached, an exceptional extension to the law was granted to couples who requested further storage of their embryos by a particular deadline. Our requests for a further delay to try to save some of the unwanted cryopreserved embryos fell on deaf ears, and 3.000 were accordingly destroyed on order from the HFEA on pain of imprisonment or the closure of the clinics that refused (Edwards and Beard 1997). The importance of these embryos – even 10 per cent of them – for urgent research to help IVF patients cannot be overstated. Embryos are urgently needed, for controlled trials to improve embryo growth in vitro, or to identify disease or cancer genes in them. This example shows how the importance of research is simply not apparent to the state authority. Embryos are in desperately short supply since most clinics cryopreserve those not transferred for later use by the patients. Virtually none are left for research, so this supply of cryopreserved embryos was an invaluable and irreplaceable source. This example shows how the HFEA has the wrong standards, and is more intent on threatening punishment on scientists and doctors and even closing their clinics (as seen even in unseemly episodes on television!) rather than trying to improve conditions for their patients. Legal authority won, and the embryos were destroyed in an action almost incomprehensible to many onlookers outside the UK.

Similar restrictive laws may be introduced in some countries over other aspects of IVF. The establishment of pregnancies in post-menopausal women could be one target. Yet many of these couples have been trying to establish their family for many years without success, and now discover they can try again. Other couples have met in their 50s and wish to raise their family. They should have a right to the benefits of modern medicine provided no harm is being done and they conceive under close medical care. Women live to an average age approaching the 80s today, and the menopause at 45 years is merely an evolutionary relic of our past genetic history. Its onset is decided by the number of eggs formed at birth and their rate of utilisation in the woman, and may be quite unrelated to the women's ability for motherhood. It has an extremely poor marker for ethics and law.

Law has recently become more capricious in France. Embryo research and preimplantation genetic diagnosis are now under close restrictions, apparently based on groundless fears of abnormal embryo growth or risk of eugenic experiments. The astonishing German law is based on totipotency of embryo cells when we do not know what totipotency is or even if it exists in humans! A powerful legal lobby passes laws which are uninterpretable or are designed to interfere with patient's rights or their access to the benefits of scientific research. The surprising thing about many of these laws is that they are often concerned with lesser problems than those left to practising IVF professionals.

What have existing forms of legislation taught us about the ethical control of IVF? In my opinion, we have learned that more responsibility for ethical and counselling should be returned to doctors and scientists practising assisted procreation. They are the ones most closely in touch with patients and the practicalities of each situation. They need more training in ethics and morals, but this could be done quite easily. It is time to end the need for these professionals to be told by a central ethical authority what they should and should not do. Giving more responsibility to professionals for patient care could increase the chances of legal actions in common law, but this possibility is a fact of all human interactions, and medicine has been no exception in the past. When IVF was practised under the control of its practitioners, ethics witnessed no major disasters (table 3). No-one was cloned, few outlandish practices were reported and these were quickly brought under control, new techniques were assessed responsibly and in great detail, fresh concepts designed to help patients were examined thoroughly and new advances passed around the world with amazing speed.

Table 3. What has happened in the ethics of IVF since its introduction?

- IVF shown to be as safe as natural conception
- The major remaining problem is multiple births
- ICSI is safe but its associated genetics requires analysis
- Embryo cryopreservation is safe but more studies on babies are needed
- Genetic diagnosis of preimplantation embryos is probably safe, but more studies still needed
- Surrogacy is becoming more common and acceptable
- No cloning has occurred
- Legislation has been passed in many countries
- IVF is practised equally responsibly in countries with no legislation

And what of the original purposes in introducing IVF (table 1). Have the restrictions of legislation caused us to lose sight of the vision which initiated this field? It has resulted in much joy for infertile couples, despite the restrictions placed on embryo research in so many countries. I believe that enthusiasm and determination to help patients are as strong as in the earlier years, and that highly novel and inspiring advances lie just around the corner. IVF still remains more of a hobby than a profession to its best practitioners.

Practitioners in assisted human reproduction should be very proud of their achievements for their patients. They have placed human conception firmly within the province of medicine, acted within acceptable ethical guidelines, dealt firmly with their own colleagues who transgressed acceptable limits, and kept the patients and the public fully informed of their work. Some individuals have perhaps been grossly overpaid, but that is hardly a matter for IVF alone. It is time to recognise this professional responsibility, to return more ethical authority to it and to use law as sparingly as possible.

References

Adams, C.E. (1956), *Preimplantation Stages of Pregnancy*, Churchill: London.

Austin, C.R. (1969), *Adv Biosci*, Vol. 4, p. 5.

Chang, M.C. (1955), *J Exp Zool*, Vol. 128, p. 379.

Chang, M.C. (1969), *Adv Biosci*, Vol. 4, p. 13.

Cole, R.J. et al. (1966), *Devel Biol*, Vol. 13, p. 385.

Dulioust et al. (1994), *Proc Nat Acad Sci*, Vol. 92, p. 589.

Edwards, R.G. (1965a), *Nature*, Vol. 208, p. 349.

Edwards, R.G. (1965b), *Lancet*, Vol. 2, p. 926.

Edwards, R.G. (1974), *Quart Rev Biol*, Vol. 49, p. 3.

Edwards, R.G. and Beard, H.K. (1997), *Hum Reprod*, Vol. 12, p. 3.

Edwards, R.G. and Brody, S.A. (1995), *Principles and Practice of Assisted Human Reproduction*, WB Saunders: Philadelphia.
Edwards, R.G. and Fowler, R.E. (1959), *J Exp Zool*, Vol. 141, p. 299.
Edwards, R.G. and Gardner, R.L. (1968) *Nature*, Vol. 214, p. 576.
Edwards, R.G. and Sharpe (1971), *Nature*, Vol. 214, p. 576.
Edwards, R.G. et al. (1966), *Amer J Obstet Gynec*, Vol. 96, p. 192.
Edwards, R.G. et al. (1968), *Amer J Obstet Gynec*, Vol. 102, p. 338.
Edwards, R.G. et al. (1969), *Nature*, Vol. 221, p. 632.
Edwards, R.G. et al. (1970), *Nature*, Vol. 227, p. 1307.
Edwards, R.G. et al (1996), *Hum Reprod*, Vol. 11, p. 917.
Fowler, R.E. and Edwards, R.G. (1957), *J Endocr*, Vol. 15, p. 374.
Fragenheim, H. (1964), *Geburts Frauenhilfe*, Vol. 24, p. 470.
Gardner, D. (1997), *Hum Reprod*, Vol. 12, Suppl., in press.
Gardner, R.L. and Edwards, R.G. (1968), *Nature*, Vol. 218, p. 346.
Gates and Beatty (1954), *Nature*.
Gemzell, C.A. (1967), 5th World Cong. Obstetrics Gynecol., p. 240.
Greenblatt et al. (1961), *JAMA*, Vol. 178, p. 101.
Hammond, J. (1949), *Nature*, Vol. 163, p. 28.
Hayashi, M. (19), 7th Int Conf. IPPF, Excerpta Medica, p 506.
Heape, W. (1890), *Proc Roy Soc Lond B*, Vol. 48, p. 457.
Hendersons S.A. and Edwards, R.G. (1968), *Nature*, Vol. 218, p. 22.
Lessey, B. (1997), *Hum Reprod*, Suppl 12, in press.
Lewis, W.H. and Gregory, P.W. (1933), *Science*, Vol. 69, p. 226.
Lewis, W.H. and Hartman, C.G. (1933), *Carnegie Inst Public*, Vol. 24, p. 187.
Lunenfeld and Donini (1969), in Thomas, C.C. (ed.), *The Ovary*, Springfield.
Paul, J. (1961), *Cell and Tissue Culture*, ES Livingstone: Edinburgh.
Menezo, Y. et al. (1992), *Hum Reprod*, Vol. 7, Suppl. 1, p. 101.
Menkin, M.F. and Rock, J. (1948), *Amer J Obstet Gynecol,* Vol. 55, p. 440.
Palmer (1946), *Acad Chir*, Vol. 72, p. 363.
Pincus, G. and Saunders, B. (1939), *Anat Rec*, Vol. 75, p. 357.
Psychoyos, A. (1993), *Proc 7th Int IVF Conf*, Kyoto.
Shettles, L.B. (1955), *Fert Steril*, Vol. 6, p. 287.
Simon, C. (1997), *Hum Reprod*, Vol. 12, Suppl., in press.
Steptoe, P.C. (1969), *Laparoscopy in Gynaecology*, ES Livingstone: Edinburgh.
Steptoe, P.C. and Edwards, R.G. (1970), *Lancet*, Vol. 1, p. 683.
Steptoe, P.C. and Edwards, R.G. (1976), *Lancet*, Vol. 1, p. 880.
Steptoe, P.C. and Edwards, R.G. (1978), *Lancet*, Vol 2.
Steptoe, P.C. et al. (1971), *Nature*, Vol. 229, p. 132.
Testart, J. et al. (1997), Proc. 12th ESHRE Annual Meeting, *Hum Reprod*, Vol. 12, Abstract, Book in press.
Yanagimachi, R. and Chang, M.C. (1964), *J Exp Zool*, Vol. 156, p. 361.

2 Two decades of IVF: A critical appraisal

Lene Koch

Some years ago, in 1990, I participated in an international conference on in vitro fertilisation (IVF). It was organised by the World Health Organisation (WHO), who wanted to discuss and reach conclusions on the future place of IVF in the treatment of infertility. The idea was to discuss IVF, which at that time was a rather new technology, from a medical technology assessment point of view. The aim of the conference was to reach agreement on a set of recommendations for rational and appropriate use of IVF (Stephenson and Wagner 1993).

In this spirit, the first day of the conference was dedicated to debating and reaching agreement on a definition of infertility. Many proposals were put forward by the interdisciplinary group of participants but the venture failed. According to the principles of medical technology assessment, appropriate use requires a clear definition of the condition to be treated, but at the conference it turned out to be impossible to define infertility. When we think of infertility until recently most people would intuitively think of a situation where a heterosexual couple actively try to have children without success because one of the parties suffers from a pathological condition in their reproductive organs, e.g. blocked tubes, impaired semen quality or lack of ovulation. This would be in agreement with standard medical definitions of infertility as 1 or 2 years of futile attempts to obtain pregnancy. But already in 1990 such medical definitions were crumbling – perhaps also because the uses of IVF had already, by that time, redefined classical medical concepts of infertility.

IVF was allegedly developed to treat one particular form of infertility i.e. blocked tubes. But gradually IVF was used on a much broader range of indications. These include infertility caused by endometriosis, ovulation disorders and even unexplained infertility. IVF is also used to treat male infertility, even though this means that women are exposed to the risks of IVF as they are treated for their partner's condition. Also conditions that may or may not be associated with infertility are treated with IVF. The broadening range of indications thus includes the use of IVF by women who already have children (if only with their previous partner), or by women who want siblings for their only child – i.e. as an instrument in family planning. Combined with egg or sperm donation IVF is increasingly used by menopausal women and by lesbians who do not have intercourse with men, or by single women who simply have not found a suitable partner. This use of IVF to make procreation possible outside the established heterosexual family and by those considered unfit for parenting – because of their sexual orientation, economically or otherwise – has long been opposed by medical and legal authorities. But even if it is possible to uphold such restrictions in publically financed clinics, it seems difficult to do so on a long term basis, and especially in privately financed clinics. One illustration is the recent American case of a couple who sought a surrogate mother to carry the fertilised frozen egg of their recently deceased daughter, because they deserved grandchildren. Not a medical indication nor an example of childlessness but rather a wish to exploit the options that technology offers.

Also today infertility is understood as temporary infertility (cf. the numbers often given when the proportion of infertile in a population is estimated). It is often stated that 10, 15 or even 20 per cent of the population experience infertility at one or more times in their lives but when we keep in mind that less than 5 per cent are involuntarily infertile at menopause, this seems to indicate that the prevalence of infertility is not as high nor rising. Instead the demand for infertility services must be understood as a demand for control over the timing and spacing of reproduction, as well as asserting the genetic relations between parents and child.

The growing interest in using IVF from women who are not infertile in the traditional medical sense of the word is one of the major characteristics of the development of IVF in the past two decades. Thus, partly because of the introduction of the new reproductive technologies, infertility should now be recognised to be a social construct rather than a clear cut medical category or diagnosis. It has become more and more difficult to draw the line between fertility and infertility. But as most today will recognise, if IVF was ever intended to be a strictly medical technology, it very quickly ceased to be so. Today IVF is used on the basis of a subjective, socially shaped experience of infertility which very often has no objective clinical correlate.

The WHO conference mentioned above took place 6 years ago, but somehow it seems like decades. This conference attempted to understand IVF as a public health issue and regulate IVF in the spirit of rational health planning, but the extremely rapid development since then has changed everything. Not only has the range of indications giving access to IVF expanded quickly since the early 1980s, but to facilitate this, a whole new array of technical options have been developed over these two decades.

New technical options

We may divide these into 4 different types.

One type aims to substitute, repair or circumvent deficient physical elements of the reproductive process (e.g.blocked tubes, lack of eggs):

- IVF + egg transfer (simple IVF)
  variants: gamete intra Fallopian transfer (GIFT) and zygote intra Fallopian transfer (ZIFT)
- IVF with intracytoplasmic sperm injection (ICSI)

Another type aims to exchange actors in the reproductive process (donation)

- IVF with (anonymous or identified) donor egg
- IVF with (ditto) donor sperm
- IVF with both donor egg and donor sperm
- IVF with a surrogate mother (womb)

A third type, freezing, aims to space out the elements of reproductive process

- IVF with frozen egg
- IVF with frozen sperm
- IVF with frozen fertilised egg

And a fourth type include

- IVF with preimplantation diagnosis
- IVF with germ line gene therapy.

Even though all of these options are not yet technically feasible, the fourth type is perhaps the most complicated of them all, because it moves us closer to the world of designer babies. The technique of preimplantation diagnosis together with the possibility of germ line gene therapy raises the spectre of eugenics, or to be more precise, of quality control of the reproductive result of IVF. Only now – in contrast to the old eugenics – based on complete voluntariness and using highly sophisticated technology. Here the prophesies of the very early critics of IVF are close to coming true. Some of the earliest criticisms that were put forward by feminist researchers was that IVF would be step one on the way to complete control of the quality of the child through a combination with genetic diagnosis and selection. I remember vividly my disbelief when a biologist tried to explain to me 10 years ago how one cell in an 8 cell embryo could be diagnosed and the rest used for a child if the quality was acceptable (Spallone 1989). This is now becoming reality, and the medical purpose – to limit suffering – is the legitimation.

In several European countries preimplantation diagnosis is considered legal and in others, such as Denmark, it is proposed to extend the use of IVF treatment to include fertile women with a known genetic risk. With this development IVF has left its original expressed purpose of being an infertility technology and is now on the verge of becoming an accessory technology in the war against genetic disease (Lovforslag nr. L5 1996).

Whether it is possible to keep this within the borders of medical indications remains to be seen. Looking at the development of IVF there is no reason to believe that genetic control will not be demanded as a commercially marketed service rather than being based exclusively on medical indications. The history of IVF is not encouraging in this respect, but is rather an illustration of the risks of departing from the treatment of traditional medical conditions. A couple of years ago, an American journal provided a similar example from the world of gene therapy. The journal discussed the first positive results with gene therapy in cystic fibrosis (CF) and quoted a survey of the British population probing how the successful experiment influenced people's expectations. It turned out that the interest in applying gene therapy on non-medical conditions such as homosexuality, alcoholism and low intelligence had increased substantially after the experiments with gene therapy became publicly known. Where only 2-3 per cent had expressed an interest in such non-medical uses before publication of the results, the interest after publication grew to encompass 10-15 per cent. Though such figures should not be interpreted too rigidly, such figures might throw light on the development that may occur once the medical control over new genetic technologies is loosened.

Documented effect?

Another characteristic feature of the impressive technical development of IVF is that it was presented as a medical improvement but without any documentation of its effects. In medicine the randomised trial comparing a new method of treatment to the old is the ideal requirement before a new method is introduced in the clinic. In other words, the movement from experiment to approved treatment should follow certain norms, i.e. those of the randomised controlled clinical trial. In infertility treatment this could include comparison of pregnancy rates between study groups and controls. Control groups should be generated at random to avoid selection bias. One of the standard setters in such trials is the British epidemiologist A. Cochrane. Though it has been estimated that very few standard medical treatments have ever been subjected to randomised clinical control, in 1979 Cochrane found obstetrics and gyneacology to be the specialty most deserving of the not very flattering prize of the wooden spoon for implementing unproven therapies. Recently however an international meta analysis of infertility studies suggested that this prize should be reallocated to infertility specialists who were strongly criticized for not using randomised studies before introducing new treatment methods. (Cochrane 1979, Vandekerckhove et al. 1993). This feature of IVF has not been very visible in the public and ethical debate – people obviously demand IVF, regardless of the fact that its efficacy has not been sufficiently proven. And in spite of its deficiences, the expansions I have described above suffice to describe IVF as a success. But rather than being a medical success – as the comments above have illustrated – I would suggest that IVF be considered a success with the consumers. This commercial success as it were, is expressed by the quick shift in the scope of socially acceptable indications and gradually a larger and larger circle of women have become potential candidates for IVF. By the early 1990s it was clear that IVF was not a medical technology proper, but rather an instrument to provide children to the generation of self-supporting women who found no time nor space to wait for pregnancies that might occur at unfortunate points in a tight career schedule.

There are many explanations for the rapid expansion and acceptability of IVF but this new reproductive technology may definitely be seen as a response to the changing conditions of women in society after the Second World War. The increasing tension in women's lives between the demands of the work place and the desire to reproduce has been articulated by the women's movement and coined as political demand for greater influence over women's reproductive biology. Access to abortion and (relatively) safe contraceptives was obtained in the 1960s and 1970s and in one sense for women the new reproductive technologies represent a further and very substantial step towards a more complete emancipation from the ties of their reproductive biology.

Feminists disagree vehemently in their evaluation of IVF but in spite of the often voiced claim that IVF oppresses women it should not be forgotten that the widespread use that women actually make of IVF is strongly legitimised by the liberal feminist ideology which has characterised the modern women's movement. This movement has strongly emphasised women's reproductive biology as a major reason for women's oppression. And even if most women have not been affiliated with the women's movement no doubt exists that the difficulty of reconciling reproduction and work remains one of the major problems for modern women, and IVF is a welcome solution.

But regardless of the fact that women line up for IVF everywhere simply because IVF seems necessary to make the ends of a modern woman's life meet, IVF has reconstructed the female body fundamentally and the female body may today be seen as an allegory of modernity. It has been disconnected from its traditional ties and its various parts are now bought and sold in the market place. Eggs and uteri are today objects of commercial transaction and bought or hired according to individual need and requirement. The growing commercialisation of the female body is the natural extension of the rights-oriented ideology of the liberal feminist movement's attitude to the female body and one of the most important features of IVF that characterises the last two decades of new reproductive technologies.

As I mentioned earlier, abortion, which was legitimised as a woman's right to control her own body was an important precursor to the establishment of IVF as an ethically acceptable technology. For most liberalists it is difficult to both argue for abortion and against a woman's right to use her uterus or her eggs as she sees fit. The egg seller or donor uses her professed right to treat her body as a commodity. But this commercialisation on the terms of the market is contradictory, also seen from the female point of view. It is marketed as creating control through an increase of reproductive choice – but the question remains if choices are increased and if control is really extended. It seems as if control and choice are only available in the context of a highly developed technological medical system which reduces women's reproductive organs to spare parts, where control is actually ceded to the medical profession, where it has not been possible to exclude serious risks to the women's health (Koch 1993), and where the baby-take-home-rate per cycle – even in the better clinics – rarely reaches 20 per cent (Andersen and Ziehe 1994). This is the price for the increasing use of IVF – the weapon to obtain control recoils on the individual and very few clinics have yet provided psychological and social support to the majority of treated women who fail to give birth to a child (Schmidt 1996).

Egg donation is an illustration of this. Most ethics reports on reproductive technology have gone out of their way to argue that commercialisation should be avoided at all costs, but in most countries egg donation is a transaction that may only take place between anonymous parties. The true gift implied in the metaphor is only possible between friends and relatives, but in many countries, strangely enough, this is the only structural setting that is prohibited. The choices we are left with are market choices, and as such the new reproductive technologies *do* create choices. But when having a child becomes a choice, and when this choice includes the time, genetic features and spacing of children have more dramatic consequenses than we would believe at first glance. By making family relations the object of detailed personal choice they are reconstructed from being traditional systems that were taken for granted and not for human beings to change into exchangeable relations that we may accept or reject, just as we do with other marketable commodities (Strathern 1992). In this way, IVF changes basic cultural points of reference by undermining what Western ethics consider taboos, unsurmountable limits between that which is human and that which is holy, not for humans to touch. Death and birth used to be such limits but today dead men and women may become parents and birth is now only an incidental point in the development of a human being.

As our traditional points of reference are being undermined by the new reproductive techniques, simultaneously they produce new and still more difficult ethical issues – both for those who want children, and for all of us who live in the society which allows these techniques. On which ethical basis should we make decisions on all the new questions that reproductive technology has created: How do we select the embryos to be replaced in the uterus, how do we dispose of surplus embryos, how do we provide donor eggs for those who do not have eggs of their own? How are people influenced by having been frozen as an embryo, or having a frozen sister or brother? How will the shaping of the identity of future generations take place when all traditional limits are broken down.

One point here is, that the consequenses of IVF are not simply private, do not only concern those who use or buy the technologies, but the consequenses are social in that they change our society and culture by forcing us to gradually develop new concepts, practices, discourses. An example may illustrate: the old philosophical question, what is a human being, now has a completely different meaning as the genetic make up of a human being is controlled by humans. The use of techniques such as cloning, twinning, ICSI, fetal reduction, preimplantation diagnosis break with the concept that a human being is a unique individuality created by an incidental combination of genes – a concept which has all-encompassing social and cultural consequenses.

Problem and solution

Features of IVF such as those mentioned above are often understood and discussed as examples of scientific progress in the struggle to prevent infertility, in spite of the many unacceptable additional effects. This is probably the greatest success of all the successes of IVF, that it has managed to convince us that IVF was developed to relieve the suffering of the infertile. A new relationship has been established between the technology and the condition which is not a linear cause-effect relation, but rather a relation of reciprocal legitimation. We have been persuaded to believe that infertility was the problem that IVF set out to solve, but now infertility has taken upon itself a new task, namely to legitimise IVF.

The broader and more inclusive our concept of infertility is constructed – to some extent independently of people's ability to reproduce – the stronger the legitimation effect becomes and the more obvious our need for IVF seems. The problems of the WHO conference in 1990 were not incidental, but an integral part of the technological development. We may say that the success of IVF comes from its ability to rearrange the world – in this case the understanding of fertility – in order to ensure its own efficacy. By constructing infertility in the setting of science and technology and as a problem that only medicine can solve, a range of types of childlessness becomes excluded from the discourse and from medical and social interest. By equalising the differences between infertility and childlessness the interest in types of childlessness that have social causes such as poverty, housing problems, difficult working hours, etc. are excluded, even though their suffering may be just as severe. At the same time the voices of the voluntarily childless couples which might modify the theory of a natural urge to reproduce are never sought. And much worse, the broad range of social options that are open to relieve childlessness are excluded from our vision. Adoption and foster-children, which are so obviously more ethical than IVF because they deal with the sufferings of existing already born children, are somehow left standing in the wings in the discourse, and the wishes of many infertility patients to receive balanced information about these options in the clinic are rarely met. This relates directly to the global problem of overpopulation which somehow seems to be an issue of such immense dimensions that most people prefer not to mention it when debating infertility, and leads me to my final section on the social regulation of IVF which is where ethical considerations may be implemented.

Regulation

How should IVF be regulated? And how have the regulatory attempts developed over the last two decades? The development has definitely been very different in most European countries. Some have shown a restrictive attitude, such as Germany and Austria, others a more liberal one, such as France and Sweden and some have adopted a complete laissez-faire attitude, such as Italy, Greece and, of course, The United States. The willingness to let ethical issues govern national legislation may constitute one way of structuring the differences in regulatory practice. I shall however propose a different approach, namely a more historical one.

Using the regulatory development in Denmark as my starting point I have found it natural to divide the two previous decades into three phases which I believe may cover, at least to some extent, the broader European experience even though these phases occur at different times and with different duration in the various countries.

The first phase was characterised by the authority of the medical doctors, the second by ethics committees and the third by statute law. Initially, when IVF and the new reproductive techniques were introduced, no legal framework existed to regulate their use, and as these techniques were introduced as medical techniques, by medical doctors in medical research settings such as hospitals and laboratories, it was more or less natural that medical doctors acted as the prime authority and also as gatekeepers controlling access to these technologies. Gradually in most countries medical doctors and medical authorities simply introduced IVF treatment in the hospitals as they would any medical treatment, without waiting for further assessment, be it of an ethical or any other nature. In Denmark this phase of professional medical regulation lasted from before 1983 when the first IVF child was conceived in a research programme, until 1986 when IVF was introduced as standard treatment for certain types of infertility in some public hospitals without any controlled clinical trial to document its effect. At the same time the first private clinic was established, and this probably gave impetus to the initiation of the second phase.

In 1987 a law was passed which established the Danish Ethical Council, composed of laymen and medical experts, to advise the health authorities in ethical matters concerning, among other issues, IVF. Though this act regulated certain aspects of embryo research, the authority to decide on clinical issues concerning indications and access to infertility treatment remained in the hands of the medical experts.

In Denmark, this second phase is now coming to a close as a bill regulating the treatment of infertility has been proposed in 1996 and will probably be passed in 1997. This situation has been reached gradually through a number of feeble attempts by authorities to limit the complete freedom of medical professionals to do as they pleased. A number of media scandals releaving how medical professionals had abused the trust that had been invested in them as they were allowed the liberty of regulating this new area helped this gradual emergence of a statutory regulatory practice. Also a number of socially unacceptable practices have been revealed, illustrating the limits of the authority of the medical profession on issues which have turned out to be social and ethical rather than medical. Thus the original exclusion of lesbian and single women was strongly attacked and shown to rest on discriminatory attitudes rather than on the allegedly best interest of the child. Such moral gatekeeping is not in line with the ideology of the nineties and is not upheld by the proposed bill.

It is not difficult to understand the reason why IVF treatment could not remain in the hands of medical doctors for ever. The general interest in increasing patient and user autonomy in the health services has clashed with the more authoritarian and paternalistic practices of the medical profession, also in the area of reproductive services. It is harder to grasp why these technologies were not directly subjected to parliamentary control rather than to the assessment of ethical committees with only advisory powers. Of course it has to do with the way reproductive and genetic issues have been constructed as ethical issues rather than as social issues – which might have been just as appropriate. By institutionalising the reflection on genetic and reproductive technology in ethics committees, these issues have, at least to some extent, been placed outside the realm of those with an obvious vested interest - the medical profession – but also outside the established political forum – probably because the issues are felt to be of a different nature than those which political parties are organised to deal with. Thus the debate about these issues is opened up to include a broader group of participants, and we are now witnessing a broader and more democratic debate where all have a natural competence as human beings. In this way ethics committees helped the process of dissolving the monopoly of medical professionals on these issues and prepared the field for a later political take-over. Ethics and ethical committees have become a form of regulation – at least they have been for a while. Whether we are approaching a period where the elected politicians will take more direct responsibility for the new technology and its social impact remains to be seen.

References

Andersen, A.N. and Ziehe, S. (1994), *Årsrapport 1994. Fertilitetsklinikken, Amtssygehuset i Herlev*, Herlev.

Cochrane, A. (1979), 'A Critical Review With Particular Reference to the Medical Profession', in Teeling Smith, G. (ed.), *Medicines for the Year 2000*, Office of Health Economics: London, pp. 1-11.

Koch, L. (1993), 'The Risks of IVF', in Stephenson, P. and Wagner, M. (eds), *Tough Choices. In Vitro Fertilisation and the Reproductive Technologies*, Philadelphia.

Lovforslag nr. L5 (1996), 'Forslag til Lov om kunstig befrugtning i forbindelse med lægelig behandling, diagnostik og forskning m.v.', *Folketinget 1996-97*, København.

Schmidt, L. (1996), *Psykosociale konsekvenser af infertilitet og behandling*, Copenhagen.

Spallone, P. (1989), *Beyond Conception*, London.

Strathern, M. (1992), *Reproducing the Future. Essays on Anthropology, Kinship and the New Reproductive Technologies*, New York.

Vandekerckhove, P. et al. (1993), 'Infertility Treatment: From Cookery to Science. The Epidemiology of Randomized Controlled Trials', *British Journal of Obstetrics and Gynaecology*, Vol. 100, pp. 1005-36.

3 Interdisciplinarity and the specific responsibility of ethics towards science and technology

Paul van Tongeren

As in other fields of applied ethics, also in biomedical ethics often an interesting paradox can be seen. On the one hand the importance of a multidisciplinary or even interdisciplinary approach will be stressed; in biomedical ethics that means especially the collaboration between biomedical scientists, medical practicians and ethicists. On the other hand, however, in discussions on ethical aspects of biomedical developments, one very often gets the impression of an antagonism between the two parties in this multidisciplinary collaboration: exceptions excluded, the scientists and medical practicians will generally be in favour of the application and development of new technologies, whereas – to put it shorthand – the ethicists usually will point to the risks and the costs and be inclined to put strict limits to the development and application of the technology.

Undoubtedly there are several explanations for this paradox, which shows that interdisciplinary research, at least this kind of interdisciplinarity, is not as easy to perform as is sometimes suggested. In this short contribution I would like to focus primarily on one part of the paradox: the antagonism. One might be inclined to explain this from the different interests of scientists on the one hand and ethicists on the other. If this were correct, it would suggest that the parties are not so much engaged in one common effort to improve the quality of human life or something like that, but rather are pursuing their own profit. To the extent to which this would be the case, one almost has to believe in some kind of an invisible hand to remain confident of the results of interdisciplinary efforts. Moreover, this explanation suggests that especially the scientists have a partial and biased perspective whereas the ethicists are the defenders of the common good.

A somewhat more thoughtful approach acknowledges (or assumes) that scientists and physicians as well as ethicists all do aim at human well-being, but have different conceptions of it, the one stressing other aspects of this well-being than the other, or having a more inclusive conception of it than the other, or feeling more strongly about the constraint of an equal distribution of this well-being than the other; or – to view it from the opposite position – the one being less confident on the success and safety of the scientific approach than the other. I have the feeling that such (partly inevitable) differences with regard to the perspective taken or to the conception of the good aimed at, do not necessarily have to lead to the above-mentioned antagonism, and that, as far as they do produce this antagonism, this might have to do with the way in which ethicists often conceive of their task.

Ethicists often feel urged or forced, so it seems, to evaluate a specific event or conduct or development as e.g. the technology of IVF. Even if they themselves do not wish to do so, they are often by others put in a position of having to either approve of or refuse or set limits to a particular technology or its application. And since (among other reasons) they do not want to be the ones that provide an alibi for a questionable practice or for what sometimes seems to be an autonomous development, they often are biased in a direction opposite to the direction which this more or less autonomous developing technology takes.

I certainly do not want to condemn this characteristic of ethical reflection. But I do want to point to the risk of a certain myopy when ethics focuses too strongly on a particular event or development to be evaluated. Apart from giving way to the antagonism I referred to, it runs the risk of making ethics itself dependent on the technological (as well as the economical or political) framework from which the request for an evaluation emerged. It forces ethicists to go deeply into the scientific and technological details, and suggests that interdisciplinarity means that ethicists become quasi-scientists themselves.At least as a complement to this approach I would like to suggest that it is the task of ethics to broaden our view. And this broadening of one's view is usually done through taking distance. From this perpective it is not so much the task of ethics to judge or set limits to what technologically or otherwise is being done to 'make things better', to improve the conditions of our existence or to overcome its imperfections, but rather to make explicit and to question what is being assumed as being self-evident and to remind ourselves of what we threaten to forget in all these efforts. In our efforts to enable people to have children if they want to, we presuppose that we know what it actually is that people desire, if they want to have children. This might, however, be less obvious than we expect it to be as long as we do not think about it (I refer to my other contribution to this volume, cf. van Tongeren 1997). When we do want to reflect on this desire for children, we should not do so under the pressure of evaluating the technology which enables us to realise this desire. Or better: ethicists might contribute more to such an evaluation, by putting the technology to be evaluated in a wider perspective. Reminding ourselves that we are finite beings is important not so much because it would set limits to our efforts to overcome it, but because it indicates that we should do more than just what we do in those technological efforts. That human beings are finite beings does not mean that they should (nor that they should not) try to improve their condition. It does mean that, in order to be what they are, they will have to learn to deal with their finiteness. In other words: it is not so much a question of setting limits to our activity, but reminding us of the importance of developing our appropriate passivity. As we all know: the more we get to know, the more we discover how much we do not know. I would like to implement this as: the more we manage to get a grip on the fulfillment of our desire for children, the more we should invest in efforts to learn how to deal with what in this desire escapes from our grip.

Ethics is a philosophical (or theological) discipline. Philosophy is not so much a problem-solving activity, but rather a way of raising questions towards what is taken for granted. An interdisciplinary collaboration of scientists and ethicists should therefore not been confined within the limits of the problems as they are defined by science or technology. When all collaborators take their own perspective and their own responsibility, this might complicate the interdisciplinarity but it will reduce the danger of a fruitless antagonism.

References

van Tongeren, P. (1997), 'To an Ethics of Desire', this volume, Part Two.

4 Different ethical perspectives in IVF discussion

Dietmar Mieth

This book may bring the saying to mind: 'If you have a lot of trees before you, you cannot see the forest for the trees'. Perhaps to see the forest you need distance and a higher point of view on a philosophical mountain. The following remarks try to concentrate the very rich and manifold perspectives in this book on infertility, indications for in vitro fertilisation (IVF), success rates, multifetal pregnancies, embryo destiny and embryo status, IVF-psychology, freedom and participation of patients, on legal diversity and consensus in Europe, on misuse and limits, on crucial questions about human dignity and nature as criteria, on the special problems of intracytoplasmic sperm injection (ICSI) and preimplantation diagnosis (PID). In view of all these different aspects I would like to point out some main questions: Is there a common language for interdisciplinary discourse? – and if it is philosophy, what kind of philosophy? What are the main contested points?

A common language for interdisciplinary discourse?

The language of interdisciplinarity is a philosophical language. From biology to theology we need philosophical discourse to understand one another even if this only succeeds in describing our disagreements. For an efficient exchange of information and argumentation, some conditions for a common philosophical ethical language must be fullfilled:

(a) It is necessary to avoid some fallacies in ethically relevant arguments. These include the empirical fallacy, the motivational fallacy and the genetic fallacy.

The *empirical* fallacy or the fallacy 'from is to ought' consists in replacing questions of ethically right or wrong action with questions of empirically validated acceptance rates in a relevant population. The belief that ethical problems can be *solved* by technical solutions belongs to this fallacy. But it is correct to say that an ethical conflict can be *avoided* by technical imagination and flexibility.

The *motivational* fallacy is given if we evaluate an argument by reducing the reasons to the motive we attribute to the arguing person and to his or her role and interests. An argument is not automatically valid or invalid when the motivation to make it may be ambiguous.

The *genetic* fallacy lies in judging the validity of an argument by suggesting that when you accept a situation you must also accept the conditions that brought this situation about. (I do not believe, for example, that it is necessary to accept embryo research because I accept that IVF had first to be constituted by embryo research.)

(b) Another aspect which may be a hindrance to a common philosophical-ethical language is a hermeneutical one. Do we accept that we cannot argue – step by step, without contradiction and comprehensibly – without having social roles, standpoints, interests, intuitions, perspectives which greatly differ from each other. For example, as a social ethicist I have, similar to social politicians, a preference to see the problems of the decline of conscience in society: too much individualism, too many rules of the free market, too many options for linear progress without regard to contexts and the ensuing problems. But I know very well that this perspective of social ethics is not the only perspective, and that there is a danger in emphasising collective goods at the expense of individual goods. With regard to IVF, I see very well that there are different approaches in ethics: the ethics of individual option, which in IVF risks denying that there are not only the adult persons making decisions but also the interest of another human being whose moral status remains controversial. Then there is the ethics of the patient-physician relationship. In this kind of approach, once we are inside the systems of IVF, we accept the conditions and we must follow the consequences. It makes no sense to introduce arguments from the outside to the functional situation inside. If you accept IVF you expect high quality, high success and minimal risks. This includes frozen embryos after a quality control, supernumerary embryos as well as the given alternatives of donation for IVF or embryo wasting research.

We have to exchange our perspectives: social perspectives, individual perspectives, treatment perspectives, to recall only some of the main possibilities. We can help to develop a common language by practising role-taking.

Even if we agree that there are some principal criteria for all of us in all situations such as the Principle of Generic Consistency (PGC), i.e. the mutual recognition of rights and obligations as moral agents (Beyleveld 1997, Steigleder 1997), it may be very difficult to apply them in different situations. Nevertheless, I hold that, besides the PGC, there will be two other fundamental norms: first, the principle of not resolving problems by a method which produces more problems than existed previously; second, I suggest that there are not categorical but plausible reasons for insisting on the protection of the embryo as well as of the fetus. The abortion regulation in Europa is not a demonstration that there is no protection for the fetus, but that there are other perspectives and circumstances in which we tolerate abortion in our laws, without pretending that in these conditions the abortion is morally right. What I do not find acceptable in this situation is a mentality which transforms the legal tolerance into a moral right, and even, in the case of prenatal diagnosis (PND), into a moral obligation. Many people feel that something has gone wrong and some researchers regard this feeling as a motivation or a reason for PID. When the women who have a genetic risk of thalassemia in Sardinia were asked what choice they would make between PND and PID, they voted 70 per cent for PID (Ludwig 1996). Even if I am not sure that this vote was based on a wide and sufficient information concerning IVF and, for example, concerning the obligation to undergo a PND later on, it shows that abortion in a late phase of the pregnancy process is taken as a great burden.

It may be that the idea of protection is relative and not a strict rule, when proportionality and potentiality or indirect obligations are taken into account, or it may be that these different aspects can be reduced to the PGC; nevertheless, I have never heard a proposition to treat all human (pre-)embryos in the same way as, for example, mouse embryos. Even if we recognise only a participation of the embryo in human rights, it may be further discussed what kind of participation is available. Someone may propose that this is not a participation founded on the embryo her- or himself, but only in its inclusion in the process of procreation treatment.

The main points of controversy

With the discussion about the moral status of embryos we have touched a main point of controversy. But there are others too. Connected to the embryo discussion is the disagreement on whether the infertility situations belong to a culture in which prevention is weak and repair is strong. Then the inside-perspective of researchers and physicians is not sufficent for an ethical analysis. Another perspective is also too restricted, too narrow: to see IVF only as an individual treatment of a woman or a couple without taking into account that other human beings are involved. The danger of a reduction of moral approaches to the agents in a strict sense has to be seen. We need better explanations of the distinction between functional and substantial, or symbolic, ontology.

IVF remains an offer of medical treatment with a burden, with risks – which, for example in the case of ICSI, will need further assessment – with a more or less low success rate and with more or less instrumentalisation of the early embryos. We are in a dilemma: if we see the goods and values in a wider social perspective, IVF remains a moral challenge. If we see value only as a function of individual options we risk replacing the question of what is morally right or wrong in the offer of treatment with the question of who decides what? Whose option and what choices are to be not only respected but accepted as legitimation for social solidarity; a social acceptance which alone makes research, clinical institutions and paid treatment possible. I will now summarise the remaining moral dilemmas. It is likely that the list is not complete:

- What are we allowed to do with early embryos?
- Are there more problems created than solved in IVF-treatment?
- Is there an equal access for all interested persons or only a strict control of indications?
- What are the priorities in the face of growing infertility, due to cultural reasons, in our society?

Indeed, there are more special questions within the treatment, such as counselling (cf. part 4 of this volume); I only wish to open up the macro-perspective. Society's penchant for responding to the social and moral dilemmas that arise from technological progress has the negative consequence of dividing the discussion into, on the one hand, a legal and institutional problem, and, on the other hand, into a public debate on individual and communtiy preference. Ethics degenerates into a separation, not merely a distinction, of regulation from social and individual counselling. The regulation then gives the space but does not resolve the moral problems. But there are nevertheless some aspects that require regulation:

- good technical and medical practice restricted only to research centers;
- no free commercialisation of IVF, ICSI and later on PID;
- clear and strict indications instead of equal unqualified access;
- the obligation to clear, complete and adequate information to the patient;
- a good distinction between the right to know and the right not to know;
- the obligation to counselling with good professional practice;
- the need of bodies/committees to prove research programmes;
- the adequate protection of embryos;
- a programme of social education.

I am convinced that the PID-discussion – which in Germany is only beginning – has to include the additional aspect of negative eugenics by individual choice. 'Negative' indicates the avoidance of genetic disease, and individual choice can be understood as an indirect selection of existing beings by offering the way for it: individual choice under the condition of social offer!

I have often heard that the ethical definition of problems is not 'realistic' because ethics has to follow the dynamics of autonomous development. I think that we need more than a very near-sighted realism. We also need to base our reflections on a broader notion of our field and our time. I think that this question of 'realism' is highly relevant when I, for example, as an ethicist propose a moratorium for new kinds of genetic diagnosis without therapy, like PID, not with categorical arguments, but with the addition of relative argumentation about the burdens, selections and the development of a so-called non-curative medicine. I do not deny that there are other, also ethically relevant arguments, but I do not accept 'realism' as an argument on the level of definition of right or wrong action, even though it might be prudent to integrate this argument in political decision-making. The conscience of an ethicist and the conscience of someone who is involved in medical or in political practice and strategy are not essentially different but they must remain distinct. This distinction may help for an efficient cooperation and for a better understanding.

References

Beyleveld, D. (1997), 'The Moral and Legal Status of the Human Embryo', this volume, Part Seven.

Ludwig, M. (1996), 'Preimplantation Diagnosis in Germany? – Statement', *Biomedical Ethics*, Vol. 1, No. 2, pp. 30-1.

Steigleder, K. (1997), 'The Moral Status of Potential Persons', this volume, Part Seven.

Part Two
INFERTILITY

1 A personal account of infertility

Phil Taylor and Kathie Taylor

Background

Kathie and I were born, brought up and still live and work in Liverpool, England. We have been married for twelve years – although we have known each other since the age of five or so.

Like most contemporary couples we wanted to buy our own house, buy items to furnish it, and generally get used to living togther. We were both happy in our chosen careers; Phil as a company director and Kathie until recently as an assistant bank manager. Never was there any talk of whether or not we would have a family – just when.

Try, try and try again...

In late 1989 we decided that the time was right to start trying for a family. We ceased to use any form of contraception and expected nature to take its course. After a several months we began to think that something should have happened. After all we had both been brought up being told that 'getting pregnant was as easy as falling off a log'.

By October 1990 Kathie had become increasingly anxious as she was aware that being already in her early thirties time was against her. I suppose I was content to carry on trying a little longer. However, Kathie decided that it would be best to see a female doctor at our General Practitioner (GP) Practice to ask her advice. Having discussed the situation with Kathie, the doctor suggested that we should continue to try for a few more months but this time trying to have intercourse at the optimum time. The doctor showed Kathie how to keep basal body temperature charts to try and predict ovulation and therefore the best time for intercourse.

How do you break bad news...?

By the New Year of 1991 still nothing appeared to be happening. So, after another visit to the GP, the doctor suggested that I should submit a semen sample for analysis. In February 1991 Kathie was told that the results of the test had been received back from the laboratory and so she arranged to visit the doctor. The doctor told Kathie that my semen analysis showed that it was unlikely that I would ever be able to father children and... by the way, had we thought about adoption? She then went on to inform Kathie that there was no treatment for male infertility and she knew of no other doctor to whom she could refer us for treatment.

The distress that this caused Kathie was unimaginable. After returning from the GP she telephoned me at work to ask me to come home. She would not tell me why; and I could not understand why she was so upset. Upon returning home from work, Kathie explained what had happened that morning. Beside the fact that I was extremely angry about the way the doctor had treated her, I could not believe that the doctor had given my test results to Kathie without me being present or without my permission.

Despair

The effect this news had upon both of us was devastating. We had never considered not having children. Our respective families, and almost all our friends, already had children. We had not been prepared to consider the situation in which we now found ourselves. We felt isolated, and feeling that we could not tell anyone about our predicament made the situation worse. Anything to do with children became an emotional issue; walking past a school at playtime, watching parents give comfort to their children when they had fallen over playing, the birthday parties of our sibling's children.

As the doctor had been so unhelpful in offering us any other point of reference Kathie tried to look for information for herself. That was when Kathie contacted CHILD – The National Infertility Support Network, they were very helpful and able to send us information about male infertility. This information gave us hope that there was something that could be done to help us have our own children. Kathie returned to see the GP and asked her to try and find a doctor that could help. After a little while the GP came up with the information and we arranged to pay privately for an appointment to see him.

Reassurance

In April 1991 Kathie and I met with Mr Desmond. He is a Consultant based in Liverpool who has a special interest in male infertility. Mr Desmond examined me carefully, requested that they carry out a further semen analysis, and that I arrange to have an ultrasound examination to ensure that he had not missed a varicoceles that may have been giving problems in the scrotum. There then followed a period of a few months until they had carried out all the tests, the results received and another appointment to see Mr Desmond came around.

The second appointment, towards the end of 1991, with Mr Desmond was more reassuring. He was able to tell us that I had nothing physically wrong with me and that the semen analysis showed that the sperm, although low in number and quality, was not as bad as first made out by our GP. Mr Desmond then prescribed 'Tomoxifen' for me to take. Tomoxifen is a drug shown to affect sperm production. After taking the Tomoxifen for three months further semen analysis was to be undertaken to see if it had affected sperm production. In tandem with this Mr Desmond arranged for Kathie to see a consultant gynaecologist to ensure that her reproductive tract was functioning and that she was ovulating.

The months and years fly by!

Just before Christmas 1991 we met with Mr Richmond, a consultant gynaecologist also based in Liverpool. He arranged for Kathie to undergo a laparoscopic dye (Lap & Dye) test. This was to ensure that Kathie's Fallopian tubes were open and that the rest of her reproductive tract was functioning correctly This is a procedure which is carried out under general anaesthetic. It is an extremely uncomfortable procedure as the gas used to separate the organs within the pelvis during laparoscopic investigation eventually travel up the body and in to the shoulders where it becomes extremely painful for two to three days.

During January and February 1992 Kathie also had regular blood tests to obtain detailed hormone analysis. This ensured that she was ovulating and that her hormone levels were within acceptable levels.

Treatment at last!

After further consultations it was decided to try using a technique known as intra uterine insemination (IUI). This involved Kathie having injections of follicle-stimulating hormone (FSH) to increase production of egg-bearing follicles on the ovaries. Then undergoing regular trans-vaginal ultrasound to measure the growth of the follicles, and then, following an injection of luteinising hormone having a prepared specimen of my sperm injected, via a catheter tube, directly into her uterus.

Three IUI treatment cycles were carried out in May, June and July 1992. Unfortunately, Kathie's response to the drugs was poor and so it was decided, in August 1992, to abandon further IUI treatment in favour of in vitro fertilisation (IVF) treatment. However, they told us, the waiting time for National Health Service funded IVF treatment would be not less than twenty months!

The effect of these events upon Kathie was particularly acute and she began to suffer from a prolonged period of reactive depression. She was away from work for fifteen weeks only returning to work part time from Christmas until February 1993.

Support

One evening in February 1993 we attended the first meeting of a local patient support group formed for patients undergoing infertility investigation or treatment. The group was, and still is, run by patients for patients. I am really not quite sure what would have happened to us if we had not had this support group with which to share our situation. The knowledge that there were other people that felt the same as us; that shared the same, or similar medical conditions, other people that were waiting the same length of time for IVF treatment as us, was a real source of strength for both of us.

Talking within the support group to other couples made us realise that not being open about our situation was creating additional stress for both ourselves and our families and friends. It also meant that the problem of infertility was not being brought out into the open so that the stigma could be removed. Therefore, Kathie and I resolved to tell our families, friends and anyone else that wanted to know why it was that we did not have children. It was quite amazing to find that many of them said things like 'Oh, we thought there must have been a problem, but we didn't like to say anything', or 'We just thought you didn't want children, we thought you were career people'.

Waiting... and waiting...

By August 1993 we felt we could wait no longer for IVF treatment and so we borrowed money to privately fund one IVF treatment cycle. However, this was to prove disastrous as no fertilisation took place between the eggs and sperm in vitro. Nothing had prepared us for this situation. At the back of our minds we remembered the words of our consultant saying that only one sperm function test matters and that's the one when the sperm is put with the eggs in vitro. It seemed to us that our worst nightmare had become a reality – that my sperm and Kathie's eggs were incompatible, and that we probably would not have our own children.

At a following consultation, the doctor was not able to give us any reason why fertilisation had failed, and this made us even more anxious. To add to the situation, we then had to consider that the only way for Kathie to achieve a pregnancy may be to use donor fertilised eggs. (This was before intracytoplasmic sperm injection had become a widely practised technique.) We then had to wait for another attempt at IVF until November 1994 when our names had come up to the top of the National Health Service waiting list. However, the intervening time did allow us, and especially me, to come to terms with the situation that we may have a baby that was not genetically mine.

Second attempt

Prior to the IVF commencing, it was suggested by our consultant that if there were enough eggs, some would be used with my sperm to see if fertilisation would take place. It transpired that four eggs were collected from Kathie's ovaries. They fertilised the best two eggs with donor sperm and they fertilised the other two eggs with my sperm. As the donor fertilised embryos looked the best to return to Kathie's uterus, it was agreed to use them. Unfortunately, no pregnancy occurred. This left us upset and disappointed on one hand yet on the other happy to know that my sperm could, after all, fertilise Kathie's eggs.

As we reflected upon this treatment cycle, we realised that, for us, it had been successful IVF. Embryos had been created and had been returned to Kathie's uterus. We were just unfortunate that on this occasion it was not to develop into a pregnancy.

Third attempt

Our third IVF treatment took place, almost a year after the second, in August 1995. Again four eggs were collected, but this time all fertilised with donor sperm as it was hoped to be able to return three embryos (the maximum permitted under UK law) to Kathie to give the best chance of a pregnancy. They returned three and the one remaining embryo was frozen so that it could be used again at a later date if needed. As time was to tell, it was needed as no pregnancy resulted from the IVF treatment. So in November 1995 Kathie took a course of drugs to prepare her for the transfer of the frozen embryo. Unfortunately, the embryo disintegrated as it thawed and the treatment was abandoned.

Final attempt

Over the Christmas and New Year Holidays we decided that we could only contemplate trying IVF one more time. Neither of us felt able to continue with treatment – with both of us now in our late thirties and, aware of the effect that this would have upon Kathie's chances of conceiving, together with the emotional and physical stress that the treatment placed upon us. We also decided to look further into the possibilities of adoption.

We had considered this earlier while waiting for treatment, but the chances of adopting a baby in our area were negligible so we had not actively pursued it. However, it became clear to us that as we had been married for over ten years by this time it would be reasonable for us to consider adopting an older child. Thus it was with this in mind that we undertook to have one final attempt at IVF treatment.

In March 1996 Kathie started to receive the fertility drugs and in April egg collection took place. Eight eggs were collected with four fertilised with my sperm and four with donor sperm. This time the best embryos were those fertilised by my sperm and so it was decided to return those to Kathie's uterus. The four embryos created with donor sperm were frozen so that they could be used at a later stage if necessary.

Two weeks of agony

There then followed the two agonising weeks that we had become familiar with during which we had to wait to see if Kathie would start to menstruate - indicating that there was no pregnancy. During the second week of our wait Kathie started to have what looked like a menstrual period together with the associated 'period' pains. The bleeding stopped, then started again, then stopped again. We spoke to a nurse at the hospital and she told us not to give up hope, but to be realistic that it may not have worked.

By the end of the second week there was only very slight bleeding and so we decided to return to the hospital to have a pregnancy test. This was mainly to put our minds at rest and show that the treatment had not worked. However, we were completely astounded when two of the nursing staff returned to the room in which we were waiting to tell us that the pregnancy test was positive. 'Positive' we asked, 'as in being pregnant'! The pregnancy test showed a very strong response and so we were also advised that it could be a multiple birth!

A conclusion

So it was that a few weeks later we were able to return to the hospital and see, for the first time, an ultrasound picture of not one baby but two. An almost incident free pregnancy followed until thirty-five weeks when Alexandra Frances and Elizabeth Fern were born by caesarian section on 13 December 1996. The babies are perfectly healthy and beautiful in every way. We feel incredibly privileged and thankful that the IVF treatment worked for us.

We earnestly hope that by talking about our experience others may understand the profound effect infertility has upon the quality of life.

2 Different kinds of infertility, possible reasons for infertility

Hans-Rudolf Tinneberg and Ulrich Göhring

Introduction

Infertility (sterility) is a worldwide problem with a prevalence of 10-17 per cent in western countries and China with exceptionally 5 per cent. Infertility is diagnosed when pregnancy did not occur in a couple after 2 years of unprotected intercourse.

Reasons for infertility are subject to regional differences. Whilst for instance in countries with a relatively low standard of living the rate of primary infertile women is fairly low and high for secondary infertility we find the opposite in industrial countries (Thonneau et al. 1992).

Established reasons for infertility are anatomical like cervical, tubal and uterine factors. Hormonal reasons for infertility include severe cases such as ovarian insufficiency and thyroid gland dysfunction as well as hyperprolactinemia and luteal insufficiency. Endometriosis is quite controversially discussed as possible cause for infertility as well as environmental factors and psychosomatic reasons. Of increasing importance are male factors in explaining infertility as meanwhile the male factor has become as important as the female factor. Only vage knowledge exists about the role of immunological factors relevant for infertility.

Anatomical reasons

Anatomical reasons can be differentiated into cervical, uterine and tubal factors. It is assumed that in 10 per cent of all infertility cases cervical factors are relevant. These can be a consequence of surgical interventions like cone biopsies, cauterisation or cryotherapy. In addition, hormonal and immunological factors can impair ascension of sperm through the cervical mucus.

Changes of the endometrium due to infections or hormonal dysbalance are uterine factors which can impair implantation. Also, intrauterine polyps and submucous fibroids can be relevant inhibitors for implantation. The Asherman syndrome with massive intrauterine adhesions can inhibit sperm migration as well as implantation of the embryo. In severe cases no significant endometrium can be detected.

Tubal disease makes up for the most common cause of infertility. Reasons for tubal damage can be operations, infections and congenital malformations. Hypoplastic tubes are controversially discussed as cause for infertility as it is very difficult to analyse the dynamics of a tube. Even operations on other organs, such as an appendectomy, can cause tubal sterility by peritubal adhesions. Infections of the tubes, the most commonly the Chlamydia infection, can lead to thickening of the wall and rigidity of the tube, rarification of the intaluminar epithelium and tubal block.

Endometriosis

Endometriosis is defined as ectopic endometrium with the histological stucture and function of the uterine endometrium. Several hypothesis try to explain endometriosis: (1) Retrograde menstruation, (2) Lymphogenic dissemination, (3) Hematogenic dissemination, (4) Coeloma hypothesis.

It has been estimated, that 80 per cent of all women in the reproductive age have an endometriosis. Out of these 30-40 per cent are infertile. Reasons for infertility through endometriosis can be tubal or periovarian adhesions, excessive production of prostaglandins as a periinflammatory effect which would inhibit tubal motility and/or ovulation.

Hormonal reasons

In over 25 per cent of cases ovarian dysfunction is the reason for infertility. The primary symptom usually is menstrual disorder. As the most common disorder, luteal insufficiency can be diagnosed in over 20 per cent of all patients seeking advice. Luteal insufficiency however is only a very mild disorder and can easily be overcome by luteal phase support with gestagens.

Hyperandrogenic ovarian insufficiency is a common cause of oligomenorrhic women. These women often suffer from hirsutism and acne. The most important reason for hyperandrogenemia is exessive production of androgens in the paranephric glands. The polycystic ovarian disease is also associated with hyperandrogenemia and often anovulation. Small follicles are arrested in the subcapsular area and under stimulation very often hyperstimulation occurs.

Laparoscopic electrocautery of the ovarian surface can quite effectively treat these conditions.

Environmental reasons

The reproductive capacity of men and women can negatively be influenced by various environmental factors. Environmental factors causing infertility consist of stress, noise, choice of food, environmental pollutants, *Genußgifte* ('social' drugs, such as coffee and alcohol etc.), other drugs and finally socio-economic factors. The mode of action can be quite different. Endocrine disruption can be just as important as impairment of gametes, gamete interaction, implantation or continuation of a pregnancy. This is not surprising as the range of influences and substances is immense.

Of major interest are substances known as environmental pollutants. Such pollutants can be accumulated in the human organism and its reproductive organs. Due to the socio-economic profile of industrial countries, the ages of couples having children have risen and in such couples a higher concentration of environmental pollutants can be expected.

The effect of reducing fertility is discussed for many chemicals that are already prohibited because of their toxicity. However, only relatively few substances are of proven reproductive toxicity which has in most cases been documented in animal studies. For humans only in very few cases has reproductive toxicity been clearly proven and the action mechanism solved. This is difficult as not only the actual pollutant but also its metabolites can be toxic (e.g. n-hexane: 2.5 hexadione or acrylamide: n-methyleacrylamide). Very little is known about the low dose range and synergistic effects of different substances have not been tested at all (Heinzow and Hanf 1995).

The list of possibly toxic agents would be too long for this chapter. The Reproductive Toxicology Center at the Columbia Hospital for Women Medical Center, Washington D.C., USA provides up to date information on the current scientific knowledge, since the disaster of Seveso in Northern Italy where massive amounts of mainly tetrachlorodibenzodioxin (TCDD), a highly lipophilic substance with a long half-life, were released into the air. Dioxins are unintentional byproducts produced primarily in the synthesis of certain chemicals and combustion processes. The chemicals involved consist of chlorphenoxy herbicides such as 2,4,5-trichlorophenoxyacetic acid, the disinfectant hexachlorophene and polychlorinated biphenols (PCBs) which were used as dielectric fluids in capacitators and transformers. High levels of dioxins have also been found in technical grade pentachlorophenol (PCP) used primarily as a pesticide and wood preservative.

In test animals, polychlorinateddibenzodioxin (PCDD) and polychlorinated-dibenzofurans (PCDFs) have produced adverse reproductive effects including congenital malformations and fetal lethality. In humans, the situation is less clear as can be seen by the Ranch Hand Study Group which consisted of Vietnam war veterans exposed to Agent Orange, a military defoliant used in South Vietnam. The neonatal death rate was reported to be significantly increased from the death rate prior to the application of this substance in Southeast Asia. The Center for Disease Control (CDC) however, was unable to uncover any striking findings regarding veterans fathering babies with serious congenital malformations.

Meanwhile increasing evidence suggests that halogenated hydrocarbons such as PCBs and PCDFs have an adverse effect on the reproductive system

Table 1. Reproductive toxicity of halogenated hydrocarbons PCB, PCDF and dioxins

PCB / PCDF	Dioxin
antispermatogenic	low pregnancy rate
reduced fertility	increased malformation rate
chromosomal aberrations	antiestrogenic

As demonstrated in table 1 environmental pollutants can also have hormone-like effects. Of major concern are substances that have an estrogenic effect. As it could be demonstrated in fish, in sexual differentiation there is a period that is sensitive to xenoestrogen compounds as could be shown by the appearance of female xenotypic characteristics (oviduct) in the gonad of the genetic male carp (Gemeno et al. 1996). Along these lines it is surprising to note that in Denmark a change in male-female ratio among newborn infants has been described which was attributed to possible environmental or other agents with toxic influence on the male reproductive system that might have led to the low male-female ratio (Möller 1996). In a Spanish study of risk factors for cryptorchidism it was concluded that an association between exposure to xenobiotics with hormone disruptive activity and increased risk of cryptorchidism was possible. So far, studies of risk factors for cryptorchidism have rarely analysed the role of overexposure during pregnancy to substances with endocrine disruptive activity (Garcia-Rodriguez 1996). A list of so-called endocrine disruptures with estrogenic activity is given below.

Table 2. Xenobiotics with potential estrogenic activity

Group	Substances
Pesticides	Aldrine, Atrazine, Chinalphos, 2,4-Dichlorphenol, Dicofol, DDT, Dieldrine, Endosulfan, Heptachlor, HCH, Kepone, Methoxychlor, Mirex, Phosmet, Toxaphene
Chemicals	Alkylphenols, Benzophenone, Bisphenol A, Butylbenzol, Nitrotoluol, Phenolred, Phtalats, PCB
Phytoestrogens	Butine, Citral, Coumestrol, Daidzeine, Formononetin, Genistein, Luteolin, Naringenine, Panoferol, Quercetine, Tetrahydrocannabiol
Mycotoxins	Zearalenone

References

Garcia-Rodriguez, J. et al. (1996), *Environmental Health Perspectives*, Vol. 104, No. 10, pp. 1090-5.

Gemeno, S., Gerritsen, A., Bawmer, T. and Komen, H. (1996), *Nature*, Vol. 384, pp. 221-2.

Heinzow, B. and Hanf, V.(1995), in *Moderne Fortpflanzungsmedizin*, Thieme Verlag.

Möller, H. (1996), *Lancet*, Vol. 348, pp. 828-9.

Thonneau, P. et al. (1992), 'Infertility in France. Results of Multicenter Survey in Three Regions of France', *Contracept. Fertil. Sex.*, Vol. 20, No. 1, pp. 27-32.

3 Accepting infertility

Ian D. Cooke

Not all patients (note the difference in terminology where sociologists refer to these individuals as clients) wish to have their infertility investigated because they are not sufficiently highly motivated, because of guilt, because of fear, or a simple unwillingness to have medicalised such an intimate area of their lives. This may be much worse in some ethnic groups which demand female-only medical staff involvement which may not be organisationally feasible. Some men decline investigation or examination which causes them to default from further attendance, amounting to 5-10 per cent.

Couples require adequate basic investigation and explanation of the data relevant to themselves. Their attitudes to this information can be significantly altered by the nature of the pathology or negative factors influencing prognosis such as female age, duration of infertility, a major male factor or combined abnormalities that they may perceive apportion 'blame' equally. In addition to these medical factors there are major social qualifications at the present time in the UK where restrictive funding has led Health Authorities only to fund in vitro fertilisation (IVF) on a basis of 9.3 per 100,000 population ranging from 0-29.3 (Report 1996). Qualifications vary among Authorities but range from strict age criteria e.g. only ages 25-35, no previous attempts at assisted conception, no previous living children in the present or any previous relationship and exclusion of those who have previously had a sterilisation (male or female). Further, the Human Fertilisation and Embryology Authority's Code of Practice (HFEA 1991) stipulates that due consideration must be given to 'the welfare of the child' and many aspects of this are laid down. All these criteria may militate against the couple's access to funded National Health Service treatment and forces them to approach any investigational treatment in the private sector, impossible for many.

Factors that influence the acceptance of infertility are the patients' perception of the adequacy of investigation, the explanation given by the professionals, the perceived expertise of those offering investigation and explanation and access to second opinions if requested. Indeed, such a request may be inhibited. It is also influenced by access to all available treatments which may not be possible depending upon the geography. In the UK this has been influenced significantly by the HFEA's recent annual publications of 'The Patient's Guide' which provides standardised data on a variety of treatments compiled from regular returns by individual licensed clinics. All clinics practising assisted conception must be registered.

Access to trained counsellors is important as professionals, both nurses and doctors, apart from providing a sympathetic ear and a caring manner, are not trained in non-directive counselling. Furthermore, such counselling requires a considerable amount of time and is more appropriately given by those with relevant skills. Apart from taking time to get over the emotional distress engendered by information that treatment cannot be offered or that the prognosis is poor and the subsequent bereavement process, there needs to be a willingness to discuss opportunities for alternative expression of their childbearing aspirations. Opportunities for such expression depend on the social structure, their age, economic situation and the nature of their partnership. Recent problems have highlighted the patients' perception of the adequacy of their previous investigation and treatment and with developments occurring in the field, some may be too old to receive techniques that have only recently been introduced, but which may have given them a reasonable prospect of success if offered earlier. Alternative strategies depend on the family structure, their relationship support and the development of their coping strategies. Counselling appears to be an important element but there is little discussion of the cost of counselling and if couples cannot afford private IVF, can they afford the counselling that would help in their adaptation to not obtaining it?

The above problems are compounded by frequent long waiting times for initial consultation and for individual investigations or treatments. They are exacerbated by professionals who are less than expert in the area, doing inappropriate investigations, being unaware of the importance of certain aspects, particularly age and duration of infertility and not knowing of technical developments in the field. There is a good argument for sensitising all family practitioners to the issues, co-ordinating centres of excellence for efficient investigation and treatment and providing an early realistic assessment of the probablity of success as defined by live mature birth of a singleton baby. Professionals frequently overestimate the probability of success and indeed define success in complex terms that are not understandable to the lay person and which do not relate to the probability of taking home a baby. National problems such as poor National Health Service funding, training situations where multiple staff members are seen sequentially and variable geographical service provision all make the process of treatment or ultimate acceptance of infertility much more difficult than it need be.

References

Human Fertilisation and Embryology Authority (1991), *Code of Practice*, Paxton House, 30 Artillery Lane, London E1 7LS.

'Report of the Fourth National Survey of National Health Service Funding of Infertility Services for the National Infertility Awareness Campaign' (1996), London.

4 Social aspects of infertility

Agneta Sutton

Parenthood has become increasingly a matter of choice and planning, almost like the choice and planning involved in purchasing a new motor car; and this observation applies to the infertile as well as the fertile. Not only is it assumed that whether or not to have a child should be a matter of choice, but increasingly people seek to make sure that any child they have is born with as few disadvantages as possible.

Prenatal diagnosis is a double-edged tool. It can be used to monitor pregnancy and ensure as far as possible the safe delivery of a child in a good state of health. Alternatively, it may be used to avoid the birth of gravely – or not so gravely – disabled children. And, as the American writer Barbara Katz Rothman has pointed out in her book, entitled *The Tentative Pregnancy*, because of prenatal diagnosis, many mothers today 'put their feelings on hold' until they have reassuring test results. That is to say, they refuse to recognise their pregnancy until the health of the child has been assessed.

That the technologisation of pregnancy is altering the woman's – as well as society's and the medical profession's – approach to pregnancy is equally evident in the case of women who have difficulties in conceiving. Being increasingly able to control nature, human beings turn to technology when nature fails, seeking either to correct it or circumvent it. Many of our new technological inventions are marvellous. But we must be aware that with new powers come new demands and new attitudes.

Today, people sometimes talk as if they have a right to a child, and so they demand services. Demands for services create new opportunities for providers of services. The availability of services calls out for custom. Couples who do not have children know that services for assisted conception are available. Not only may they feel that they have a right to them, but they may even feel that they are expected to make use of them.

The way in which our new powers in the area of reproductive medicine have fostered new attitudes, new demands and new expectations is well illustrated by the way we talk about assisted reproduction. The statistics of fertility treatment are couched in terms of success rates, frozen embryo transfers, micromanipulation techniques etc.

Language of its nature is always significant. Often it signifies more than is consciously apprehended or intended. The language of assisted reproduction, which is referred to by some feminists as 'repro-speak', tells a story of its own. Even the word 'reproduction' tells a story if we remember that people used to speak of 'procreation'.

'Repro-speak' promotes a reductionist way of thinking. Of course, much medical jargon has a tendency to reduce the patient to an object – but none more so than 'repro-speak'. Women undergoing fertility treatment are sometimes talked of as if they were aggregates of pieces that may be taken out and apart and put in or together again, sometimes in the same, sometimes even in another, woman. 'Repro-speak', tends to reduce the woman to a functional or non-functional baby-machine.

'Repro-speak', in other words, has a tendency to reduce the human person to biological raw material and biological product. Human procreation becomes a mere biological process, or in the context of the new techniques, a bio-technological process. Yet, both doctors and patients know that this is precisely what it is not.

But language is seductive. Thus, we are well advised to remind ourselves now and then that we must not let either language or technology dehumanise us. Language like technology can reinforce desires, fears and attitudes, and, perhaps nowhere more so than in the context of reproductive medicine. This is an area of medicine touching as much upon the human psyche as upon the human body. Assisted conception has not only physical implications but psychological and, of course, familial and social, implications. The desire for a child is a deep-seated desire in the human heart. And the way in which it is satisfied calls for careful consideration.

We are talking about an issue that concerns both the human soul and the foundations of society. Medicine alone does not suffice to deal with this. For a start, assisted reproduction demands proper counselling. To offer these techniques without proper psychological assessment of their consequences is irresponsible. In some countries, there are stories about women who have become obsessed with the idea of having a child and seek treatment after treatment despite the odds.

The success of modern medicine, and not least in reproductive medicine, can lead to an over-reliance on medical interventions of the technical kind, with the result that women or couples turn to the man in the white coat and to his technology seeking help for not only medical but even psychological and social problems.

In a world were God has been declared dead by men such as Nietzsche, Marx and Freud, it is not surprising that the doctor has taken over many of the roles reserved for the priest, pastor and rabbi. The rumour of God's death has left a vacuum in our society. But this is not a vacuum that medicine is necessarily well equipped to fill. Indeed, medicine cannot solve all ills and both patients and doctors must recognise its limitations. This is particularly pertinent in the area of assisted conception, where in many cases the childless woman would do better to accept remaining childless than to seek at all costs to have a child.

Despite the enormous achievements that we have seen the last decade, many women go away disappointed. There is no denying that sometimes the treatment for infertility creates more problems than it solves. It is it time-consuming, tiring and often painful and embarrassing for the patients. Even if clinicians are careful, it might promote obsession in some patients. It may certainly lead to depression if it is unsuccessful.

Yet, if a woman does become obsessed, this sad state of affairs should not be attributed solely to her doctor or to medicine but must be located within the wider framework of her own psychological make-up and social conditions. In fact, all these conditions will by nature be mingled and inter-twined. Often there is a social pressure, in a wider sense, on the woman to have a child. And, as argued above, often this pressure is magnified by the availability of medical services.

Together the technological advances and the prevailing consumerist attitude within modern western society, can sometimes make it hard for people to accept that there are times when the goods cannot be delivered. Thus both doctors and patients may be inclined to say: 'let's try just once more'. In other words, while the patients focus on their own desires, the doctors do all they can to satisfy their patients, with the result that neither of them see that there might be other ways of coping with the situation than that of producing a child.

Of course, infertility treatment should aim at helping the infertile patient. However, it is important to realise that successful treatment might be of two kinds. The birth of a child is the most obvious of the two. But learning to live with infertility can also be seen as a successful outcome.

5 Psychosocial aspects of infertility and treatment

Lone Schmidt

Epidemiology

About 10-28 per cent of 25- to 45-year-old women who have tried to conceive a baby experience infertility one or more times (Gunnell and Ewings 1994, Schmidt and Münster 1995, Schmidt et al. 1995, Sundby and Schei 1996). Only about 5 per cent of the women in western countries will remain involuntarily childless because of infertility problems (Schmidt and Münster 1995). Not all infertile couples seek medical treatment: only about 25 per cent have sought treatment in USA (Hirsch and Mosher 1987), 50 per cent in Denmark and England (Gunnell and Ewings 1994, Schmidt et al. 1995), and around 90 per cent in Scotland (Templeton et al. 1991). The modern reproductive technologies are effective in contrast to earlier methods of treatment. They offer a realistic possibility for the infertile couple to become parents. Results from all the public fertility clinics in Denmark (1994) show that about 50-60 per cent with in vitro fertilisation (IVF) or intracytoplasmic sperm injection (ICSI) treatment and about 80 per cent with donor insemination will become parents. The female patients' mean age was 34 years and mean duration of infertility was five years.

Infertility and psychosocial research

Two decades ago emotional factors were presumed to be a cause of infertility in 30-50 per cent of the non-organic infertile cases (Stanton and Dunkel-Schetter 1991). The possibilities of finding medical causes of infertility have improved and in the 1980s the emotional distress experienced by many infertile couples was seen as a consequence of the infertility problem rather than the cause. Infertility was described clinically as a crisis with predictable stages but no study has confirmed this description. During the last years many of the researchers including myself regard infertility as a stressful experience which the infertile couples have to cope with (Stanton and Dunkel-Schetter 1991).

All scientific knowledge about psychosocial consequences of infertility is based on empirical studies which only include infertile couples who have sought treatment. In other words, there is no scientific knowledge about the thousands of infertile couples who choose not to seek medical solutions. Most of the studies are cross-sectional and are therefore not adequate to discover and describe the long-lasting process of infertility. Many of the studies use standard scales for e.g. psychiatric morbidity as SCL-90. These kinds of standard scales of psychopathology are not suitable tools to identify and describe the psychosocial distress of either infertility or the medical treatment process (Berg and Wilson 1990).

This text is based mainly on the results of longitudinal studies which include both the women and the men from the infertile couples and involve repeated investigations of the same study group. I also include results from in-depth interview studies including my own study with 16 infertile couples (Schmidt 1996).

Stressful experience

Infertility is a stressful life-event (Freeman et al. 1985) which can be described as the blockage of one or more major life goals. Infertility is a process which often continues for many years (Lalos 1985, Möller 1985, Wirtberg 1992). Infertility involves loss of potential and expectations, e.g. loss of a hoped-for baby, loss of the possibility of the transition from non-parenthood to parenthood, loss of the image of having a healthy body, loss of the possibility of giving your parents grandchildren (Mahlstedt 1985).

Repeated losses

The infertility process is a process with repeated losses. Every month the menstruation is the sign telling that a conception has not occured. Every test is possibly a diagnosis of the cause of infertility. Every treatment attempt may fail.

Longitudinal studies have shown that the reactions to infertility do not follow the well-described stages of a traumatic crisis (shock, reaction, adaptation, reorientation) (Lalos 1985, Möller 1985, Wirtberg 1992). Emotional reactions to infertility can be described as a prolonged process with repeated periods of crisis. The model of the traumatic crisis does not fit as infertility is a process of repeated losses and not one traumatic loss as e.g. divorce or the death of a close family member. The model also claims that every individual has to experience identical stages after a traumatic loss. The coping research shows that every individual has different potential and different ways of handling crisis.

Psychosocial consequences of infertility

Emotional responses

Many individuals from infertile couples suffer from emotional responses such as grief and depressive feelings, anger, guilt, denial and anxiety (Golombok 1992). Many of these individuals experience periods of low self-esteem (Abbey et al. 1992a).

Doubt and ambivalence

The reasons for the desire to have children are not different between infertile and fertile couples (Lalos et al. 1985). People want children because children express the meaning of life and it is a way to express feelings of love between spouses (ibid.). Infertile couples have years with periods of doubt and ambivalence as they do not succeed to become parents when they make an effort. They question for example whether they really want to become parents; whether they will become adequate parents; whether a divorce is a possibility; whether the taxing medical treatment is worth continuing.

Marriage

Infertile couples often estimate their life-quality as high (Hearn et al. 1987). In quantitative questionnaire studies there are no differences between infertile and fertile couples in estimations of satisfaction with marriage and sexual life (Freeman et al. 1983, Abbey et al. 1991). However, in qualitative studies infertile couples express that the infertility problem is a serious threat to the existence of the marriage (Lalos 1985, Wirtberg 1992, Schmidt 1996). At the same time the infertility problem can strengthen and deepen the couples' relationship (Stanton et al. 1991, Schmidt 1996). The sexual life will often be impaired with periods of rare, scheduled intercourses which focus on conception rather than joy and pleasure (Möller 1985, Schmidt 1996).

Social relations

Some infertile couples experience changes in social relations such as periods of isolation and feelings of not being accepted and not being understood by family and friends (Lalos 1985, Miall 1985). Others experience emotional support from family and friends (see later). Infertility can lead to an unwanted but mutual withdrawal from the company of friends with children (Lalos 1985, Schmidt 1996).

Women and men

Most studies conclude that women from infertile couples report more intense emotional reactions than the men (Andrews et al. 1991, Greil 1991, Wright et al. 1991). However, men with reduced semen quality seem to react just as intensely as women (Nachtigall et al. 1992).

Ways of coping

Women and men in infertile couples use several ways of both problem-focused and emotion-focused coping at the same time (Schmidt 1996). Problem-focused coping means, for example, seeking information, seeking treatment, or stopping treatment and seeking adoption. Emotion-focused coping means, for example, finding positive aspects of being childless, weeping and grieving, and expressing emotions when talking with others.

Women often take the initiative by visiting the medical doctor and making appointments for treatment (Collins et al. 1992, Wirtberg 1992, Schmidt 1996). Women often find it more pleasurable and supportive than men to talk with other infertiles (Berg et al. 1991, Greil 1991). Men from infertile couples often use more passive ways of coping, for example, trying not to get emotionally involved, not talking with others and not looking for information (Schmidt 1996).

In my own study the participants managed their infertility in three different ways in relation to other people:

1. *secrecy,* when the participant did not share the infertility experience with others;
2. *formal*, when sharing only formal information (e.g. date of treatment, number of eggs retrieved);
3. *open-minded*, when both formal information and emotional feelings of the infertility experience were shared with others.

The male participants were equally distributed in the three groups. Only a few women were in the secrecy group and most of them were open-minded.

Only the open-minded group experienced emotional support and understanding from family and friends. Hynes et al. (1992) found that women in IVF-treatment who used avoidance coping reported a lower degree of well-being than the women who used active ways of coping.

Modern reproductive technology and the infertility process

For decades women from infertile couples have sought medical treatment. However, in earlier periods the treatment offered seldom resulted in births. In contrast modern medical infertility treatment offers a realistic possibility for the infertile couples to become parents. In Denmark about 60 per cent will have at least one live-born child after treatment of high quality.

On the one hand treatment is a relief. The couple's infertility problem is treated seriously. The couple has an opportunity to have the cause of infertility explained and a fair chance to become parents. In my own study treatment was experienced as a relief among the couples who had told friends and relatives of the forthcoming pregnancy at the moment when the couples had begun to have unprotected intercourses (Schmidt 1996).

On the other hand, for most of the couples, treatment is experienced as an additional burden (Koch 1989, Collins et al. 1992). To choose treatment is to choose a loss of privacy, to choose periods of great hope alternating with despair and deep sorrow. The infertile couples often experience treatment as an automatic process with one examination which leads to the next one and different diagnoses automatically leading to the different kinds of treatment. In spite of the automatic process the patients themselves have to make repeated decisions with unknown consequences. After every failed treatment attempt, the couples have to decide if and when they want to continue treatment; if they want to quit; if they want to adopt a child, or want to live a life without becoming parents (Schmidt 1996).

Treatment in the health care system focuses on the biological aspects of infertility and treatment. Infertile patients are in general satisfied with the technical aspects of treatment offered by the medical staff (Sabourin et al. 1991, Halman et al. 1993). However, the patients are often dissatisfied with the communication (Sundby et al. 1994). Infertile patients express a great need for psychosocial and sexual aspects of infertility to be included in the health services provided. The patients wish to discuss, to have professional advice and counselling, and want the opportunity to participate in support groups (Lalos 1985, Möller 1985, Daniluk 1988, Sundby et al. 1994, Schmidt 1996). Some patients want the possibilities of other solutions like adoption to be discussed with the medical staff during the treatment period (Halman et al. 1993, Schmidt 1996).

New medical reproductive technologies can prolong the treatment process. In Denmark, for example, infertile couples have to wait one to two years for an initial visit to a public fertility clinic. The different treatment attempts often last for two to five years as well. Some couples will try all the treatment options available at the public fertility clinics. Some of them will pay themselves at private clinics either during the waiting period for public treatment or if public treatment has been terminated without a live-born child. Some couples decide to stop treatment before all available options are tried, not forgetting the fact that still many infertile couples do not seek treatment at all.

Medical treatment can in this way prolong the couples' process of deciding to seek another solution such as adoption. We know that, at least in Denmark, couples rarely apply for adoption without having tried some medical treatment initially.

However, the psychosocial process related to infertility is a longlasting process whether medical treatment is an option or not. From clinical experience we know that many women from infertile couples describe the infertility process as not stopping before the women feel too old to have a baby or before the women are postmenopausal.

On the basis of the scientific knowledge of what infertile patients are missing in the health care system it is maybe possible to improve the professional skills. My hope is, that in the future medical treatment can fruitfully contribute to the infertile couples' psychosocial process. A fruitful contribution requires that:

1 infertility treatment is offered at clinics where the couples have to meet only a few different staff-members;
2 the treatment proceeds without waiting times;
3 the treatment follows a plan which is known to both the doctor and the couple;
4 the man in the infertile couple is actively involved in the investigations and in the treatment process;
5 the infertile couples are involved in treatment plans and decision-making;
6 the staff shows empathy and the clinic offers counselling about psychosocial and sexual consequences of infertility and treatment;
7 from the beginning of the treatment process the staff mentions that treatment attempts can fail;
8 the staff actively supports couples in stopping treatment if they experience several unsuccessful treatment attempts;
9 the staff has knowledge about alternative ways to become parents, i.e. adoption and fostering;
10 the staff invites the couple to discuss alternative solutions to treatment.

References

Abbey, A., Andrews, F.M. and Halman, L.J. (1991), 'Gender's Role in Responses to Infertility', *Psychol Women Quarter*, Vol. 15, pp. 295-316.

Abbey, A., Andrews, F.M. and Halman, L.J. (1992a), 'Infertility and Subjective Well-being. The Mediating Role of Self-esteem, Internal Control, and Interpersonal Conflict', *J Marr Fam*, Vol. 54, pp. 408-17.

Abbey, A., Halman, L.J. and Andrews, F.M. (1992b), 'Psychosocial, Treatment, and Demographic Predictors of Stress Associated with Infertility', *Fertil Steril*, Vol. 57, pp. 122-8.

Andrews, F.M., Abbey, A. and Halman, L.J. (1991), 'Stress From Infertility, Marriage Factors, and Subjective Well-being of Wives and Husbands', *J Health Soc Beh*, Vol. 32, pp. 238-53.

Berg, B.J. and Wilson, J.F. (1990), 'Psychiatric Morbidity in the Infertile Population: A Reconceptualization', *Fertil Steril*, Vol. 53, pp. 654-61.

Berg, N.J., Wilson, J.F. and Weingartner, P.J. (1991), 'Psychological Sequelae of Infertility Treatment: The Role of Gender and Sex-role Identification', *Soc Sci Med*, Vol. 33, pp. 1071-80.

Collins, A., Freeman, E.W., Boxer, A.S. et al. (1992), 'Perceptions of Infertility and Treatment Stress in Females Compared With Males Entering In Vitro Fertilization Treatment', *Fertil Steril*, Vol. 57, pp. 350-6.

Daniluk, J.C. (1988), 'Infertility: Intrapersonal and Interpersonal Impact', *Fertil Steril*, Vol. 49, pp. 655-65.

Freeman, E.W., Boxer, A.S., Rickels, K. et al. (1985), 'Psychological Evaluation and Support in a Program of In Vitro Fertilization and Embryo Transfer', *Fertil Steril*, Vol. 43, pp. 48-53.

Freeman, E.W., Garcia, C.-R. and Rickels, K. (1983), 'Behavioral and Emotional Factors: Comparisons of Anovulatory Infertile Women With Fertile and Other Infertile Women', *Fertil Steril*, Vol. 40, pp. 195-201.

Golombok, S. (1992), 'Psychological Functioning in Infertility Patients', *Hum Reproduc*, Vol. 7, pp. 208-12.

Greil, A.L. (1991), *Not Yet Pregnant. Infertile Couples in Contemporary America*, Rutgers University Press: New Brunswick.

Gunnell, D.J. and Ewings, P. (1994), 'Infertility Prevalence, Needs Assessment and Purchasing', *J Publ Health Med*, Vol. 16, pp. 29-35.

Halman, L.J., Abbey, A. and Andrews, F.M. (1993), 'Why Are Couples Satisfied With Infertility Treatment?', *Fertil Steril*, Vol. 59, pp. 1046-54.

Hearn, M.T., Yupze, A.A., Brown, S.E. et al. (1987), 'Psychological Characteristics of In Vitro Fertilization Participants', *Am J Obstet Gynecol*, Vol. 156, pp. 269-74.

Hirsch, M.B. and Mosher, W.D. (1987), 'Characteristics of Infertile Women in the United States and Their Use of Infertility Services', *Fertil Steril*, Vol. 47, pp. 618-25.

Hynes, G.L., Callan, V.C., Terry, D.J. et al. (1992), 'The Psychological Well-being of Infertile Women After a Failed IVF Attempt: The Effects of Coping', *Br J Med Psychol*, Vol. 65, pp. 269-78.

Koch, L. (1989), *Ønskebørn. Kvinder og reagensglasbefrugtning* (Desired Children. Women and In Vitro Fertilization), Rosinante: Copenhagen.
Lalos, A. (1985), *Psychological and Social Aspects of Tubal Infertility*, Department of Obstetrics and Gynaecology, Umeå University, Medical Dissertation.
Mahlstedt, P.P. (1985), 'The Psychological Component of Infertility', *Fertil Steril*, Vol. 43, pp. 335-46.
Miall, C.E. (1985), 'Perceptions of Informal Sanctioning and the Stigma of Involuntary Childlessness', *Dev Behav*, Vol. 6, pp. 383-403.
Möller, A. (1985), *Psykologiska aspekter på infertilitet* (Psychological Aspects of Infertility). Department of Psychology, University of Gothenburg, Dissertation.
Nachtigall, R.D., Becker, G. and Wozny, M. (1992), 'The Effects of Gender-specific Diagnosis on Men's and Women's Response to Infertility', *Fertil Steril*, Vol. 57, pp. 113-21.
Sabourin, S., Wright, J., Duchesne, C. et al. (1991), 'Are Consumers of Modern Fertility Treatment Satisfied?', *Fertil Steril*, Vol. 56, pp. 1084-90.
Schmidt, L. (1996), *Psykosociale konsekvenser af infertilitet og behandling* (Psychosocial Consequences of Infertility and Treatment), FADL's Forlag: Copenhagen, PhD-Thesis.
Schmidt, L. and Münster, K. (1995), 'Infertility, Involuntary Infecundity, and the Seeking of Medical Advice in Industrialized Countries 1970-1992: A Review of Concepts, Measurements, and Results', *Hum Reprod*, Vol. 10, pp. 1407-18.
Schmidt, L., Münster, K. and Helm, P. (1995), 'Infertility and the Seeking of Infertility Treatment in a Representative Population', *Br J Obstet Gynaecol*, Vol. 102, pp. 978-84.
Stanton, A.L. and Dunkel-Schetter, C. (eds) (1991), *Infertility. Perspectives From Stress and Coping Research*, Plenum Press: New York.
Stanton, A.L., Tennen, H., Affleck, G. et al. (1991), 'Cognitive Appraisal and Adjustment to Infertility', *Women and Health*, Vol. 17, pp. 1-15.
Sundby, J. (1994), *Infertility – Causes, Care and Consequences*, Department of Epidemiology, National Institute of Public Health and Section for Medical Anthropology, Department Group of Medicine, University of Oslo, Medical Dissertation.
Sundby, J. (1992), 'Long-term Psychological Consequences of Infertility: A Follow-up of Former Patients', *J Women Health*, Vol. 1, pp. 209-17.
Sundby, J. and Schei, B. (1996), 'Infertility and Subfertility in Norwegian Women Aged 40-42', *Acta Obstet Gynaecol Scand*, Vol. 75, pp. 832-7.
Sundby, J., Olsen, A. and Schei, B. (1994), 'Quality of Care for Infertility Patients. An Evaluation of a Plan for a Hospital Investigation', *Scand J Soc Med*, Vol. 2, pp. 139-44.

Templeton, A., Fraser, C. and Thompson, B. (1991), 'Infertility – Epidemiology and Referral Practice', *Hum Reproduc*, Vol. 6, pp. 1391-4.
Wirtberg, I. (1992), *His and Her Childlessness*, Department of Psychiatry and Psychology, Karolinska Institute Stockholm, Dissertation.
Wright, J., Allard, M., Lecours, A. et al. (1989), 'Psychosocial Distress and Infertility: A Review of Controlled Research', *Int J Fertil*, Vol. 34, pp. 126-42.
Wright, J., Bissonette, F., Duchesne, C. et al. (1991), 'Psychosocial Distress and Infertility: Men and Women Respond Differently', *Fertil Steril*, Vol. 55, pp. 100-8.

6 Is the desire for a child too strong? or Is there a right to a child of one's own?

Walter Lesch

The double title of this paper points to my uneasiness concerning the ethical approach appropriate to normative problems in connection with the phenomenon of infertility. Can an ethicist sincerely presume to decide whether the desire for a child is too strong? I am convinced that no arrogance of moral speculation will be able to destroy the strength and authenticity of an *ethics of desire*. Leaving the sphere of privacy, the philosopher moves to an *ethics of rights* in order to repeat the disturbing question in a different, more objective voice: is there a right to a child? A child of one's own? Having explored the right-based approach the ethicist discovers that this path leads to some structural clarifications which are useful for the public debate. But the puzzle of desire will continue to irritate our moral investigation. The paper wants to offer nothing more than some tentative comments on the oscillating movements between an ethics of rights and an ethics of desire. They represent a mutual challenge and a necessary ambivalence in the foundation of applied ethics.

Infertility and the desire for a child seem to be first of all medical and psychological problems (Auhagen-Stephanos 1991) – independent from ethical and legal considerations. Can there be an impartial moral point of view from which we might pronounce judgements upon the reasons and justifications for such a strong wish? I suppose that a liberal moral philosophy is not authorised to comment on these personal wishes. We can discuss the means for reaching an end. But this end is not controversial; the motivation in itself should not be part of a moralising public debate. Infertile couples already have to suffer from the contradictory attitudes by which there is an enormous pressure on couples without children; at the same time these people have to face the suspicion that they seem to need children as a sort of artificial limb (Winkler 1991, Delaisi de Parseval 1990). Whatever they do, they have already been forced to expose their intimate desire in the public of experts.

Desires can never be strong enough and often go beyond the necessity of deciding what is right or wrong. This may be the reason why wishes are often considered as irrational and uncontrollable. But we also know about the negative consequences of a constant repression of strong desires. Therefore the public discussion of problems associated with infertility has at least the chance to break a taboo, to eliminate prejudices against a growing minority in our society and to contribute to a more careful argumentation in matters of reproductive behaviour.

Taking into consideration the dynamics and the value of dearest wishes our ethical approach should take a less emotional starting point: the question whether there is *a positive right to a child of one's own*. In order to analyse this right I am going to have a closer look at three aspects of the problem. First of all I give a short description of the main characteristics of a right-based moral theory as far as the analysis of our subject is concerned. Secondly this theory will be discussed in the context of human rights. Finally I want to show that even in terms of rights the concrete question of the desire for a child of one's own is not silenced and implies much more than just the interests of the infertile couple.

The requirements of a right-based moral theory

Moral reasoning in the tradition of modern liberalism can be constructed as a theory of subjective rights gained in most cases after a long and hard struggle (Almond 1991, Tugendhat, 1993, p.336): a right to live in freedom, a right to health, a right to work etc. We have to find out the logical structure of these demands. Obviously it is a basic good not to be forced to suffer from hunger and poverty. And we have the right to live under conditions guaranteeing the protection against this suffering. Is the access to in vitro fertilisation (IVF) treatment such a basic right or is it a privilege that does not necessarily have to be recognised within a system of public health?

Having a right to a child of my own would mean that the professionals of reproductive technology have the obligation to do all that is possible in order to make my wish become reality. In this way of thinking the possibility of parenthood is regarded as an essential part of human self-realisation. Infertility would therefore be an obstacle that has to be overcome if the technical means are given. Infertility treatment would not be an act of supererogation, but a moral obligation of those who are able to apply the methods of IVF. Of course this obligation implies the duty to inform the patients completely about risks, success rates and all side effects of the treatment. Even a strong and hot desire can quickly cool off when we learn about the concrete conditions of its technical realisation.

The justification of the moral right to assisted procreation implies that infertility could be regarded as a disease comparable to other pathological facts. This is partly true, partly in contradiction to our intuitions because it is a very special kind of suffering (Wiesing 1993). Someone who suffers from cancer will do everything to be cured of this disease; and no healthy person can seriously wish to be attacked by cancer. Someone who lives involuntarily without children may express the strong desire to have a child of his or her own; but on the other hand we can easily imagine people who would see no problem in living without children of their own or without any children at all. We would never call it a pathological wish when somebody wants to be cured of a disease that causes pain and death. But the desire for fertility might indeed be regarded as *too strong* and even pathological in some cases. So we have to ask again what it means to have a moral right to procreation.

There is certainly a *negative right* to a child: the right not to be prevented from having a child. This is not at all self-evident in all situations if we think about birth control in totalitarian countries or of measures of eugenics motivated by different scientific or ideological reasons. Involuntary sterilisation would thus be strictly forbidden. But even if we leave such difficult cases out of consideration we cannot conclude from the negative right to a positive right. There seems to be no positive claim to have the strong desire for a child realised at any price, but only in the case of a limited number of indications.

The fact that the object of the desire is a future human being means that the right to procreation cannot be thought in terms of property rights. The responsibility for an independent being implies another degree of obligation than, for instance, the responsibility for a transplanted organ. Nevertheless, a reproductive technology is not bad in itself, but *one* legitimate answer to the suffering of infertility (Thévoz, 1990, p.124).

The larger horizon of human rights

A right-based moral theory is to be seen in the broader context of the international human rights system which is an important instrument for defining basic needs and corresponding rights (Alexy 1994, Galtung 1994). The articles 16 and 25 of the UN Declaration of Human Rights (1948) have to be considered with particular attention. Art. 16 defines the family as the natural and basic unit of a society. Marriageable women and men are not to be kept from starting a family: neither by race nor citizenship nor religion. Art. 25 concerns the right to benefit from social security and health care. Together these two articles could serve as a moral and legal basis for the right to infertility treatment because they emphasise the high good of individual freedom and self-determination.

Both articles clearly articulate the conclusion from basic needs and essentials of human life (sexuality, health) to corresponding rights which have to be recognised and guaranteed by the state's institutions according to the doctrine of fundamental human rights. But once again this does not automatically mean that these institutions are obliged to make all dreams come true and to manage the citizens' lives in a paternalistic way.

The human rights tradition is not concrete enough to provide a sufficient legitimation for positive rights in the area of procreation (Delaisi de Parseval 1993). Again we find the structure of a negative right: the rule that no authority can keep couples from becoming parents – even in the case of sterility. Any categorical refusal of medical aid against sterility would violate the fundamental principle of non-discrimination (Thévoz, 1990, p.124).

The complexity of needs, rights and interests

The look at the key arguments of a right-based morality leaves us with a feeling of helplessness because the clarification of justified claims does not cover the whole range of the moral problems connected to the new reproductive technologies. If we only regard the infertile couple's strong desire the answer is relatively easy: there should be no restrictions of the fulfillment of legitimate wishes that do not cause harm to other people. But the interaction of basic needs and rights is not free of interests that have to be taken into account. The claim to reproductive rights implies at least the following structure*: A and B have a right to C with the help of D and including possible interests of E, F, G...*

A/B are a woman and a man with their specific dynamics of living together and having individual and shared visions of a 'good life'. Who decides whether potential parents will be 'good' parents (cf. the case of adoption)? What about special wishes of lesbian couples?

C is the desired child: a future individual with its own rights and duties. Will he or she have a right to start living with the best possible genetic heritage?

D is the physician (and other experts of the medical system). Is he or she obliged to offer IVF treatment? Is there a right to propose (or even impose) such a treatment as a therapy and to use it for reasons of research?

The description of this very complex situation is not complete without a great number of further persons and institutions being involved in the realisation of a 'medicine of desire': E, F, G, ...: relatives and friends of the couple, health care and medical research institutions, assurances ...

Let's have a closer look at these persons and their specific interests.

A/B: Nobody can better explain the motivations, fears and ethical reflections than the couples directly concerned by infertility and having decided to get in contact with IVF specialists. That is why I warmly recommend a paper of the ethicist Paul Lauritzen who has written about his and his wife's own experiences with unusual frankness and sensitivity. He knows the clinical reality of sterility treatment and decribes the expectations and deceptions a couple has to live with after once having accepted the rules of this at the same time sophisticated and insecure set of methods. He also clearly points out one of the most crucial ethical problems: 'If reproductive technology is developed because every person has a right to bear a child, does it not follow that every person has a right to bear a perfect child?' (Lauritzen, 1990, p.44, cf. Testart 1994). Must infertile couples be better parents than others in order to resist the temptation of the ideal of perfection and health? This question can partly be answered by studying the requirements in the parallel case of adoption (Ernst, 1990, pp.446-448). Anyway the serious project of parenthood should be the most important and valid indication for the beginning of a usually longer sterility treatment.

C: Sexual reproduction and assisted procreation do not only concern the parents' (sometimes narcissistic) desires. There is a responsibility for the children who will be individuals with their own rights (a dimension which is still to be better implemented in the international system of human rights!). What does the desired child really stand for? We can make the comparison with fertile couples having children they did not wish for. This must not necessarily mean that these children will have a troubled life. The decision is more complicated in the case of possible disabilities because IVF in connection with preimplantation diagnosis could open the way to selection. 'Although we consider it ethically necessary to provide treatment to keep children alive who have serious illnesses, we do not consider it ethically necessary knowingly to conceive children with those same disorders' (Cohen, 1996, p.25).

D: What about the relation between the couple's desire and research interests?

> While there is no conspiracy to gain control of the process of reproduction, there is increased control. And if one theme joins the various objections to the new reproductive technologies, it is that they increase the medical profession's control over the process of reproduction and that such control has deleterious consequences (Lauritzen, 1990, p.45).

E, F, G ....: Medical treatment refers first of all to the autonomy of patients and the competence of the physicians. But we cannot neglect community interests concerning costs of treatment, allocation of resources. In the horizon of a communitarian bioethics, ethical reflection will also have to consider alternatives to IVF including the questions of how to diminish the pressure on infertile couples and to facilitate the conditions for adoption.

Epilogue

A differentiated analysis of rights and duties in the field of sterility and treatments of infertility (cf. Baertschi, 1996, p.34) shows the limits of ethical argumentation because there can be no medical or social management of strong desires. Obviously we have to combine different types of moral philosophy: social ethics (ethics of rights) and an ethics of individual well-being (ethics of desire) (cf. Bond 1996). As far as I know an encouraging and therapeutical ethics of desire has still to be written. Will this be possible within the limits of a liberal theory of justice? Can ethics itself be a therapeutical science? I hope that the preliminary remarks and open questions of this paper illustrate some of the aspects of a double strategy that I would like to suggest. As so often the case, it will be a walk on a slippery slope because a good and strong desire can always be misused and instrumentalised for undesirable purposes. It is a special feature of new reproductive technologies that the most intimate hopes and emotions are in closest proximity to a cool rationality which has an increasing control over life and death and over the definition of the desirable and the undesirable. The only remedy that ethics can offer is the invitation to try several points of view. Usually there is more than one way of coping with a difficult situation and with the promises and limits of medical feasibility.

References

Alexy, R. (1994), *Theorie der Grundrechte*, Suhrkamp: Frankfurt a.M.

Almond, B. (1991), 'Rights', in Singer, P. (ed.), *A Companion to Ethics*, Blackwell: Oxford, pp. 259-69.

Auhagen-Stephanos, U. (1991), 'Die unerfüllte Sehnsucht nach dem Kind', in Bernauer, U. (ed.), *Kinderwunsch – Wunschkind*, Katholische Akademie der Erzdiözese Freiburg: Freiburg i.B., pp. 10-24.

Baertschi, B. (1996), *Le bonheur c'est... d'avoir peu d'enfants,* (Folia Bioethica, 18), Société Suisse d'Ethique Biomédicale: Lausanne.

Bond, E.J. (1996), *Ethics and Human Well-being*, Blackwell: Oxford.

Cohen, C.B. (1996), '«Give Me Children or I Shall Die!» New Reproductive Technologies and Harm to Children', *Hastings Center Report*, Vol. 26, No. 2, pp. 19-27.

Delaisi de Parseval, G. (1990), 'L'enfant prothèse', *Le Supplément. Revue d'éthique et théologie morale*, Vol. 174, pp. 47-56.

Delaisi de Parseval, G. (1993), 'Droit de procréer', in Hottois, G. and Parizeau, M.-H. (eds), *Les mots de la bioéthique. Un vocabulaire encyclopédique*, De Boeck: Bruxelles, p. 144.
Ernst, C. (1991), 'Künstliche Zeugung', in Fleiner, T., Gilliand, P. and Lüscher, K. (eds), *Familien in der Schweiz*, Universitätsverlag: Fribourg, pp. 437-50.
Galtung, J. (1994), *Menschenrechte – anders gesehen*, Suhrkamp: Frankfurt a.M.
Lauritzen, P. (1990), 'What Price Parenthood?', *Hastings Center Report*, Vol. 20, No. 2, pp. 38-46.
Testart, J. (1994), *Le désir du gène*, Flammarion: Paris.
Thévoz, J.-M. (1990), *Entre nos mains l'embryon. Recherche bioéthique*, Labor et Fides: Genève.
Tugendhat, E. (1993), *Vorlesungen über Ethik*, Suhrkamp: Frankfurt a.M.
Wiesing, U. (1993), 'Diagnosen und Krankheitsbegriffe in der Reproduktionsmedizin – empirische und normative Aspekte', in Eckensberger, L.H. and Gähde, U. (eds): *Ethische Norm und empirische Hypothese*, Suhrkamp: Frankfurt a.M., pp. 284-301.
Winkler, U. (1991), 'Die Not der Kinderlosigkeit', in Wacker, B. (ed.): *Die letzte Chance? Adoptionen aus der 3. Welt*, Rowohlt: Reinbek, pp. 28-40.

7 To an ethics of desire

Paul van Tongeren

Walter Lesch (1997) opens his interesting paper with some rather sceptical remarks on the possibility of what he calls with a beautiful expression: an ethics of desire. At least a liberal moral philosophy should, according to his opinion, not be authorised to comment on personal wishes. Therefore he takes another approach, and asks the question of rights: do people have a right to a child of their own? But at the end of his paper it becomes obvious that not only has this rights-based approach its limits, but that it even presupposes a further elucidation of the parents' desires and the being desired of the future child, in order to assess the relevant rights. We need an ethics of desire. In my comment I would like to discuss – briefly – the relation between liberal moral philosophy and an ethics of desire, and then give two examples of what could be elaborated on in such an ethics of desire.

Instead of suggesting that a liberal moral philosophy excludes the question of the moral meaning and value of personal desires, I would like to suggest that liberalism *needs* an ethics of desire. An ethics of desire belongs to what has been called a theory of morality in the broad sense. Liberal moral philosophy on the contrary proposes a theory of morality in the narrow sense, i.e. of this minimum of morality that is needed to provide as many people as possible with an equal freedom to develop their own life and their own moral convictions, their own morality in the broad sense. This means, however, that liberalism would be pointless, when this free space which it provides, were not been filled with the plural substance of broad moralities (which will partly be moral evaluations of our desires). Ethics should not restrict itself to a reflection on the minimal constraints to which all participants will be bound, but also help those participants (and their communities) to elaborate their part. It should not only define the stage, but also help to write the roles to be played. And since the stage will have to be arranged in such a way that it allows the actors to play their role, the relation between the minimal morality of liberalism and substantial moralities will have to be two-way.

As an illustration I would like to suggest two elements of such an ethics of desire. Some years ago, I was asked to give an ethical commentary on a report from social scientists who had done research among so called 'second-chance-mothers': women who initially preferred to work for their career, and then – at the age of about 35 – realised that, if they did want to have children, they had to decide that right now. The problem that was at the basis of this research, was that these women seemed to hesitate very long, whereas they did not have the time to hesitate. What struck me, while reading the interviews they did with many of these women, is that almost all of them did not really know why they did want to have children, and that they hardly knew that they did not know. Almost all the anwers they gave to the question, why they might want to have children, could be summarised as: 'it's good fun'. Reflecting on this, I realised that we indeed hardly know why we want to have children. The expectations of those who do not have children yet, will be rather vague. And those who already have children often talk more about the many cares and concerns they have to endure in raising their offspring rather than being always or completely conscious of the depth of the bond that exists between them and their children. One way of exploring this desire would be to attempt a phenomenological exploration of the way in which 'we' *love* our children. My own efforts to attempt such a phenomenological description (van Tongeren 1995) confirmed my expectation that we love our children in a different way compared with the way we love our partners.

Philosophical literature does not say much about the way we love our children, nor about the human desire for children. Levinas suggests a relation between this desire and a desire for immortality (Levinas, 1961, part IV). It is in our children that we continue to live, after we die. That might also be the reason why people often seem to decide to have children not because they want them now, but because they are afraid that later on, when being older, they will regret not having had children. Also this should be elaborated in a phenomenology of our desires, or a hermeneutics of our experience.

One reason why such an ethics of desire would be important, also for ethical considerations regarding reproductive technologies, would be that it could warn us against becoming caught in a possible paradox when we try or pretend to be in control of our desire at the cost of the gratuitous or maybe illusory nature of what we desire.

References

Lesch, W. (1997), 'Is the Desire for a Child Too Strong? or Is There a Right to a Child of One's Own?', this volume, Part Two.

Levinas, E. (1961), *Totalité et Infini. Essay sur l'Extériorité*, Nijhoff: Den Haag.
van Tongeren, P. (1995), 'The Paradox of Our Desire for Children', *Ethical Perspectives*, Vol. 2, pp. 55-62.

Part Three
INDICATIONS FOR IN VITRO FERTILISATION

1 Infertility treatment without consideration of differenciated indications

Hans-Rudolf Tinneberg

Numerous indications for in vitro fertilisation (IVF) are to be taken into consideration especially when other forms of infertility treatment have failed so far. Indications for medical interventions are important in order to perform a cause related therapy which at the same time is adequate in its measures. However, even though reproductive medicine has experienced probably the highest progress in medical development, most of the conditions underlying successful establishment of pregnancy still remain unknown. In light of the demand for a conscious use of financial resources the debate is justified whether in any case a causal therapy should be performed or what is established as the most successful therapy. In our own hands comparing success rates as pregnancies per embryo transfers, intracytoplasmic sperm injection (ICSI) as a special form of IVF achieves a pregnancy rate of 26 per cent while IVF shows a lower pregnancy rate of 20 per cent. Similar trends were observed in other centers. Reasons for this difference cannot be provided, however it was hypothesised that perforation of the zona pellucida could improve implantation rates as it would assist hatching. Purely treating the zona pellucida without injection of sperm could not improve pregnancy rates.

According to the task force of gynaecological endocrinology and reproductive medicine of the German Society of Gynaecology and Obstetrics, ICSI therapy is indicated in case of two IVF attempts without fertilisation or in case of azoospermia, cryptozoospermia and oligoasthenoteratozoospermia or other forms of long time male subfertility.

With respect to reduced financial resources and the traumatic effect of unsuccessful treatment for infertility it should be discussed whether to perform ICSI instead of IVF in all cases of severe infertility, especially as it could be demonstrated by Meschede et al. (1995) that genetic risk in pregnancies resulting from ICSI is negligible.

References

Meschede, D., De Geyter, C., Nieschlag, E. and Horst, J. (1995), 'Genetic Risk in Micromanipulative Assisted Reproduction', *Human Reproduction*, Vol. 10, No.11, pp. 2880-6.

2 Infertility propagated to the next generation by in vitro fertilisation

Dieter Meschede and Jürgen Horst

The reasons for human infertility are manifold and still not completely understood. However, there is increasing evidence that in a substantial percentage of affected couples genetic abnormalities cause or contribute to the fertility problem, which is particularly true for male factor infertility (Lilford et al. 1994). Sex chromosomal and balanced autosomal chromosome aberrations, congenital bilateral absence of the vas deferens, and microdeletions in the long arm of the Y chromosome (Simoni et al. 1997) are among the best known examples. The latter entity will be discussed here to illustrate how the new in vitro fertilisation (IVF) methods can contribute to the propagation of infertility genes in the next generation and in which way this might affect our outlook on assisted human reproduction.

The long arm of the Y chromosome (Yq11) carries one or possibly several genes that are essential for normal spermatogenesis. DAZ (*d*eleted in *az*oospermia) is a gene with a testis-specific pattern of expression and represents a strong candidate for being the long-searched 'azoospermia factor' on Yq11 (Reijo et al. 1995). The rate of submicroscopic deletions in DAZ among azoospermic or severely oligozoospermic infertile men ranges between 3 and 4 per cent (Vogt et al. 1996, Simoni et al. 1997). In selected patient cohorts the prevalence may be even higher (Reijo et al. 1995).

Until very recently the chances of fathering a child were dismal for patients with severe oligozoospermia or azoospermia. Intracytoplasmic sperm injection (ICSI) has completely changed the prognosis for these conditions and – as a symptomatic form of treatment – offers a realistic chance for such men to have children of their own. Even non-obstructive azoospermia is no absolute obstacle to fatherhood anymore as sperm may be retrieved directly from testicular tissue (testicular sperm extraction, TESE) and then be used for ICSI.

However, once such treatment is successful in a patient carrying a Y chromosomal microdeletion the underlying genetic defect will inevitably be transmitted to all his sons. This would most likely lead to the recurrence of the father's fertility problem in male offspring. Some intergenerational variability in the clinical presentation may occur, as the general experience with dominant loss-of-function mutations suggests.

How do affected patients cope with this situation? We have counselled two men with DAZ microdeletions that were detected before a planned course of ICSI treatment. The nature of the genetic defect was carefully explained to them, as was the 100 per cent recurrence risk for subfertility in any sons they would have. The patients achieved a clear understanding of the situation including the specific genetic risk for their male offspring. Both opted to go ahead with the planned treatment, and their partners were fully supportive of this decision.

If patients are willing to accept such genetic risks, should high-cost assisted reproductive technology (ART) then be withheld by the treating physicians? This question touches upon the more general issue of patient autonomy in reproductive and family planning decisions. Also, barring patients with heritable disorders from participation in ART programs might be interpreted as discrimination based on genetic constitution. The World Health Organisation in its recently published 'WHO Guidelines on Ethical Issues in Medical Genetics and the Provision of Genetic Services' (1995) takes an uncompromising stance on these issues:

> Reproductive decisions should be the province of those who will be directly responsible for the biological and social aspects of childbearing and childrearing. (p.3)
>
> The ethos in present day medical genetics is to help people make whatever voluntary decisions are best for them in the light of their own reproductive goals. (p.3)
>
> Alternatives for couples at genetic risk include not having children, taking their chances of having a child with a genetic condition, having prenatal diagnosis and either selectively aborting affected fetuses or carrying them to term, adopting a child without the disorder, the use of donor gametes, and/or other methods of assisted reproduction. (p.13)

These WHO-supported statements fall in line with the practice of genetic counselling in Western societies, where most institutions favour a 'non-directive' approach.

For the medical geneticist it is everyday work to deal with conditions that have a high recurrence risk in the counsellees' offspring and to offer individuals or couples at genetic risk support in achieving their reproductive goals. The situation in infertile men carrying a DAZ microdeletion or any other kind of heritable disorder is particular insofar as the patient has a chance to act upon his reproductive decision only if massive support is granted from the medical system. For the physician who carries out the IVF treatment this may create a difficult situation in that on the one hand he wants to help the patient, on the other hand he is expected to guard against diseases in the patient's offspring. While this dilemma is to be fully acknowleged and critically discussed in each single case, we think that barring patients from ART programs based on the presence of or a predisposition to a genetic disorder would be harmful (Meschede et al. 1995). Acting in this way would introduce into assisted human reproduction a note of genetic discrimination that may indeed carry some eugenic undertones.

References

Lilford, R., Jones, A.M., Bishop, D.T., Thornton, J. and Mueller, R. (1994), 'Case-control Study Whether Subfertility in Men is Familial', *British Medical Journal*, Vol. 309, pp. 570-3.

Meschede, D., de Geyter, C., Nieschlag, E. and Horst, J. (1995), 'Genetic Risk in Micromanipulative Assisted Reproduction', *Human Reproduction*, Vol. 10, pp. 2880-6.

Reijo, R., Lee, T.-Y., Salo, P., Alagappan, R., Brown, L.G., Rosenberg, M., Rozen, S., Jaffe, T., Straus, D., Hovatta, O., de la Chapelle, A., Silber, S. and Page, D.C. (1995), 'Diverse Spermatogenic Defects in Humans Caused by Y Chromosome Deletions Encompassing a Novel RNA-Binding Protein Gene', *Nature Genetics*, Vol. 10, pp. 383-93.

Simoni, M., Gromoll, J., Dworniczak, B., Rolf, C., Abshagen, K., Kamischke, A., Carani, C., Meschede, D., Behre, H.M., Horst, J. and Nieschlag, E. (1997), 'Screening for Deletions of the Y Chromosome Involving the DAZ (Deleted in Azoospermia) Gene in Azoospermia and Severe Oligozoospermia', *Fertility and Sterility* Vol. 67, pp. 542-7.

Vogt, P.H., Edelmann, A., Kirsch, S., Henegariu, O., Hirschmann, P., Kiesewetter, P., Köhn, F.M., Schill, W.B., Farah, S., Ramos, C., Hartmann, M., Hartschuh, W., Meschede, D., Behre, H.M., Castel, A., Nieschlag, E., Weidner, W., Gröne, H.-J., Jung, A., Engel, W. and Haidl, G. (1996), 'Human Y Chromosome Azoospermia Factors (AZF) Mapped to Different Subregions in Yq11', *Human Molecular Genetics*, Vol. 5, pp. 933-43.

World Health Organisation and Wertz, D.C., Fletcher, J.C. and Berg, K. (1995), *Guidelines on Ethical Issues in Medical Genetics and the Provision of Genetic Services*, WHO: Geneva.

3 What shall we do with the unexplained infertility?

Urban Wiesing

In this short text I want to focus on the moral question: what shall we do with the so-called[1] idiopathic infertility or the unexplained infertility? Shall we treat unexplained infertility with reproductive technology, especially when this kind of infertility is interpreted as a physiological protective reaction caused by stress, as a wise reaction of the body? More generally put: how should the teleology of the body be dealt with ethically? And the so-called unexplained infertility raises the question whether active intervention is useful if this kind of infertility is not interpreted as a disease.

Specialists in psychosomatics and psychoanalysis stress that, at least in some cases, the unexplained infertility must be seen as a physiological protective reaction. Should we treat a physiological reaction that is not a disease but can be interpreted as a kind of wisdom of the body? If the answer is 'no, we should not', then I think a kind of avoidance strategy is at work which is not tenable. This kind of argumentation mentioned before tries to avoid a moral judgement by giving a definition. This common avoidance strategy can frequently be found in medicine despite its inadmissibility as an argument. Let me explain:

Since medicine lacks a binding definition of disease, the question whether infertility is a disease or not does not get us any further. The deontological quality of the definition of disease is ignored as well as the preceeding value judgement which declares 'We only want to treat what we describe as a disease'. Couples undoubtedly suffer because of their childlessness and why should this suffering not be treated?

If we speak of the wisdom of the body, we must admit that it is an interpretation of the reactions of the body. And in this case we should not think of the wisdom of the body only but also of the stupidity of the body. Both interpretations of a reaction are possible. Or, spoken in term of the Evolutionary Theory: Reactions of the body can be functional as well as dysfunctional, and a functional reaction might become dysfunctional when the surrounding conditions have changed. Therefore, it is not easy to decide whether an unexplained infertility, or an infertility caused by stress, is a wise reaction of the body or a stupid one. It might have been a wise reaction in former times, but is it still a wise reaction under the conditions of modernity?

However, in my opinion, with this veiled teleological argumentation it is necessary to make very exact distinctions: I think it is inadmissible to use teleological argumentation in order to refuse treatment. The argument 'I do not treat unexplained sterility because it is a protective reaction of the body' is not tenable. On the other hand, one cannot avoid considering the fact that unexplained infertility might be a protective reaction if one wants to treat such a disease intelligently (Koch 1927).

Other options in therapy are possible: considering unexplained infertility as a protective reaction can help to avoid defining the aim of therapy solely as the birth of a child, but to reduce the stress. If this kind of infertility is interpreted as caused by stress, one would at first refrain from interventionary measures and try to create conditions under which the organism becomes fertile. In practice: Instead of intervening immediately, one could recommend a holiday or relaxation measures, which are – by the way – the most effective treatments in the case of unexplained infertility. Statistics show that the number of pregnancies after a holiday or during breaks in treatment is many times higher than the success rate of reproductive medicine (Stauber 1988).

Let me summarise: The alleged teleology of the body, the alleged wisdom of the body, cannot substitute the moral question whether this kind of suffering should be treated or not. Moral arguments must be stressed to answer that question. On the other hand: Prudent medicine should always have a look at the teleology of the body. The question how to treat this kind of suffering cannot be answered intelligently without considering that it might be a protective reaction of the body.

Note

1 In order to get an impression of the confusion in terminology see Wiesing 1990.

References

Koch, R. (1927), 'Ärztliches Denken und Zweckmäßigkeit im Organischen', Die Schildgenossen, Vol. 7, pp. 449-73.

Stauber, M. (1988), *Psychosomatik der sterilen Ehe* (Fortschritte der Fertilitätsforschung 17), Grosse: Berlin.

Wiesing, U. (1990), 'Ist die idiopathische Sterilität eine Indikation für die In-vitro-Fertilisation?', *Geburtshilfe und Frauenheilkunde*, Vol. 50, pp. 417-20.

4 Alternative, non-IVF therapies

Aldo Campana and Dilys Walker

The ultimate goal for any couple seeking treatment for infertility is to achieve a pregnancy. In the case of infertility, as with other medical conditions, the physician must first correctly identify the problem, investigate the cause of the problem, and then propose the appropriate treatment plan. The most important step in the infertility investigation is to identify the cause or causes of infertility; which is not always a simple task. To assist in this evaluation, our department follows a straight forward, step by step approach to the infertility evaluation which is illustrated by the flow chart shown in figure 1 (Campana et al. 1995).

Although in vitro fertilisation (IVF) may have achieved popular notoriety, it is certainly not the only option, nor is it necessarily always the best option for treating infertility. Other treatments including timed intercourse, ovarian stimulation, and artificial insemination, are important alternatives to IVF. It is important to appreciate the relative contribution of these alternatives in helping the couple achieve a pregnancy. In our department, IVF or intracytoplasmic sperm injection (ICSI) is responsible for only about 20 per cent of pregnancies among infertile couples. This means that in most cases, pregnancies are obtained through non-IVF therapies. It is interesting to note that more than 20 per cent of all pregnancies are spontaneous, achieved during the course of infertility investigations (table 1).

The occurrence of spontaneous pregnancies during the infertility work is well known and has been documented in a study conducted by the World Health Organisation (WHO), with pregnancy rates ranging from 12 to 16 per cent (Cates et al. 1988). Another recently published study (Gleicher et al. 1996) showed that the cumulative rate of spontaneous pregnancies in women seeking infertility treatment was 20 per cent after one year. This data illustrates the importance of a thorough investigation that can be helpful not only for determining a diagnosis, but also may result in a pregnancy.

What are the possible explanations for spontaneous pregnancies occurring during the infertility evaluation? The first explanation lies in the fact that, in the general population, monthly fecundability is variable and depends upon a variety of factors. The woman's age is a typical example. For a woman throughout her 30s, there is natural progressive decline in fecundability (Frank et al. 1994). This decline explains why a woman in her later reproductive years might become spontaneously pregnant *after* more than one year of unprotected intercourse. One year is generally accepted as the cut off for the period of time after which a couple is considered infertile. Another important issue related to the occurrence of these spontaneous pregnancies is the inherent variability of each couple's fertility. For example, sperm quality is influenced by many factors such as stress, illness, or medical treatments (Campana et al. 1995). Therefore, temporary, transient abnormalities in sperm quality occur often. The same is true for the ovulatory function. Furthermore, spontaneous pregnancies occurring after some years of infertility may be explained by a number of 'subfertility' factors, affecting one or both partners. And finally, perhaps the most important explanation for these spontaneous pregnancies is that they may be the result of careful counselling and dialogue between the couple and physician.

Treatment of female infertility

Female infertility can be due to a tuboperitoneal, ovulatory, uterine, cervical or vulvovaginal factor (Campana et al. 1995). The most frequently encountered female factor is tuboperitoneal, followed by the ovulatory. Uterine and cervical factors are less frequent, and a vulvovaginal factor is rarely identified as the cause of infertility.

Tuboperitoneal factor refers to damage to the fallopian tubes and/or intraperitoneal adhesions and scarring. This problem is usually caused by prior pelvic infection, endometriosis, or surgery and often results in partial or complete blockage of the fallopian tubes, making spontaneous pregnancy unlikely. Some cases of tuboperitoneal factor infertility can be successfully treated by surgery. Most of these surgeries are performed by laparoscopy, with their success dependent upon the underlying severity of the problem. In our experience, the pregnancy rate after tubal surgery is about 30 per cent. In the majority of cases however, a tubal factor cannot be successfully treated by surgery. It is for these cases that IVF provides the best therapeutic alternative.

Ovulatory disorders account for about 15 per cent of all infertility factors (Speroff et al. 1994). In some cases it is possible to treat the cause of the disorder and in this way restore the normal ovulatory cycle (see table 2). These disorders may originate outside the hypothalamic pituitary axis and therefore may require the correction of other associated endocrinologic problems, behavioural changes, or surgery. After ruling out or treating other problems, a pharmacologic treatment is indicated to induce ovulation. The choice of hormone therapy depends on the underlying cause of the disorder or imbalance (table 3). Clomiphene citrate is the most commonly used drug to induce ovulation and acts by stimulating the hypothalamic release of GnRH (Gonadotrophin releasing hormone). In some cases, clomiphene is not effective in inducing ovulation and other drugs have to be considered. Gonadotrophins are often the next line of therapy and directly stimulate ovarian function. All of these treatments have important side-effects, but the most important complication, at least for clomiphene and gonadotrophin therapy, is the risk of multiple pregnancy: This risk is about 5 per cent for clomiphene, and 10 to 40 per cent for gonadotrophin therapy, depending on the quality of the monitoring and good medical judgment (Speroff et al. 1994).

Overall, how effective is hormone therapy in achieving a pregnancy? According to various studies, patients undergoing clomiphene treatment have cumulative pregnancy rates ranging from 25 to 49 per cent (Hammond 1996). The cumulative pregnancy rates for gonadotrophin therapy range from 40 to 90 per cent, and again, depend on the underlying cause of the ovulatory disorder (Speroff et al. 1994).

Uterine causes for infertility include congenital anomalies, submucous fibroids, uterine polyps, and intrauterine synechiae (Campana et al. 1995). These uterine factors can be a cause of both infertility and recurrent spontaneous abortion. All of these conditions may be successfully treated by hysteroscopic surgery.

Cervical factor infertility accounts for about 5 per cent of all infertility cases and refers primarily to abnormalities in the cervical mucus. In case of a cervical infection, antibiotic treatment is advised. In most cases, however, the quality of the cervical mucus cannot be improved by medical treatment, and intrauterine insemination is considered the treatment of choice (Campana et al. 1996).

Treatment of male infertility

If the semen analysis is abnormal, further investigations should be performed according to the specific type of sperm anomaly: azoospermia, aspermia or another sperm abnormality (Campana et al. 1995). Azoospermia may be due to a primary testicular failure, a hypogonadotrophic hypogonadism, or to an obstruction of seminal pathways. Primary testicular failure is a condition which cannot be reversed by medical or surgical treatment. In some cases, it is possible to aspirate spermatozoa directly from the testes, and to achieve fertilisation and subsequent pregnancy by ICSI (Silber et al. 1995). In contrast, hypogonadotrophic hypogonadism can be treated with gonadotrophin therapy (Martin-du Pan and Campana 1993). Obstructive azoospermia can be treated in some cases by surgery, or, as an alternative, by sperm aspiration from the epididymis with subsequent ICSI (Silber et al. 1995). As is the case for azoospermia, other categories of semen abnormalities such as oligozoospermia, asthenozoospermia, and teratozoospermia require an etiologic diagnosis before suggesting either a medical or surgical treatment. In some cases a medical or surgical treatment may improve sperm quality. For example, prostatitis causes sperm abnormalities that may be successfully treated with a combination of antibiotics and anti-inflammatory agents. Patients with varicoceles may benefit from surgical revision. The most important therapeutic approaches for male infertility are listed in table 4.

Unfortunately, most causes of sperm abnormalities cannot be significantly improved by either medical or surgical treatment. In such cases, it is important to accurately quantify the number of normal spermatozoa present in the ejaculate. This will allow one to estimate the chances of obtaining a pregnancy with artificial insemination. A recent evaluation of the insemination program at our hospital provides some important information (Campana et al. 1996). Pregnancy rates for insemination cycles are directly related to both sperm counts and the age of the woman. Table 5 illustrates the dramatic drop in pregnancy rates when the woman is over the age of 40. Another important factor in predicting the success of insemination is the number of motile spermatozoa (table 6). In our study the pregnancy rate was significantly lower when less than 0.5 million total motile sperm were used for the insemination. Even when the number of total motile sperm inseminated was between 0.5 and 1 million, pregnancy rates tended to be lower than when more than 1 million motile sperm could be used. Consequently, couples in which the male displayed severe asthenozoospermia or a combination of oligozoospermia and asthenozoospermia with a total motile sperm count of less than 1 million sperm, failed to obtain a pregnancy.

Treatment of unexplained infertility

The prevalence of unexplained infertility ranges from 3 to 14 per cent of all investigated infertility cases (Cates et al. 1988). Many empiric treatments have been proposed for unexplained infertility, the most popular one is pharmacologic treatment with clomiphene. According to the results of randomised studies clomiphene is more effective than placebo, with a cumulative pregnancy rate of about 20 per cent after 3 or 4 treatment cycles (Fisch et al. 1989, Glazener et al. 1990). Insemination both with and without ovarian stimulation has also been suggested for the treatment of unexplained infertility. Overall, the highest pregnancy rates for unexplained infertility are reported in cycles treated with clomiphene, with or without insemination, or in gonadotrophin stimulated cycles with or without insemination (Nulsen et al. 1993).

Conclusion

Although some may believe that IVF is the 'ultimate' endpoint, or 'gold standard' in infertility treatment, we have seen how this may not be the most appropriate choice. However, there is also another important consideration in this day and age of rising medical costs. Clearly, the economic impact of IVF with both direct and indirect costs must be acknowledged. Considering only direct costs, the price of IVF is more than 10 times that of clomiphene treatment or insemination. The indirect costs (premature babies, complications related to the procedure, etc.) are also very important and must certainly be added to the direct costs for a correct assessment of overall costs attributable to IVF. It is then up to society as a whole to determine the relative costs and benefits for IVF in the context of other therapeutic options.

Table 1. Infertility treatments and subsequent pregnancies (N=444).

	Pregnancies	
Treatment	No.	%
Spontaneous pregnancies	99	22.3
Hormone treatment		
· *Female*	56	12.6
· *Male*	5	1.1
Antibiotic treatment of the couple	42	9.5
Surgical treatment		
· *Female*	38	8.6
· *Male*	2	0.5
Artificial insemination with husband semen	58	13.1
Artificial insemination with donor semen	56	12.6
IVF or ICSI	80	18.0
Pregnancies after IVF or AIH failure	8	1.8

Table 2. Etiologic treatment of ovulatory disorders.

I. Treatment of extragonadal endocrinopathy
   A. Adrenal dysfunction
   B. Thyroid dysfunction

II. Psychotherapy in cases of psychogenic amenorrhea

III. Dietary means
   A. Weight loss
   B. Obesity

IV. Moderation of exercise and fulfillment of optimal nutritional needs in exercise-related amenorrhea

V. Change of treatment in case of iatrogenic ovulatory disorders

VI. Surgical treatment
   A. Prolactinoma
   B. Craniopharyngioma

Table 3. Symptomatic treatment of amenorrhea and infertility.

Etiology	Treatment
Hypogonadotrophic normoprolactinemic amenorrhea, failure of estrogen production	1. Gonadotrophin treatment 2. Pulsatile GnRH
Polycystic ovary syndrome and hypothalamic amenorrhea with estrogen production	1. Clomiphene citrate 2. Gonadotrophin treatment 3. Pulsatile GnRH
Hyperprolactinemic amenorrhea	1. Dopamine agonists

Table 4. Medical and surgical treatment of male infertility.

Infertility causes	Treatment
Hypogonadotrophic hypogonadism	Gonadotrophin therapy GnRH therapy
Prolactinoma	Surgical or medical treatment
Epididymal or vas deferens obstruction	Microsurgical anastomosis
Ejaculatory duct obstruction	Endoscopic surgery
Epididymal cyst	Microsurgical resection
Varicocele	Surgical treatment Transvenous embolisation of the internal spermatic vein
Prostatitis, vesiculitis	Antibiotics, anti-inflammatory drugs
Immunologic infertility	Corticosteroids
Erectile dysfunction	Sex therapy
Retrograde ejaculation	Sympathicomimetics
Anejaculation	Sex therapy Electroejaculation Parasympathicomimetics
Premature ejaculation	Sex therapy

Table 5. Pregnancy rates (a) per patient and (b) per insemination cycle with reference to the age of the woman.

(a)

Age (years)	No. of patients	No. of pregnancies	Pregnancy rate per patient (%)	Mean no. of cycles per patient
< 30	55	9	16.4	2.6
30-34	116	25	21.6	3.1
35-39	104	23	22.1	3.6
40-44	47	5	10.6	4.3
> 44	10	0	0.0	3.6
Total	332	62	18.7	3.4

(b)

Age (years)	No. of cycles	No. of pregnancies	Pregnancy rate per cycle (%)
< 30	143	9	6.3
30-34	357	25	7.0
35-39	377	23	6.1
40-44	202	5	2.5
> 44	36	0	0.0
Total	1115	62	5.6

Table 6. Pregnancy rates after intrauterine insemination with respect to (a) total motile sperm count per insemination and (b) total motile sperm count before sperm preparation.

(a)

Total motile sperm count per insemination (millions)	No. of cycles	No. of pregnancies	Pregnancy rate per cycle (%)
≤ 0.5	164	3	1.8
0.51 - 1.0	116	3	2.6
1.1 - 5.0	520	37	7.1 a
> 5.0	315	19	6.0 b
Total	1115	62	5.6

a : χ^2=5.4, P=0.02 compared to the ≤ 0.5 group
b : χ^2=3.6, P=0.06 compared to the ≤ 0.5 group

(b)

Total motile sperm count (millions)	No. of cycles	No. of pregnancies	Pregnancy rate per cycle (%)
≤ 1.0	37	0	0.0
1.1 - 10.0	209	8	3.8
10.1 - 20.0	169	8	4.7
20.1 - 40.0	170	15	8.8
40.1 - 100.0	259	9	3.5
> 100.0	271	22	8.1
Total	1115	62	5.6

Figure 1. Evaluation of the infertile couple.

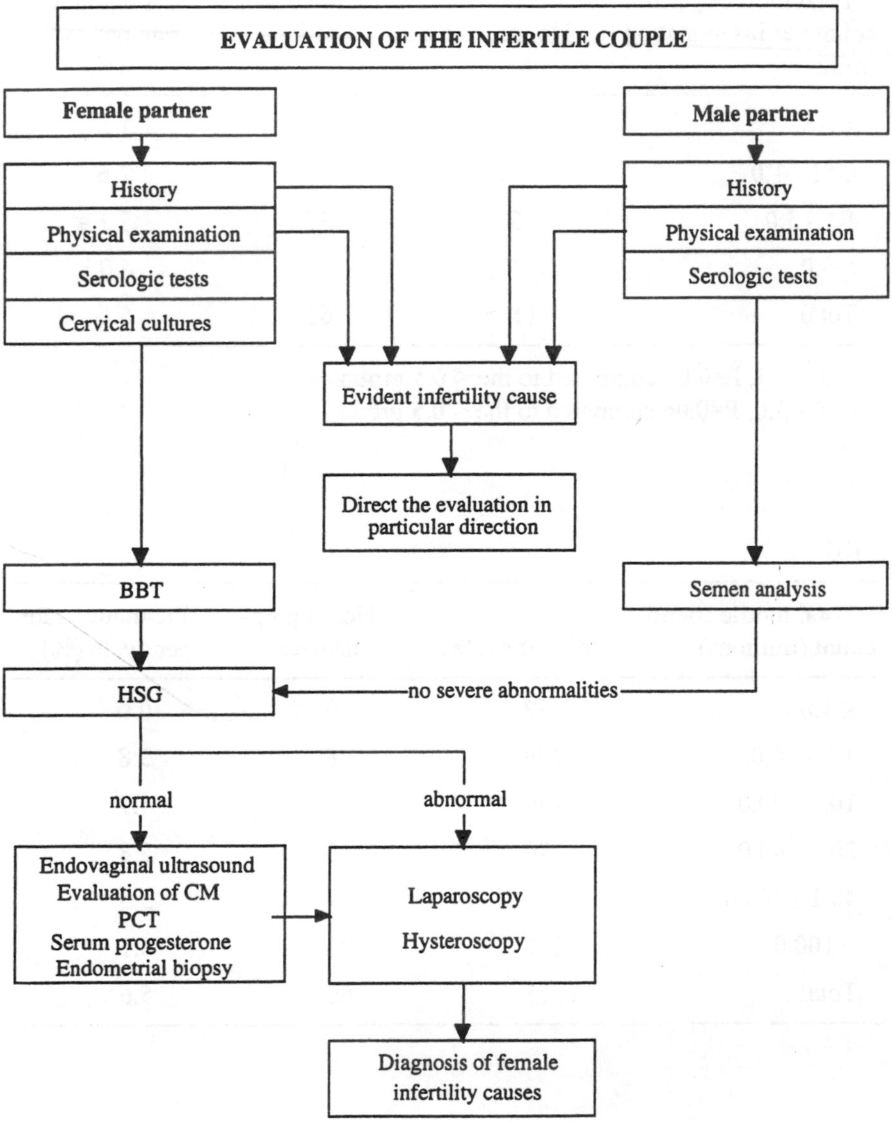

References

Campana, A., de Agostini, A., Bischof, P., Tawfik, E. and Mastrorilli, A. (1995), 'Evaluation of Infertility', *Hum Reprod Update,* Vol. 1, pp. 586-606.

Campana, A., Sakkas, D., Stalberg, A., Bianchi, P.G., Comte, I., Pache, T. and Walker, D. (1996), 'Intrauterine Insemination: Evaluation of the Results According to the Woman's Age, Sperm Quality, Total Sperm Count per Insemination, and Life Table Analysis', *Hum Reprod,* Vol. 11, pp. 732-6.

Cates, W., Farley, T.M.M. and Rowe, P.J. (1988), 'Patterns of Infertility in the Developed and Developing Worlds', in Rowe. P.J. and Vikhlyaeva, E.M. (eds), *Diagnosis and Treatment of Infertility*, Hans Huber Publishers: Toronto, pp. 57-67.

Fisch, P., Casper, R.F., Brown, S.E., Wrixon, W., Collins, J.A., Reid, R.L. and Simpson, C. (1989), 'Unexplained Infertility: Evaluation of Treatment with Clomiphene Citrate and Human Chorionic Gonadotrophin', *Fertil Steril*, Vol. 51, pp. 828-33.

Frank, O., Bianchi, P.G. and Campana, A. (1994), 'The End of Fertility: Age, Fecundity and Fecundability in Women', *J Biosoc Sci*, Vol. 26, pp. 349-68.

Glazener, C.M., Coulson, C., Lambert, P.A., Watt, E.M., Hinton, R.A., Kelly, N.G. and Hull, M.G. (1990), 'Clomiphene Treatment for Women with Unexplained Infertility: Placebo-controlled Study of Hormonal Responses and Conception Rates', *Gynecol Endocrinol*, Vol. 4, pp. 75-83.

Gleicher, N., van der Laan, B., Pratt, D. and Karande, V. (1996), 'Background Pregnancy Rates in an Infertile Population', *Hum Reprod*, Vol. 11, pp. 1011-2.

Hammond, M.G. (1996), 'Induction of Ovulation with Clomiphene Citrate', in Sciarra, J.J. (ed.), *Gynecology and Obstetrics*, Vol. 5, Lippincott-Raven Publishers: Philadelphia, Chap. 68.

Martin-du Pan, R.C. and Campana, A. (1993), 'Physiopathology of Spermatogenic Arrest', *Fertil Steril*, Vol. 60, pp. 937-46.

Nulsen, J.C., Walsh, S., Dumez, S. and Metzger, D.A. (1993), 'A Randomized and Longitudinal Study of Human Menopausal Gonadotrophin with Intrauterine Insemination in the Treatment of Infertility', *Obstet Gynecol*, Vol. 82, pp. 780-6.

Silber, S.J., Nagy, Z., Liu, J., Tournaye, H., Lissens, W., Ferec, C., Liebaers, I., Devroey, P. and van Steirteghem, A.C. (1995), 'The Use of Epididymal and Testicular Spermatozoa for Intracytoplasmic Sperm Injection: The Genetic Implications for Male Infertility', *Hum Reprod*, Vol. 10, pp. 2031-43.

Speroff, L., Glass, R.H. and Kase, N.G. (1994), *Clinical gynecologic endocrinology and infertility*, Fifth Edition, Williams & Wilkins: Baltimore.

5 Ethical considerations concerning alternatives to IVF therapies

Monika Stuhlinger

What are to be thought of as alternative, non-IVF therapies? In my opinion there are different alternatives we could consider.

Firstly, following the scientific medical point of view, alternatives could avoid creating embryos and thus avoid normative problems – we could improve endoscopic tubal surgery or transcervical balloon tuboplasty, we could experiment with hormonal treatment of insufficient spermatogenesis, we could further evaluate the immunological cause and treatment of male infertility and so on. In this way, we would rely wholly on scientific progress in treating infertility. In this context we should thoroughly consider the underlying concepts of health, treatment and medical care. And we should solve the problems related to the techniques themselves, *before* they become standard routine (see for example the debate 'Rewards and Risks in ICSI' 1995).

Secondly, following a psychosomatic and psychosocial perspective, some of the money spent on IVF therapies should be used to pay for ten-week holidays for infertile couples, or should be used for psychological counselling about motives for child-bearing, about wishes for a child of one's own, about ambivalence toward parenthood or the possibility of adoption. This position gives attention to the psychology, social context and meaning of infertility and even emphasises the ability of individuals to cope with infertility by altering their life-plans and self-expectations. The much-cited right to a child of one's own – in contrast to the wish for a child – might be uncovered as the inability to accept human limitations.

Thirdly, we could insist on a feminist position and demand female control over all reproductive technologies and welfare programs to raise children – and we could plan a huge follow-up study to document the outcome of this experiment: which preferences and which choices in matters of reproduction would be altered, which means of treating infertility would still be used? Seriously, there *is* a need to discuss the position that the social construction of ideals about family and motherhood, combined with problems of equal respect for both sexes are the main factors to be treated by alternative, non-IVF therapies.[1]

Finally, we could once again change our point of view and adopt an ecological perspective, considering pollution, chemicals and life-style as causes for infertility. Changes in individual habits and industrial legislation possibly would not only cure some infertile couples, but also contribute to the prevention of infertility, an alternative, which is – not only in this area – not often considered.

None of these four alternatives, which I have outlined very roughly, promise a comprehensive understanding of fertility and infertility. However, the medical perspective, with and without IVF, is dominant. The average career of an infertile couple very quickly leads to IVF and related techniques. Psychological support is not routine. Research efforts concentrate on medical-technical treatments. It is not much to conclude that the non-medical ways to treat or integrate infertility are to be taken much more seriously than they are, which indicates serious deficits in research.

The use of reproductive technologies – IVF and their alternatives – is commonly said to be a territory held by individuals; it is said to be a question of individual choice. This is the line of argumentation of most gynecologists, geneticists and also ethicists. For instance, the ethics committee of the American Fertility Society works on basis of this assumption in the 'Ethical Considerations of Assisted Reproductive Technologies' (1994).

I hold that simply relying on the individual woman's or couple's autonomous decision is a fiction for several reasons. First of all, the social impact on decisions concerning fertility therapies is usually ignored and emphasis is given only to personal counselling between doctors and patients to achieve a certain degree of autonomy. This is necessary but not sufficient. Furthermore the implicit value choices inherent in medical indications to IVF are overlooked, and the influence of professional interests in certain technologies is played down. As a consequence, women or couples exploring their options have to deal with a hidden twofold impact on their decisions.

This is important for considerations about informed consent. Even more important, in reflecting on the possibilities of fertility treatment, we do not enter an area of solely individual evaluative choices. Although very few biomedical ethicists rely on the possibility of normative consensus in pluralistic societies and even fewer do rely on agreement concerning evaluative choices, questions in the field of reproductive medicine often leave us with strong feelings of uneasiness when they are answered from an exclusively individualistic perspective. What is at stake is a society's ability to strive for consensus in important value questions. Matters of how we should procreate and which children we should bear are not to be separated from anthropological considerations about human dignity and human need to be cared for, even, and above all, as imperfect individuals.

Questions about the use of technologies and the sort of medicine we want, in order to improve our health and happiness, must be to a large extent a collective choice, not only an individual one. Many perspectives are necessarily involved in considering and evaluating alternatives to IVF therapy and, as I tried to show, the non-medical perspectives have to be emphasised. The consequences of developments in reproductive technologies have to be borne by all, especially by women. Thus, decisions about alternatives should not only involve the proponents of one perspective.

Note

1 For a thorough discussion of the feminist discussion about reproductive technologies see the whole issue of the *Journal of Medicine and Philosophy*, Vol. 21, No. 5, October 1996.

References

Ethics Committee of the American Fertility Society (1994), 'Ethical Considerations of Assisted Reproductive Technologies', *Fertility and Sterility*, Vol. 62, No. 5, Supplement 1.

'Rewards and Risks in ICSI' (1995), *Human Reproduction*, Vol. 10, No. 10, pp. 2518-28.

Part Four

COUNSELLING IN THE PROCESS OF DECISION-MAKING

1 Ethical decision-making for in vitro fertilisation in a multicultural setting

Farhan Yazdani

Guidance for science

In a short span of twenty years in vitro fertilisation (IVF) has brought satisfaction and hope to childless couples but at the same time it has challenged traditional concepts of human life, uprooting values on which social structures are grounded and inspiring distrust in societies where misuse of technology for profit has led to undiscriminating suspicion towards scientific methods.

A brilliant technician cannot be expected to be versed in all the moral expectations of society, nor can we expect the social regulators such as moral leaders, politicians and judges to fully understand the implications and side-effects of swiftly advancing techniques. In view of this, Jacques Testard in France and other members of the scientific community, aware that science is unable to determine its own course without guidance from the society that is to benefit from its services, asked for a moratorium on research work on the embryo.

Economic reality is another essential consideration for decision-making. The high costs incurred by IVF have to be taken into account in societies faced with economic recession and require rationing and choice in health programmes. The high profits in perspective, the increasing number of teams providing IVF, the swiftly advancing techniques, all make social control uncertain and tedious legislative efforts outdated before the laws are even passed.

Finally, in multicultural societies a diversity of beliefs, opinions and priorities coexist. Technicians, patients and social regulators with diverging standards can become involved in conflict and violence as it has already been the case with anti-abortion activists. Scientific reasoning and juridical rulings can by no means compensate for the moral standards which take root in the subjective elaborations of hearts and minds and provide the warp and woof of human societies. Religious and moral convictions on the other hand cannot ignore rational reality, withhold scientific development or deprive society of the advantages that science can offer to those seeking a happy family life.

Multidisciplinary decision-making

The numerous factors involved make it impossible for a single person to apprehend all aspects of such complex issues. Only a close collaboration between technicians and moral exponents of social regulation can provide solutions acceptable to citizens who have to be included in the debates on a subject they are concerned with. Grounds have to be provided for such interchange between the hyperspecialised academic structures, and when interchange does occur, technical jargon has to be simplified to allow mutual understanding.

Coping with practical problems arising in every-day medical practice, a preliminary study was opened in Lyon in 1976 under the supervision of Dr Nicole Léry. The data resulting from the cases submitted for counselling in the University Hospital in Lyon gave rise to a check-list or 'tool-box' method that breaks down complex global issues into more manageable items, making sure that all aspects of each problem have been considered. The rewarding results in various ethical issues have led in 1988 to the establishment of an Ethical Consultation 'Droit et Ethique de la Santé' which has dealt with over 2,900 ethical cases to date.

Ethical decisions and moral standards

Historically, the words 'ethics' from Greek and 'morals' from latin have been considered as synonymous and are still used as such by many thinkers. The first outcome of this experience has been to draw a clear distinction between the practical decision-making in clinical ethics, a procedure used by a practitioner or a technician seeking an *ethical decision* which leads to an appropriate line of action in his daily work, and the *moral standards* that are the general guide-lines refered to by theologians, philosophers and sociologists in identifying standards and norms considered as acceptable in each society.

To illustrate this point, we can consider a mental patient taking a class-room full of children as hostages. Shooting him down is 'wrong' by all *moral standards* but this step might well prove to be the least inappropriate *ethical decision* in that specific case. Thus decision-making can yield different results in different climes and times. The following case produced by a general practitioner (GP) illustrates this:

> A teenage girl back from a holiday with her family in North-Africa is pregnant. She has been married against her will to a man she does not wish to live with. Unaware of the legislation on voluntary interruption of pregnancy in France, she seeks for abortion after the ten-week gestational

limit. She is not adult and her family is opposed to an abortion. The GP does not know what to do.

The discussion reveals that if this marriage is valid in her country, it may not be the case in France. Can it be established that she had been subject to pressure? Would that be considered as assault? How would her family react to an abortion against the parents' consent? The GP did not tell us how his story ended, nor would we feel entitled to publish such a decision. The case shows how uneasy cross-cultural ethical cases can be.

In societies that integrate cultural plurality, the framework of laws regulating medical practice allow some latitude for moral standards upheld by various citizens within a legislative framework. There are limits beyond which no member of that society can transgress. A general consensus will for instance allow freedom of religious practice but might exclude female genital mutilation or the death of a child through parental rejection of blood transfusion. For obvious reasons, ethical counselling will often provide the necessary information for all parties concerned to reflect upon, without suggesting a decision that ultimately belongs to those involved.

All societies, however primitive, are structured on moral standards that inspire laws and regulations upholding a specific social order. These standards derive their legitimity from values that the individual acquires from his social environment. Immigration causes a mingling of such values and the migrant may feel as inadapted as a British driver driving on the continent or a football player trying to play football in a team that is playing rugby.

The affective connotations involved in all value systems explain the distress and chaos that can result when such rules are questioned or changed. Alvin Toffler foresaw this in 'Future Shock' and the Nobel Prize winner, Jacques Monod in his very rational 'Hazard et la Necessité' admitted that 'No system of values can pretend to be a true ethic unless it proposes an ideal that transcends the individual to the point that he or she becomes prepared to sacrifice him- or herself for it if necessary'.

Hence ethical decision-making not only involves taking 'right' decisions, but also decisions in conformity with what society is ripe to appreciate, aware that these decisions may in turn foster new values or deleteriously modify social behaviour.

The first step in decision-making is to collect relevant data for a benefit/risk/cost equation. This will require collecting up to date technical data, information on legal and deontological rulings, various recommendations, cultural factors and moral and religious convictions of those involved.

Up to date technical data

The first and foremost requirement for decision-making is reliable and up to date technical data that must be in conformity with the currently accepted scientific facts. Some 30 per cent of problems that are submitted for counselling in Lyon can be solved by providing reliable technical data. For Jean Bernard, the first president of the Comité Consultatif National d'Ethique (CCNE), two thirds of the ethical problems encountered today might be solved by technical advances in years to come. This does not mean that technology will overrule ethics, but that science and technology will have to submit to social requirements and provide new means for prevention and therapy that will comply with moral standards. This concept was once memorably illustrated in Lyon:

> An absent-minded elderly lady set fire to her kitchen for the second time. No one really wished to send her to a nursing home but neighbours could not risk a third accident. Her blunt refusal to leave her flat led psychiatrists and social workers into legal and ethical considerations on medical certificates, responsibility issues and consent. Finally the fireman who was politely listening to the knowledgeable assembly timidly interrupted, suggesting a smoke detector and the replacement of the gas stove by an electrical induction plate.

No one had imagined submitting a complex ethical problem to a technician. Ethical decision-making aims at practical solutions and not intellectual accomplishments. When a Jehovah's witness is prepared to let his child die by refusing blood transfusion, the long-term technical response is research work for blood substitutes, and the prompt legal response can be a call to the judge to see if he wishes to overrule parental decisions.

Many ethical problems in IVF could be solved by technical advances on oocyte conservation. This, for the moment seems to require an initial research work on embryos resulting from frozen oocytes. Such research being prohibited, other technical solutions may have to be considered. This interaction between technology and the social regulators requires a constant dialogue and collaboration and enough time for society to understand and integrate such advances. Doing the right thing at the wrong time can yield adverse results and hinder further progress.

Legal framework

Ethics is not law, but ethics can in no wise avoid reference to laws which are the codified expression of norms and standards assembled and adopted by the representatives of the social structure of each state. They express a firm consensus that clearly defines the limits and boundaries that each citizen can readily identify and respect. These established standards define a legal framework that can be refered to by all citizens and transgressions imply punishment if a mistake, neglect or a criminal behaviour is established.

In Europe, law has defined medical practice as a 'symmetrical and tacit contract' between patients and health professionnals as 'free and equal partners'. It is law that reminds us that all citizens are born free and equal in rights. The law itself has made provisions for regulating procedures in specific legislation. Laws function as a set of collective landmarks prior to all action and which can be brought to bear by whoever needs justice. Laws and the time consuming debates that precede their adoption represent efforts made by society to establish binding norms and values that can be identified by all and considered as universal.

Again some 30 per cent of the cases presented in the ethical consultation in Lyon are solved through arguments calibrated within pre-established juridical standards. Legal implications of each issue should be listed and carefully studied before decision-making.

In France IVF procedures are covered by the 'bioethical law' of 29 July 1994 which prohibits all experimentation on the embryo and fixes a penalty of 7 years imprisonment and a fine of 700,000 FF. Exceptional studies after consent from the parents are acceptable by Art. L. 152-8 and L. 184-3. A revision of this law is expected in 1999 and we will see below that the CCNE has already suggested some amendments.

If we considered the embryo without a parental project as being a human subject with no hope for survival if support is withdrawn, organ removal and cell cultures could be envisaged. In France the 'Caillavet law' of 22 December 1976 regulating organ donation and the 'Huriet-Sérusclat law' of 20 December 1988 controling medical experiments on human volunteers could well cope with these situations after parental consent. It should, however, be remembered that all children at birth have no hope of survival if support is withdrawn.

In 1993 the Court in Créteil rejected a request from a widow for post-mortem insemination with her husband's sperm on the grounds that a child could not be conceived without the parental project of a living couple. Laudable as this might be, a naturally conceived child does not benefit from the same degree of protection. The same court accepted the request in another similar case. It is understandable that the legislators should be baffled by technical data and should over-protect embryos conceived through technical procedures compared to children conceived naturally for which they are not invited to legislate.

The rapid technical advances are a challenge to legislative efforts and would suggest that some of the more versatile guidelines in IVF should be entrusted to one of the more readily amendable structures listed below.

Deontological or professional codes

The next step in decision-making is the study of deontological rules. The word 'deontology' was first introduced into French through the translation in 1825 of the work of the utilitarian English philosopher Jeremy Bentham. It stems from Greek 'deon' (binding), 'logos' (discourse) and means 'the science of duty'. Here the norms are established by professionals and brought to bear in codes that define the standard of 'good behaviour' required from the members of that profession. Hippocrate's sermon and Maïmonade's prayer are historical examples of medical codes. Most countries have a deontological medical code and a European medical code has now been established. In France there is a professional deontological code for lawyers, dentists and midwives and nurses now have an international code.

These standards of reference result from long experience and express accumulated wisdom. Although not as binding as laws, the French Deontological Code is enforced by the Medical Council who controls all medical practice. It is adopted after a parliamentary vote and transgressions can lead to sanctions, including professional exclusion inflicted by the Medical Council which can in addition report offenders to court. Magistrates also refer to these codes when assessing malpractice. Much more maleable and easier to amend than laws, deontological codes are a necessary intermediate step between technical practices and the legal framework.

The 1995 version of the French Medical Deontological Code submits research work (Art. 15), IVF procedures (Art. 17) and abortion (Art. 18) to legal restrictions. This means that a practitioner violating the rules will be liable to penalty from both the Medical Council and the public prosecutor.

Recommendations and consensus

The research work for decision-making must also seek recommendations, resolutions and reports from sources such as the Council of Europe. Recommendation 1046 (1986), for example, deals with the use of human embryos and foetuses for medical purposes. Resolution (78) 29 harmonises the legislations of member states on removal, grafting and transplantation of human substances. Recommendation R (90) 3 deals with research work on human beings, R (90) 13 on prenatal genetical screening and the 1993 report gives the principles of human artificial procreation.

Other international efforts such as the UNESCO meetings in Varna in 1975 and Venise 1986, the Helsinki-Tokyo declaration published by the World Medical Association in 1975, the Manila declaration in 1981 directed by the World Health Organisation, all contribute to a better understanding of the ethical challenges facing humanity and can be a help in grasping and debating difficult ethical issues.

An authoritative source of ethical proposals in France is the CCNE which was established by President Mitterand in 1983 in order to face the multiple dilemmas introduced by the rapid advances in scientific techniques. Bringing together a multidisciplinary and multiconfessional team of 37 eminent personalities amongst physicians, philosophers, moral leaders and other specialists, the CCNE has provided valuable guide-lines that inspire seachers and legislators.

These opinions and proposals are not laws, but guide-lines. Researchers in good standing cannot ignore them, magistrates refer to them in their rulings and legislators use them as a basis for laws.

In France, associations such as the Federation of CECOS (Centers for the Conservation and Study of Human Oocytes and Semen) who are authorized to conserve and supply human semen and the FIVNAT association (National Association of IVF Centers) establish consensus, codify their procedures and publish their own rules, providing professional guide-lines for technicians. This data is a valuable source of information for all searchers and would deserve a wider audience than the small group of specialists to whom they are made available.

Cultural and moral guide-lines

Medical practice is frequently confronted with the patient's beliefs and public acceptance. Organ transplants are uncommon in Japan due to the belief that the soul lingers in the organs for seven days after death. Moslems may reject organ donation on the grounds that the body has to be complete for resurrection or refuse porcine heart valve replacement.

Authoritative references

In some countries religious rules are directly enforced, but in multicultural settings, technicians might ignore their patients feelings and the patients might dissimulate or misunderstand their own religious teachings. Within a same tradition, interpretations may differ greatly and it can sometimes prove difficult to obtain authoritative views. The Judeo-Christian and Islamic traditions being well represented in Europe, we will take as examples the Hindu, Buddhist and Baha'i views.

Throughout Asia, folk belief regards the embryo as coming alive at the time the mother senses movement, notions similar to the idea of 'quickening' in the West. This implies a ready acceptance of all technical procedures involving IVF. At closer study however, the classical teachings of both Hindu and Buddhist traditions, as preserved in texts, hold that conception occurs during intercourse. In the pan-Indian idea of conception based on an agricultural model, a seed (semen) is planted in a paddy (menstrual blood), the two elements conjoining with a third, namely the spirit of a recently deceased person.

The Baha'i position is on the contrary precise with abundant references to authenticated writings and authoritative interpretations dating between 1844 and 1957. In addition to these, clear provisions have been made for an elected body called the 'House of Justice' which legislates on matters not explicitly dealt with in the writings and abrogates previous laws according to the needs of each day and age. Since science and religion are considered as complementary, no technical procedure is irrevocably condemned but applications may be restricted, aiming at the well-being of humankind.

For the Baha'is spiritual parenthood is considered more important than the biological one. Adoption is highly recommened and should be considered as a serious alternative to IVF. At present IVF procedures not requiring surrogacy or gametes from outside a married couple are permitted and the Baha'is are encouraged to assume personal responsibility by taking ethical decisions with respect to the laws of the country where they reside and after consulting competent physicians.

For the Baha'is the soul is the essential part of human reality and remains unharmed by disease or injury afflicting the body. It is subject to progress, appearing at conception and developing gradually, by stages, as the perfections of the spirit are reflected therein. Its evolution is held in abeyance when the embryo is frozen and it will resume its spiritual progress after death through other worlds on its way to perfection, without a physical return into this world.

Filiation

In France, the word 'procreation' which conveys the idea that sexual reproduction creates a new being has replaced the word reproduction. Procreation transmits genetical information and education imparts a spiritual (immaterial) information from one generation to the next. Attitudes towards IVF reflect the ideas prevailing in each culture on conception, filiation, inheritance and birth. In studying different religious representations of filiation Czyba (1988) notes that before IVF normal inheritance was represented as a *biological filiation*, although the father, 'semper incertus', sometimes doubted on his biological participation. Adoption was represented as a *symbolic filiation.*

Protestants value the representation of *symbolic filiation*, whereas the Catholic Church insists on the importance of the natural settings of *sexual filiation*. Both the Jewish and Islamic traditions value representations of *biological filiation*. In the Jewish tradition however, inheritance is from the mother and sperm donation which is officially practised in Israel is only acceptable from a non-Jew; masturbation being prohibited, it is improper for a Jew to donate in this way.

In the Islamic representation of filiation, all IVF procedures are acceptable as long as there is no gamete donation from outside the couple. This attitude results from the Islamic prohibition of adoption; a donated gamete being assimilated to a form of adoption. The dilemma can be very painful in Islamic culture that considers a woman's fertility as an important asset.

Universal diversity

Plurality renders decision-making complex but diversity in cultural practices can provide valuable data for comparison. In some cases, local particularities need to be respected, in others, a universal consensus is required. For example, research work on embryonic stem cells holds a promise of high profits. This can encourage more lenient legislations in some states in order to facilitate research work and financial benefits, thus leading to competition and abuse. Only a harmonisation of international legislation can control such potential misuses. Besides, if a state produces scientific data obtained through illegal research, could other states manage to ignore such information?

Efforts towards a 'Global Ethic' have been made by The World Council of Religions and projects such as that of Hans Küng in Germany and Leonards Swidler in the US. A general denominator of all moral systems is the 'Golden Rule' which consists in doing to others as we wish to have done to ourselves.

This concept may be insufficient for solving diverging interests between individuals or between individuals and society, but all efforts towards an oecumenical dialogue should be applauded if religion is to be a means for harmony and well-being and not a source of conflict. Interreligious consultation and exchange in multidisciplinary ethical meetings is an important step towards this goal and most religious groups in France participate enthousiastically and some are represented in the CCNE.

In short, ethical decision-making should enquire into the moral engagements of those involved with reliable information and contact with religious authorities whenever necessary, bearing in mind that even the so-called secular societies are impregnated by pre-existing religious values and that Greek philosophy founding Western secular democracies was inspired by the prophets of Israel.

Establishing a benefit/risk/cost equation

Once the necessary data and competence has been collected, decision-making can take place by establishing a benefit/risk/cost equation. As times and conditions change, the equation is modified. The economic factor has become an ever present aspect of ethical debates. Health is priceless, but healthcare costs a lot and it is essential to consider the sacrifices that are ultimately borne by taxpayers. It should also be remembered that each equation reflects a certain situation. Who knows what our equations would look like tomorrow if a small part of the ten thousand billion dollars expended by the planet in armament each year and the immense fortunes wasted through lack of collaboration were directed to health?

Genetic and spiritual inheritance

Besides the risks of oocyte collecting for the mother and moral objections, we must remember that each attempt at IVF costs 20,000 FF. The French Social Security refunds three attempts at IVF and spends one billion FF on 4,000 births, bringing the cost of each birth by IVF to some 250,000 FF. To this must be added the high costs of premature births resulting from multiple pregnancies. In 1990, of the 800,000 births in France, 2,500 were conceived by IVF, the procedure being seven times more common than in the US where it is not state-funded.

Recently a promoter of IVF contended that the human species was hypofertile; let us not in our attempts at justifying a superb technique forget that the 'demographic explosion' was used as a plea for the right to abortion, by the same technicians. Since the depenalisation of abortion by the 'Veil law' in 1975, some 165,000 voluntary abortions are performed in France each year.

This means that the humans are socially 'dysfertile' with some families getting more children than they can cope with and others not enough. This brings up the obvious question: why not donate from families who have too many to those who have too little? It is true that the ideal ingredients for family making combine biological, sexual and symbolic filiation, but why not facilitate adoption procedures to the great satisfaction of orphans and parents?

This would promote the symbolic or spiritual representations of filiation over the genetic one and lead to loving a child which is not the 'flesh of my flesh and blood of my blood'.

My Will be done...

A side effect of fertility control is the idea that children are consumer products belonging to parents. Already apparent in divorce cases where children are torn apart by adults, irrespective of the child's interests, this trend overlooks the principle that the well-being of future generations should overrule the personal wishes of adults. The claim of a 'right to a child' should be replaced by the child's claim of a 'right to a happy family life'. Antoine de Saint Exupéry wrote: 'We do not give the earth as a heritage to our children, they lend it to us during our life-time'.

Here we touch another adverse effect of IVF: the fostering of the illusion that science is an all-powerful source of satisfaction for all our wishes. A popular joke says that the difference between God and the IVF technician is that God knows that He is not a technician, while the technician believes that he is God.

Let us also remember that in some cases the 'right to a child' dissimulates an unconscious urge to normality, to 'possessing' the physical capacity for procreation. This reflects a society where human value is calibrated on what one might 'possess' rather than on the service one might 'produce' during the short span of life on this planet.

Guarantee of 'normality'

This leads to another potential misuse of IVF, the eugenic temptation. All those privileged by working with handicapped children know that they are happy to live and only unhappy about the way 'normal' people treat them. Disease cannot be eliminated by eliminating the diseased without undermining social cohesion. The following personal experience illustrates this:

> As an intern I was called to the pedriatric department for a handicapped 14 year old boy with severe pneumonia. His physical appearance was misfortunately repulsive and as I went in, the nurse explained that he was aggressive, difficult to care for and unwanted by his family, implying that he could be left without treatment. As I approached the gasping and feverish child, he took hold of my gown, his imploring eyes unmistakenably begging for treatment. Antibiotics were administered and he was soon well and up to his pranks again. I do not know how his life ended, but I know that had I withheld medical treatment on that day, I would not feel the person I am today.

It is true that a severely handicapped child can be an unbearable strain to parents and endanger the development of other children in the family. Social institutions can compensate through a helping hand, but they lack necessary funds for doing so. Again, even though it is morally wrong to eliminate the handicapped before birth, it could be in some cases the least inappropriate solution in our present situation.

Eliminating a Down's syndrome before implantation will cause less stress for the mother and the practitioner than abortion later on. The unpleasant work will be done by the biologist and not the gynaecologist. Will he or she be sued if he or she misses a preimplantation diagnosis, as has happend to gynaecologists? How will future generations judge our decisions? Would they frown on us as we do on those who applied euthanasia to mental patients during the famine-stricken years of the second World War? Could not rejecting the handicapped result in the loss of biodiversity and a growing intolerance towards other handicapped, weakening the social fabric? Would not the process of caring for the handicapped be a spiritually rewarding exercise for our societies?

The ethical decision

Most decisions in IVF do not require this elaborate process of decision-making. Technicians providing and patients applying for these techniques have usually matured their projects and legislators have already provided the necessary legal grounds for the social contract.

However, when problems arise and dilemmas occur, it may prove necessary to seek further competence. Interrelations may become complex and multiple tensions can bear on decision-makers. To face such situations, it is customary in Lyon to draw a sociogramme or chart which is called a 'relational flower' representing all the actors involved and the nature of their interrelations. The drawing is included in the patient's case history and can be reviewed as the situation evolves, providing a comprehensive vision of the various stages of the issue and making sure that no party or tension has been neglected.

The resulting decision is a compromise that is neither a 'good' solution, nor one applicable to other cases; it is the least unfavorable decision in a specific case at a given time. The persons demanding help are provided with the necessary data for assuming their own responsibilities.

The use of a consultative process, whatever the results may be, provides evidence that no arbitrary action has been enforced and that all feasible solutions have been considered, making the final decision more acceptable to those involved. The data resulting from this interdisciplinary collaboration is highly instructive for all participants, but confidentiality that is essential for decision-making impairs the free use of this data for teaching purposes.

References

Aspects éthiques et juridiques de la procréation médicalement assistée (1994), Colloque organisée par l'ordre des Avocats à la Cour de Paris et l'Ordre National des Médecins, 5 Mars 1994.

Baha'i documents available at http://www.bcca.org/~cvoogt/writings.html.

Buddhist documents available at http://www.psu.edu/jbe/jbe.html.

Czyba, J.-C. (1988), 'Les représentations de la filiation et les procréations artificielles', *Psychologie Médicale*, Vol. 20, No. 5, pp. 661-3.

Hughes, J.J. and Keown, D. (1995), 'Buddhism and Medical Ethics: A Bibliographic Introduction', *Journal of Buddhist Ethics*, Vol. 2, pp. 105-24.

'Human Embryo Freezing: Statement in France (1985-1993)' (1996), *Contraception, Fertilité, Sexualité*, Vol. 24, No. 3, p. 229.
Keown, D. (1995), *Buddhism & Bioethics*, Macmillan/St.Martins Press.
LaFleur, W.A. (1992), *Liquid Life: Abortion and Buddhism in Japan.*
Lipner, J.J. (1989), 'The Classical Hindu View on Abortion and the Moral Status of the Unborn', in Coward, H.G., Lipner, J.J., and Young, K.K. (eds), *Hindu Ethics,* State University of New York Press: Albany, New York, pp. 41-69.
Premières Journées de la Fédération Française d'Etude de la Reproduction (1996), *Contraception, Fertilité, Sexualité*, Vol. 24, No. 8-9.
'Research on Human Embryos' (1996), *Contraception, Fertilité, Sexualité*, Vol. 24, No. 11, pp. 800-2.

2 The process of ethical decision-making

Hille Haker

The process of a medically supported pregnancy, beginning with hormonal stimulation and possibly ending with in vitro fertilisation (IVF) or intracytoplasmic sperm injection (ICSI), has been the focus of many lectures and papers concerning the modern reproductive technology. As regards the decision-making process, however, the general concern was directed rather towards the professionals who must guarantee the free and informed consent of a couple to the medical procedure than to the couple's perspective itself. With respect to the *ethical* aspects of decision-making the recourse to the patients' autonomy as well as to the principle of beneficence seemed to be a sufficent basis for the counselling (Beauchamp and Childress 1994).

As the *beneficence* of a medically supported pregnancy seems to be obvious, namely the 'production' of a child, the physiological and psychological side effects of the treatment itself are often interpreted as in no way needing to be balanced against the good of a baby to take home. Therefore, the success rates of IVF are seen in the light of the success rates of other diseases where the risk of the therapy is being balanced against the suffering of the ill person. It is the intention of the medical treatment to reduce this suffering within the constraints of the patient's consent.

Because of the specific situation of a couple that is experiencing a non-fulfillment of their wish for a child in a situation of otherwise good physical health, the evaluation of medical treatment becomes more difficult. Whereas it seems clear that there is a right to be helped when suffering of a disease and, vice versa, a duty to help on the side of the physicians, it is not as clear whether there is a (morally positive) right to be helped in procreation and, vice versa, a duty to help on the side of the physicians. Since the introduction of IVF the medical profession has acted *as if* there is such a right without ever really discussing the moral impact of this presupposition. I cannot decide here whether the pragmatic medical view is morally right, but if it is, then it is the duty of the state to guarantee the establishment of and access to those medical institutions that can submit the treatment of IVF or alternatives.

If we hold the weaker thesis – as I prima facie do – that IVF is at least morally permissible, there still remains much to be said concerning the ethical problems that have to be faced in a decision-making process and be balanced against the possible success of the treatment. There are more and different problems in the praxis of IVF in modern societies in socio-ethical terms, but I will confine myself to those aspects relevant for the *autonomous* decision of individuals. These are:

> the *physical side effects* of the medication for woman, the *psychological effects* of a controlled sexuality for both man and woman, and the influence on the life style including the financial burden it takes in some countries to undergo the treatment of IVF;
>
> the high risk of *multiple pregnancies* with its own physical problems for the woman, the potential fetocide, and the risk of premature births. Only in a few countries these problems have led to a restriction of embryo transfers (e.g. max. 3 in Germany), although this reduces the success rate dramatically. Especially the fetocide causes serious ethical problems, concerning the moral status of the early fetus and the selection of the fetuses who are 'reduced';
>
> the *restriction of access* to IVF. Can it be morally argued that there should be a restriction to married couples, to heterosexual couples or couples at all, if the wish for a child is the basis of the treatment? How far are biological boundaries such as the menopause still relevant or, said in a different way: how is the status of the 'natural course of life' to be determined against modern medical techniques that undermine the normative force of nature?
>
> the double effect of *societal value systems and individual wishes*. The role of the desire for one's own child has to be estimated in the context of the women's identity and social role. The wish for a child may disguise the deeper wish to be 'normal' which itself is interpreted as 'good', whereas to live without children appears to be 'abnormal', interpreted as 'bad'. The evaluative power of this matrix becomes obvious when couples – or more spefically, women – feel stigmatised by their families, friends or acquaintances, if they cannot meet their expectations to give birth to a child. Whereas other single couples choose their life without children, it is the absence of choice that often produces the desperation on the side of the

couples concerned, and that intensifies the wish for a child that might have been simply one option as long as there seemed to be the choice;

the *treatment of human life at its beginning* is a question that goes far beyond the problem of the moral status of the frozen embyo. It has to be considered as a general question of the moral setting in modern culture and the attitude towards life;

the *production, selection and destruction of embryos* or pre-embryos, as given in the preimplantation diagnosis, are actions of direct ethical concern, because they are based on a decision which genetic disorders are to be 'avoided' and which are to be tolerated.

The subject of an ethical decision with regards to IVF and alternative treatment depends on the context: it is not only the *couple* who undergoes the special therapy to have a child, but the *medical staff* has to make decisions, too. Whereas the medical professionals have to judge single situations *and* the overall direction of medical treatment including health politics and financial costs, the couple has to evaluate their individual and private life, in the near and distant future.

As I am concerned with the individual decision of a couple, the two ethical guidelines: free and informed consent as a condition and counselling as support of the action referring to IVF are not questioned. I suggest the following four steps as decision-making procedure that could also serve as a guideline for ethical counselling in reproductive matters.[1]

First: Information

First, the couple has to gain all relevant medical information including possible alternatives to IVF. Financial aspects should be mentioned, especially when the patients themselves will have to pay for the treatment. Juridical information has to refer to the national legislation. Ethical information should in general be concerned with the problems mentioned above or problems occurring in the individual situation. Ethical information therefore leads to the second and third step of the decision-making process.

Second: Ethical reflection – turning to 'the good life'

In the second step a special kind of ethical self-reflection is pursued.[2] The persons concerned are invited to make their goals and purposes of the prospective actions explicit. These can be considered in the context of personal life planning, ideals for one's identity and, in general terms, in the context of the good life of a person. Through this the values and background of a person's ethical judgements can be reflected, and possible conflicts between the partners on the one hand, between patients and medical staff on the other hand, can be faced *before* the action procedure has started. If, for example, a couple wants IVF, but no cryoconservation of embryos, or the transfer of only one embryo, this must be respected.

Third: Moral reflection – the concern for the other

In the third step the couple should reflect on or be confronted with the direct moral problems concerning the moral status of an embryo. The moral impact of, for example, cryoconservation of embryos, of diagnosis and selection before embryo transfer, of 'reduction' of fetuses after transfer, and of prenatal diagnosis and possible abortion, has to be part of the decision-making process, although the answers to these problems might not be obvious. It is the task of the counsellors to inform themselves about the scientific-ethical reflection and to be able to report the discussion to the clients, if wished for. However, it is not the task of the counsellors to state directive prescriptions that might follow the moral arguments.

Fourth: Ethical integration of moral aspects

The last step is meant to gather the ethical and moral problems in a single perspective that results in the decision. Integration of the moral point of view into the personal ethical view of living one's life is the goal of this step that might not be possible in all contexts and situations. Therefore the counsellor's task will be to help the couple finding that solution that is closest to such integration. The potential compromises then will be practical. They do not, however, touch the correctness of either the ethical or the moral judgements.

Conclusion: A specific – but generally used – procedure of ethical decision-making has to be implemented in the normal course of information and counselling. The 4-phase-model I introduced could serve as a general orientation that needs further and more concrete formulation.

Notes

1 For a broader discussion of this model of ethical counselling see: Haker, forthcoming (a).
2 The discussion of an ethics of good life cf. Taylor 1989, Krämer 1992, Ricoeur 1990. For a discussion of different views cf. Haker forthcoming (b).

References

Beauchamp, T.L. and Childress, J.F. (eds) (1994), *Principles of Biomedical Ethics*, Oxford University Press: New York.

Haker, H. (forthcoming [a]), 'Entscheidungsfindung im Kontext pränataler Diagnostik', in Kettner, M. (ed.), *Beratung als Zwang. Schwangerschaftsabbruch, genetische Diagnostik und Aufklärung und die Grenzen kommunikativer Vernunft*, Leske & Budrich: Leverkusen.

Haker, H. (forthcoming [b]), *Moralische Identität. Literarische Lebensgeschichten als Medium ethischer Reflexion. Mit einer Interpretation der 'Jahrestage' von Uwe Johnson.*

Krämer, H. (1992), *Integrative Ethik*, Suhrkamp: Frankfurt am Main.

Ricoeur, P. (1990), *Soi-même comme un autre*, Seuil: Paris.

Taylor, C. (1989), *Sources of the Self*, Cambridge University Press: Cambridge.

3 Counselling practice

Ian D. Cooke

Apart from counselling for adoption, counselling was first mentioned in legislation in the Human Fertilisation and Embryology Act (HFE Act 1990) in the UK when it was stipulated that all patients for assisted conception or using donor gametes should have the 'opportunity to receive proper counselling'. When the draft legislation was published much debate ensued on what comprised 'proper counselling'. It was defined in a report by the King's Fund, subsequently adopted by the Code of Practice of the Human Fertilisation and Embryology Authority (HFEA 1991) as comprising four components:

1 Information, containing details of the pathology and prognosis in understandable terms for the couple.
2 Implications, the way these data may impact on the couple and how they may react to them.
3 Support, after having explored the coping strategies developed by the couple.
4 Therapeutic, for those instances where intervention was required for the future stability of an individual or couple.

There has been much debate by medical staff and counsellors as to where responsibilities lie and the HFEA invited the British Infertility Counselling Association and the British Fertility Society to establish a Steering Group on Training and Accreditation for Infertility Counselling which has recently reported (Steering Group 1996). A key issue was the definition and allocation of responsibilities. The Code of Practice stipulated that information and implications were mandatory for all couples. *Implications* were described as 'not necessarily requiring the role of a trained counsellor, but a practitioner would benefit from basic training and counselling skills as well as an understanding of reproductive health care in medical, social and emotional contexts'. *Support* was 'the role of the counsellor and other professional staff but should require the minimum acquisition of counselling skills' to a specified intermediate level (National Vocational Qualifications Levels 2/3). *Therapeutic* work involved the role of the independent counsellor which should be filled by someone with qualifications and experience at National Vocational Qualifications Level 4/5 (highest level) 'in counselling and/or psychotherapy'. These definitions have taken some time to emerge. A crucial factor has been that counsellors need understanding of reproductive medicine and medical practitioners require an understanding of counselling skills.

'Independence' of counsellors has also been a disputed term but is now generally accepted as meaning independence from the decision-making of the clinician. However, progressively fertility treatment has been given in multidisciplinary teams of which a counsellor is a member. In our own clinic about half the patients are introduced to a counsellor as part of the clinical consultation, but only about 5 per cent have a second or subsequent visit. Only the occasional patient requires longer term therapeutic intervention by an external counsellor referred to as 'independent'.

One of the difficulties working in clinical teams is the counsellor's ethos of confidentiality. Clinicians are much more used to working in teams and sharing clinical information to reach what is deemed the best conclusion on management for a couple. It has taken some time for the counsellors to be able to share some of their information, not necessarily all the details, and this is encouraged by their participation in group discussions of difficult clinical problems.

Although there is a widespread feeling that counselling 'is good for people' there is little substantive evidence that it is efficacious. In our own IVF unit in a careful randomised trial we were unable to show that additional counselling made any further difference to couples. This is an area requiring research. However, if one uses greater intervention, such as cognitive behaviour therapy where the evidence of efficacy is greater, it would be appropriate if this technique could be applied in the field of assisted conception (Andrews 1996).

Training in infertility counselling is currently being discussed in the UK. It has been agreed (Steering Group 1996) that the approach should be based on the development of competences upon which a documented portfolio route for accreditation of counsellors should be based. A national body has been established by the government focussing on 'advice, guidance, counselling and psychotherapy' to determine what should constitute evidence of these competences and the detail is emerging. It has been suggested that development should be supported to identify a specialised evidence route for infertility counselling. Practitioners should be advised by an accredited adviser as to how they should accumulate that evidence and there should be a national register for infertility counsellors within the currently established United Kingdom Register of Counsellors.

References

Andrews, G. (1996), *British Medical Journal*, Vol. 313, pp. 1501-2.

Human Fertilisation and Embryology Act (1990), Chapter 37, Her Majesty's Stationery Office, PO Box 276, London SW8 5DT.

Human Fertilisation and Embryology Authority (1991), *Code of Practice*, Paxton House, 30 Artillery Lane, London E1 7LS.

Steering Group on Training and Accreditation for Infertility Counselling (1996), *Report*, obtainable from the British Fertility Society, c/o the Honorary Secretary, Mr P. Wardle, Department of Obstetrics and Gynecology, St Michael's Hospital, Southwell Street, Bristol BS2 8EG.

4 Ethical neutrality in counselling? The challenge of infertility

Stella Reiter-Theil

Introduction

In this paper the role and the ethical orientation of the counsellor in the treatment of infertility are analysed. In vitro fertilisation (IVF) – like many other interventions of reproductive medicine – has received wide attention and is still provoking controversial debate. Issues such as whether the understanding of the family is threatened (Macklin 1991) or the quality of parenting and the development of the children in the context of reproductive intervention (Golombok et al. 1995) show both the concern resulting from this field of medical technology as well as the scientific effort to give answers to these urgent questions. Gynaecologists, psychologists, ethicists and other disciplines have contributed to reflection on the ethical dimensions of intervening into 'natural human procreation', but the problem of finding a consensus remains (Hepp 1994, Kuhse 1994). Therefore, the question of the ethical and professional attitude of the counsellor towards reproductive medicine and towards clients' preferences is not a trivial one. The lack of consensus and the plurality of values in this intimate domain constitutes a constant challenge to the counsellor which needs analysis and coping-strategies.

Starting with central concepts such as non-directivity and expertise, this paper studies the conditions under which ethical reflection may or shall occur in counselling and how it could be handled. Then, the question is approached, whether, or in which way, the rule of neutrality can be ethically justified and applied to practice. It is argued that neutrality is not to be regarded as an alternative to medical paternalism and that it cannot be realised in a simplified overall fashion. A model of different aspects of neutrality is suggested for counselling practice. As a result it is concluded that ethical orientation in the role of the counsellor in the treatment of infertility should not be restricted to negative or defensive concepts, even if they represent a kind of 'implicit ethics' but needs to be linked to explicit ethical principles of a general nature. The conclusions are illustrated in a case study of infertility and treatment.

Non-directivity – implicit or explicit ethics?

In the field of genetics and family planning, there has been an elaborate debate about the role and psychological competence of the counsellor dealing with difficult choices and decisions of clients or patients such as abortion (Ratz 1995, Reiter-Theil 1995a, Wertz and Fletcher 1988). On the background of the widespread consensus in genetics to abolish eugenic concepts as well as medical paternalism in counselling and to adopt rather an orientation to the respect for autonomy of the person, non-directivity became a leading principle (Wertz et al. 1990, Wolff and Jung 1994). Genetic and family counsellors, thus, often seek orientation from the concept of non-directivity and it seems that this concept influences counsellors in the field of treating infertility as well, since they too are dealing with sensitive issues related to the private sphere and even taboo zones such as procreation and sexuality (Reiter-Theil and Kahlke 1995).

Deriving from client-centered psychotherapy elaborated by Carl Rogers (1951), non-directivity is embedded in a context of humanistic values by which the professional helping relationship can be shaped (Reiter-Theil 1995a). It is also applicable to different professional groups working with people suffering, even to non-physicians. The humanistic context, together with the focus on the autonomy of the person in need for help or advice, and the professional flexibility of non-directivity contribute to the general attitude that the concept is regarded as an alternative to medical paternalism which has received increasing criticism in the recent medical ethics debate internationally (Beauchamp 1995). But avoiding medical paternalism on the basis of concepts such as non-directivity may run the risk of neglecting the ethical principles of beneficence or non-maleficence. (Clarke 1991, Reiter-Theil 1990, Yarborough et al. 1989). Simple adoption of either concept – paternalism or non-directivity – seems to be due to a lack of explicit discourse about the ethical basis of counselling. Being a technical guideline, non-directivity has ethical implications as has paternalism, and moreover, the two concepts should not be regarded as concepts lying at the same level of abstraction. Ethical implications – such as the tacit ethos of a certain communicative technique – can be helpful or even sometimes sufficient in practice, but they do not provide clarification or justification of ethical issues, nor do they solve contradictions. These goals can better be served by explicit ethical reflection and discourse.

Counselling and expertise

In order to find out which concepts might be helpful for a comprehensive professional as well as ethical orientation in the role of the counsellor, the concept of expertise deserves further study. This is particularly important in the light of criticism of medical paternalism. According to a definition of Weinstein (1993, p.59, p.62), there are two kinds of expertise: firstly, epistemic expertise – knowing *that,* and secondly, performative expertise – knowing *how.* A counsellor needs epistemic expertise in his or her field to formulate and justify opinions; he or she needs performative expertise to apply knowledge to individual cases and to conduct counselling with one or more clients. Besides the evidence that a counsellor in the medical context and also in the treatment of infertility needs expertise of both kinds, we have to look at the areas of the professional expertise as compared to the other agent of expertise in the process: the client or patient. Thompson asks the provocative question 'who is the expert – counsellor or client?'

- on how the client feels;
- on what has happened to the client;
- on what is happening to the client;
- on what has worked and what has not worked in the past for the client;
- on the interests, values, and goals of the client (Thompson, 1989, p.19).

If we compare the definition of an expert by the two components (epistemic and performative expertise) on the one hand with the areas formulated above where expertise is needed, we can see that in all these fields 'knowing that' is dominant over 'knowing how' and that in every field the professional or counsellor cannot realise the epistemic expertise without the help of the client or patient. On the other hand, it seems unlikely that any person seeking professional help or advice in the medical context would not need help to gain insight into these very personal issues. Expertise, as far as knowledge about the patient and his or her life is concerned, cannot thus be regarded as a solely professional quality; our comparison, rather, suggests an interactive and collaborative understanding. The second part of expertise, knowing how, refers more to technical skills to be applied solely on the basis of special training and experience. In a medical context such as IVF it would be impossible to ignore the exclusive access to 'knowing how' including the availability of technical facilities for the procedures involved. But we could imagine other domains in health care, where 'knowing how' to perform a particular action would again require strong assistance and collaboration from the side of the patient, e.g. physical mobilisation after an operation, withdrawal of drugs in an addict, or even taking the history of a patient for diagnosis – examples which show that experience and evaluation from patients are a very valuable, if not a necessary part of good clinical practice. Overall, there can be no successful counselling without active expertise on both sides, with a strong emphasis on collaboration at the epistemic level and a dominance of the counsellor at the level of performative expertise. In the case of treating infertility, the person involved in counselling is not necessarily the performative expert of IVF or alternative medical treatment; therefore, performative expertise may be split among a few professionals and realised within the frame of division of (medical) labour. From an ethical point of view we can conclude that

- professional counselling is the application of knowledge and skills on behalf of, or in the best interests of, the patient(s) or client(s);
- therefore, there is no special justification required for acting as an *expert* in counselling;
- on the contrary, there would have to be good reasons to defend the opinion that a counsellor should abstain from applying her or his expertise;
- patients or clients and their relatives have a claim on information and clarification, when they seek professional assistance;
- patients or clients have *expertise* themselves which has to be integrated in the counselling process.

There should, thus, be agreement that the realisation of expertise is by no means to be equated with paternalism, at least not in the sense of overriding the patient's wishes or choices. What we have to analyse in more detail is the question, whether the expertise of the counsellor comprises information and clarification about *ethical issues* as well.

Constellations of ethical reflection in counselling

As a prerequisite for analysing the conditions for neutrality of the counsellor, we need to look at different constellations of ethical awareness on both sides. Table 1 distinguishes the perspectives of counsellor and client or patient, respectively, and shows four constellations.

In the first constellation, both sides agree that there is no ethical issue involved at this stage of counselling and decision-making which would need to be discussed (A). This agreement may well be tacit and even not consciously working. Another constellation, where counsellor and client or patient can agree, is that they share the view that the treatment options have ethical implications relevant for the counselling process (D). But this agreement does not necessarily mean that there is agreement about the nature of the ethical problem, nor about the best way out. Conversation will then have to be conducted by the counsellor with special delicacy. Disagreement occurs, when the counsellor does but the client does not see an ethical issue to face (B), or the other way round (C). The latter constellation enables the counsellor to try to understand why the client has this ethical problem and to try to help him or her to cope with it. Disagreement of type B, however, is a serious challenge to the professionalism of the counsellor, who needs to integrate contradictory values – personal, professional, and the values of the client – at the same time and it might even be necessary to accept that the ethical dimension cannot satisfactorily be clarified, because the client or patient does not cooperate with this approach.

Table 1. Constellation of ethical reflection in counselling

		Counsellor sees	
		No ethical issues	Ethical issues
Client sees	No ethical issues	**A**	**B**
	Ethical issues	**C**	**D**

Options for dealing with ethics: to talk or not to talk?

The next question, whether, and if so, under which conditions, a counsellor may or shall speak with clients or patients about the ethical dimension of the treatment choices or decisions at issue and under which conditions this would be false, needs more reflection. Let us consider two radical positions: 'no, never' and 'yes, always' as well as two milder variants: 'no, except ...' and 'yes, except ...'. In table 2, these possibilities are listed together with the justifications as well as with the risks involved.

Position 1 can be seen as a radical liberal approach in not interfering with the patient's self-determination or privacy, not even questioning his or her preferences. The risks of this attitude, however, are that an important (ethical) problem might be overlooked or left out and, thus, not be treated in the best interest of the patient. Self-referentially, this approach might contribute to a professional attitude close to ethical nihilism or it may at least stimulate criticism from outside in this direction. In the humanities, there has been a growing trend to challenge the concept of value-free science. In medicine the situation seems to be ambiguous: there is still a considerable part of medical practice characterised by keeping values and ethics out, at least in direct contact with the patient.

Table 2. Talking with clients about ethics?

Position	Reasons	Risks
(1) No, never!	Respect for autonomy, privacy of patient; value free medicine	Neglect, nihilism
(2) Yes, always!	Ethics cannot be separated from health care professions; identity; transparency	Moralising, paternalism
(3) No, except in cases where the integrity of the counsellor is threatened	Self-protection of the counsellor, identity; see (1)	see (1) and (2)
(4) Yes, except in cases where client(s) refuse to	see (1) and (2), chance for better decisions	expecting too much from client(s)

Traditional hippocratic medicine as well as modern medicine with its lively ethical discussion support the view that the health care professions cannot be separated from their inherent ethical dimension. Consequently, position 2 can be justified by transparency, openness, or honesty towards the patient as well as the need to realise one's professional identity. But this brings with it the risk of moralising the medical services or even create an atmosphere of paternalism, when it is combined with the claim to moral authority on the side of the health care professional.

Position 3 can be considered as a rather defensive attitude: only if the counsellor feels severely impaired in his or her values as a professional or as a person by the ethical implications or consequences of treatment options, should he or she intervene at an ethical level. Reasons correspond to those mentioned for position 1, risks to those of positions 1 and 2.

The last option is a mild variant of position 2 saying that speaking about ethical aspects of treatment belongs to professional medicine and health care, but it should and could not be done when the patient or client is not willing to do so. Among the reasons for position 4, which correspond to those for position 1 and 2, is the effort to provide the ground for better decision-making. It is possible that this option means to expect or demand too much from clients or patients, but the risks of moralising or paternalism should be minimised by respecting patients' possible refusal.[1]

The problem of 'neutrality' as a starting point for explicit ethical orientation in counselling

Adoption of the rule of non-directivity, efforts to avoid medical paternalism, and particularly striving not to moralise patients' wishes in counselling and treatment has contributed to the rhetoric of 'neutrality' as an ideal, respectful, and superior attitude (Reiter-Theil 1989). After the analysis of constellations for ethical reflection of options (table 1), whether or not to talk with clients about ethical aspects of their treatment (table 2), there will be no doubt that ethical neutrality cannot be a simple solution for the problem. Several levels have to be taken into account and need consideration instead of 'deciding' about neutrality in general: (1) Relation between counsellor and client(s), (2) professional identity of counsellor, (3) personal identity of counsellor, (4) personal values of client(s), (5) conflicts of interests on the side of client(s), (6) difficulties with 'technical neutrality' towards client(s) on the side of the counsellor(s). The following list shows the suggestions presented for discussion developed on the basis of studies published earlier (Reiter-Theil 1989, 1994):

Table 3. Ethical orientation in the counsellor's role. The problem of 'neutrality' at different levels

1	Relation between counsellor and client(s): *no neutrality*, because accepting, warm attitude towards client(s) is necessary.
2	Professional identity of counsellor: *no neutrality*, because of the goals of health care, and because ethical principles, codes, guidelines etc. are binding.
3	Personal identity of counsellor: *no neutrality*, because personal values and goals set limits to acting in a 'neutral' way – authenticity instead.
4	Personal values of client(s): *'technical neutrality'*, because of respect for autonomy and privacy of client(s), but explicit reflection of possible consequences of choices.
5	Conflicts of interests on the side of client(s): *'technical neutrality'*, because of respect for autonomy, empathy, and fairness for everyone involved, but explicit reflection of possible consequences of decisions.
6	Difficulties with 'technical neutrality' towards client(s): *reflection, supervision, transferral* in order to avoid maleficence, judgemental response, or manipulation.

At the levels 1 to 3 there is 'no neutrality' in the counsellor's role possible, because non-neutral value-oriented attitudes are required, such as (1) an accepting, warm attitude, (2) goals, principles or codes, and (3) aspects of personal identity and authenticity of the counsellors. These levels include more of the counsellor's own person and relation towards the client than the next levels 4 and 5 do. Here, where the focus is on the client's perspective, a 'technical neutrality' is necessary in order to safeguard professional distance, privacy and respect towards the client(s). In the case of difficulties with 'technical neutrality' on the side of the counsellor, again a professional, self-reflective attitude is suggested to facilitate readjustment in the counsellor's role or to transfer the client(s).

Again, we are facing a melange of implicit and explicit ethical concepts which contribute to professional and ethical orientation in counselling. The ethical core principles are beneficence, respect for autonomy (level 1), general orientation at the ethical basis of the profession (level 2), personal ethical identity (level 3), respect for autonomy and privacy, deliberation of consequences (level 4), respect for autonomy, empathy and fairness for everyone involved, i.e. justice, deliberation of consequences (level 5), non-maleficence, non-manipulation, non-judgemental attitude (level 6). This quintessence integrates the four principles elaborated by Beauchamp and Childress (1994). But beyond *respect for autonomy, non-maleficence, beneficence and fairness* it emphasises two further components of orientation: *a general orientation at the ethical basis of the profession* and *a personal ethical identity*. Between these two components there is a strong link, because professional guidelines may support identity, as well as potential for conflict, when personal views differ from professional standards. It seems that in recent medical ethics this dimension has been neglected, maybe because there are no solutions for conflicts at hand. Professional counselling – like any other professional work – has a normative basis and inherent general ethical principles, this has to be acknowledged. At the same time, the individual counsellor has no other possibility to perform ethically and professionally than to be herself or himself, acting in accordance with her or his personal ethical identity. In this formulation, the tension between objectivism and subjectivism or between generalism and individualism becomes obvious. As with the 'neutrality' of the counsellor, there is no option of choosing either/or, but we need to construct specific answers for specific challenges according to general lines of ethical orientation. The more explicit the ethical concepts, and the more aware we are of them, the better our answers to the questions posed will be.

Case study: Counselling in IVF – right to treatment or exclusive indication?

Mrs S. (37 years) and Mr S. (41 years) ask for help, because their wish for a child has remained unfulfilled in the last four years. Two years after stopping contraception – two years ago – Mr S. underwent a physical examination with the result that the quality of his sperm was reduced. At the next control, the quality of sperm turned out to be significantly better. Mrs S. was then inseminated with the sperm of her husband. After a series of unsuccessful attempts, Mr S. is frustrated and wishes to discontinue this treatment.

As a couple with 'idiopathic sterility', they seek IVF, expecting that this treatment will be less embarrassing and stressful and they hope that treatment in a specialised IVF practice will be more personal than in the hospital. The counsellors – a gynaecologist and a psychologist – inform the couple about the procedure and explore the habits of Mrs and Mr S. in their sexual life: It seems that they have established a pattern of strictly controlled sexual intercourse centering around the days of conception, only. The counselling team tries to find out, whether the couple is willing to reconsider the situation, because it seems possible that stress and tension have reduced chances for conception so far. But the couple insists on their request to be treated with IVF. A date is fixed, but the treatment is not successful – despite the positive spermiogram.

During the following session, the counsellors try to find out with the couple, whether the IVF procedure has become a kind of way out of the strict 'regime' of sexual intercourse after calendar for both. They share – for the first time – feelings about the need to control their bodies in terms of perfect functioning and start thinking about the possibility of living a life without children (see Reiter-Theil and Kahlke 1995, pp.36-37; the case is reported by Fiegl and Kemeter ibid.).

The case study may help to clarify our suggestions for solving the problem of ethical neutrality in the counsellor's role. In the short description of the counselling and treatment process, there are a few hints of an understanding and accepting attitude towards the clients. (For a more detailed case study see Reiter-Theil and Kahlke, 1995, pp.36-37). The relationship between counsellors and clients, thus, is not neutral (level 1). The counsellors act on the basis of their professional ethics – respecting the autonomy of and informing the clients, trying to help and to offer helpful options (level 2). As far as it is reported in the case, the personal identity or the values of the counsellors were not challenged (level 3). The personal values of the couple were involved from the beginning of the counselling. In exploring the difficulties of the couple as well as in suggesting new options, these values were respected, which can be described as 'technical neutrality'. If there is reason for critical reflection, it would rather be that the counsellors may have not been explicit enough about the restrictions of indication and outcome of IVF, particularly in a case such as this couple with 'idiopathic sterility' (Hölzle and Wiesing 1990). The case report does not permit a judgement about the attitude of the counsellors in dealing with conflict of interests on the side of the clients (level 5), nor does it give information about particular difficulties (level 6). But the course of counselling (in more detail in the longer version cited above) shows that the gynaecologist and the psychologist tried to help the couple according to *their needs and preferences*, even up to the limits of the medical indication of IVF. Only when the treatment turned out to be ineffective and when more signs indicated an emotional and behavioural component of the sterility, the counsellors intervened to stimulate reflection about an alternative to IVF.

It is interesting to note that the ethical dimension of this counselling process is handled in a very discrete way as the counsellors did not elaborate on the potential conflict between the clients' wish for IVF on the one side and the doubtful medical indication on the other, but concentrated on consensus and on maintaining the counselling relationship. We do not know from the report, however, whether ethical principles such as finding the best treatment available etc., were mentioned explicitly, but it seems that the relevant values had been 'communicated' in some way and had created trust on the side of the clients. Another interesting aspect of this report is the context: a gynaecologist and a psychologist working together in counselling and treating infertility in a specialised private practice – a situation which is quite rare, but obviously has its advantages, allowing for very professional and individual work.

Conclusions: Ethical reflection may prevent problems

The question may be asked, whether ethics can be considered to be a therapeutic science (Lesch 1997). In a broad sense, ethics can be qualified as having preventive and therapeutic value. In this respect, we can speak of ethics being a therapeutic or preventive form of practice rather than being a scientific activity in the strict sense. According to the 6-level model of neutrality (table 3) we have shown how ethical reflection of the counsellor may prevent difficulties on both sides; the counsellor's and the client(s)'. In dealing with ethical conflict in the context of counselling, special training and competence will be helpful to solve – to 'treat' – problems for the good of the clients. Not all of the competence required for dealing with ethical conflicts is implied in professional medical or psychological training per se, but rests on individual efforts and study or even specialised post-graduate ethics courses or clinical ethics consultation.

Note

1 An important question, asked by Eve-Marie Engels (1997), concerns the language or terminology which may be used in conversation about ethical aspects of treatment between professional and client. It would not be convincing to restrict conversation to the patient's usual language, only, or to the technical terminology of ethics. The first would – at least with patients who have less elaborate verbal competence – not be sufficient, the second would in most cases be completely useless, because of difficulties of understanding. A compromise must be sought as a kind of (i) flexibly joining the language of the client(s) in order to enhance mutual understanding and encouraging conversation on the one hand and (ii) on the other hand using ethical concepts from ordinary language with explanations, as far as necessary. The main problem in this compromise language will be that it must frequently be adjusted within a very short period of time, without the chance of longer period of learning in the patient-counsellor-relationship. Therefore, we would like to mention a project aiming at the development of a common vocabulary, communication, and culture of discussion in health care, the 'Patients' Forum Medical Ethics' established as a model since 1993 (Reiter-Theil 1995b, Reiter-Theil and Hiddemann 1996). Patients, relatives, health care professionals, and ethicists discuss ethical issues, (e.g. informed consent) from different points of view and on the basis of personal experiences. In conferences and discussions like these it becomes evident, as well, that patients have indeed the capacity to learn how to express their opinions about ethical preferences, arguments, or problems. It becomes evident as well how difficult this is sometimes for medical staff members despite their familiarity and closeness to the ethical issues in every day practice.

References

Beauchamp, T.L. (1995), 'Paternalism', in Reich, W.T. (ed.), *Encyclopedia of Bioethics*, Macmillan: New York, pp. 1914-20.

Clarke, A. (1991), 'Is Non-Directive Counselling Possible?', *Lancet*, Vol. II, pp. 998-1001.

Culver, C.M. and Gert, B. (1988), *Philosophy in Medicine. Conceptual and Ethical Issues in Medicine and Psychiatry*, Oxford University Press: New York, Oxford.

Engels, E.-M. (1997), Personal communication at the symposium 'In Vitro Fertilisation in the 90s – Methods, Contexts, Consequences', 16-19 January 1997, Stuttgart.

Golombok, S., Cook, R., Bish, A. and Murray, C. (1995), 'Families Created by the New Reproductive Technologies: Qualities of Parenting and Social and Emotional Development of the Children', *Child Development*, Vol. 66, pp. 285-98.

Hepp, H. (1994), 'Ethische Probleme am Anfang des Lebens', in Honnefelder, L. and Rager, G. (eds), *Ärztliches Urteilen und Handeln. Zur Grundlegung einer medizinischen Ethik*, Insel: Frankfurt a.M., Leipzig.

Hölzle, C. and Wiesing, U. (1990), *In-Vitro-Fertilisation – ein umstrittenes Experiment*, Springer: Heidelberg.

Kuhse, H. (1994), 'New Reproductive Technologies: Ethical Conflict and the Problem of Consensus', in Bayertz, K. (ed.), *The Concept of Moral Consensus*, Kluwer Academic Publishers: Dordrecht, pp. 75-96.

Lesch, W. (1997), 'Is the Desire For a Child Too Strong? or Is There a Right to a Child of One's Own?', this volume, part 2.

Macklin, R. (1991), 'Artificial Means of Reproduction and Our Understanding of the Family', *Hastings Center Report*, January/February, pp. 5-11.

Ratz, E. (ed.) (1995), *Zwischen Neutralität und Weisung – Zur Theorie und Praxis von Beratung in der Humangenetik*, Ev. Presseverband für Bayern e.V.: München.

Reiter-Theil, S., (1989), 'Therapeutische Neutralität in der Paar- und Sexualtherapie', *Ethik Med*, Vol. 1, pp. 99-107; reprinted in Reiter, L. and Ahlers, C. (eds) (1991), *Systemisches Denken und therapeutischer Prozeß*, Springer: Berlin, Heidelberg, New York, pp. 66-74.

Reiter-Theil, S. (1990), '«Paternalismus» in der Reproduktionsmedizin. Ein Thema für Familienberater?', *System Familie*, Vol. 3, pp. 148-56.

Reiter-Theil, S. (1995a), 'Nichtdirektivität und Ethik in der genetischen Beratung', in Ratz, E. (ed.), *Zwischen Neutralität und Weisung – Zur Theorie und Praxis von Beratung in der Humangenetik*, Ev. Presseverband für Bayern e.V.: München, pp. 83-91.

Reiter-Theil, S. (1995b), 'Von der Ethik in der Psychotherapie zur patientenorientierten Medizinethik. Das Modell Patientenforum medizinische Ethik', *Psychosozial*, Vol. 18, pp. 25-33.

Reiter-Theil, S. and Kahlke, W. (1995), 'Fortpflanzungsmedizin', in Kahlke, W. and Reiter-Theil, S. (eds), *Ethik in der Medizin*, Enke: Stuttgart, pp. 34-45.

Reiter-Theil, S. and Hiddemann, W. (1996), 'Der Beitrag von Patienten zur Ethik in der Medizin: Problemwahrnehmung, Perspektivenwechsel, Mitverantwortung', *Ärzteblatt Baden-Württemberg*, Vol. 4, pp. 140-1.

Rogers, C. (1951), *Client-centered Therapy*, Houghton Mifflin: Boston.

Thompson, A. (1989), *Guide to Ethical Practice in Psychotherapy*, John Wiley & Sons: New York.

Weinstein, B. (1993), 'What is an Expert?', *Theoretical Medicine*, Vol. 14, pp. 57-73.

Wertz, D.C. and Fletcher, J.C. (1988), 'Attitudes of Genetic Counselors: A Multinational Survey', *Am J Hum Genet*, Vol. 42, pp. 592-600.

Wertz, D.C., Fletcher, J.C. and Mulvihill, J.J. (1990), 'Medical Geneticists Confront Ethical Dilemmas. Cross-cultural Comparisons Among 18 Nations', *Am J Hum Genet*, Vol. 46, pp. 1200-13.

Wolff, G. and Jung, C. (1994), 'Nichtdirektivität und genetische Beratung', *Med Genet*, Vol. 6, pp. 195-204.

Yarborough, M., Scott, J.A. and Dixon, L.K. (1989), 'The Role of Beneficence in Clinical Genetics: Non-directive Counseling Reconsidered', *Theoretical Medicine*, Vol. 10, pp. 139-49.

5 The illusion of neutrality in counselling practice

Walter Lesch

A competent physician is not only characterised by scientific knowledge and technological skill. In order to be recognised as a comprehensive expert of health care and despite an increasing tendency to specialisation he or she has more and more tasks in clinical counselling because the patients must give their informed consent before a treatment can be started. This shift from paternalism to the work with competent patients is one of the main reasons for the importance of ethics in high-tech medicine where physicians often have to cooperate with experts of psychology and psychotherapy.

It is a misunderstanding to mix up the counsellor's neutrality with the ideal of scientific objectivity. On the other hand there should of course be a serious effort to be unprejudiced: objective in the sense of impartial, able to listen to the interlocutor in order to establish a basis for an atmosphere of confidence and for the analysis of good arguments (Reiter-Theil 1993). The sharp contrast between neutrality (in combination with the ideal of autonomy) and paternalism gives no chance for a more benevolent interpretation of unavoidable asymmetries in situations of counselling.

The choice of the counsellor (if there is a possibility to choose) determines to a considerable degree the result of a conversation. Imagine that you contact a medical doctor who is primarily interested in scientific research. He or she will give another advice concerning in vitro fertilisation than the collegue who is inspired by the feminist criticism of the new technologies which lead to an instrumentalisation of the female body. The two cases demonstrate the necessity of an ethical orientation for the profession of counselling that would assist a delicate process with a client-centered attitude and in the direction of greater autonomy. An example of such a nondirective method is well known as the therapeutic approach developed by Carl Rogers.

But do clients/patients always want exactly this kind of help? The specific situation of a treatment in reproductive medicine is often characterised by a lack of time, the profound confusion of the couple and a strong wish for someone who can show the way out of an emotionally difficult moment (Beck-Gernsheim 1995). This is no plea for going back to a type of paternalism that fortunately belongs to the past – in theory at least. But a strictly nondirective, ethically informed counselling seems to be a contradiction in itself (Krämer, 1992, p.323). Ethicists, therapists and genetic counsellors must be aware of their duty to offer at least some elements of concrete problem solving and decision-making. If not, we do not need them.

One ethical dimension of counselling is the sympathetic assistance with value clarification. A further role of the counsellor should be that of an advocate of the interests not represented in the situation of decision-making: above all the interests of the future child. And finally the perspective of the society (Callahan 1994) has to be taken into account in the relation between the counsellor and the client(s). On this level (corresponding to the methodological approach of discourse ethics) neutrality will certainly be a good guiding principle. But again it is not a view from nowhere because the consideration of the public interests is filtered by the counsellor's partial perception of this framework. If we agree that the competence of counsellors does not depend on natural gifts and vague intuitions the society must be interested in giving future experts a good training including ethical expertise and techniques of fair communication. When a consultation fails because the clients do not accept the counsellor's point of view, they are free to find another expert (within the limits of the legal regulation and without being tempted by the possibility of 'medical tourism' in Europe).

References

Beck-Gernsheim, E. (1995), 'Genetische Beratung im Spannungsfeld zwischen Klientenwünschen und gesellschaftlichem Erwartungsdruck', in Beck-Gernsheim, E. (ed.), *Welche Gesundheit wollen wir? Dilemmata des medizintechnischen Fortschritts*, Suhrkamp: Frankfurt a.M., pp. 111-38.

Callahan, D. (1994), 'Bioethics: Private Choice and Common Good', *Hastings Center Report*, Vol. 23, No. 3, pp. 28-31.

Krämer, H. (1992), *Integrative Ethik*, Suhrkamp: Frankfurt a.M.

Reiter-Theil, S. (1993), 'Wertfreiheit, Abstinenz und Neutralität? Normative Aspekte in Psychoanalyse und Familientherapie', in Eckensberger, L.H. and Gähde, U. (eds), *Ethische Norm und empirische Hypothese*, Suhrkamp: Frankfurt a.M., pp. 302-27.

6 Genetic counselling

Ulrike Mau

In this text I would like to focus on one special counselling problem in our work with infertile couples and the resulting questions. In Tübingen we have established a pretherapeutic clinical and genetic evaluation and counselling programme especially for couples undergoing intracytoplasmic sperm injection (ICSI) treatment. After gynaecological counselling and evaluation, the couple is referred for genetic counselling. In principle two different types of counselling situations exist:

1 The sterile otherwise healthy couple without any unusual genetic risk for future offspring – which means most probably they have the same general risk as everybody (a 3-5 per cent risk of abnormalities in a child).

2 The sterile couple with unusual findings: e.g. a monogenetic disorder or a chromosomal aberration in one of the partners. They might have a reasonable, sometimes high risk for a genetic disease or abnormalities in offspring.

I would like to focus on this latter genetic counselling situation. As a matter of fact its frequency and relevance are increasing the more popular infertility treatment programmes become. Genetic counselling because of unusual findings in one of the partners is a very stressful situation for the couple. Suddenly there is not only the burden of infertility. A possible illness or mental and/or physical handicap threaten their dream of a future baby. The couple has to cope with the new information, its meaning and possible effects and risks. Feelings like guilt, shame, fear and ethical conflicts arise. The child they dreamed of and they are yearning for withdraws.

In this situation the genetic counsellor requires a great sensitivity. Apart from his or her function to provide counselling that is non-directive, supportive, and responsive to the patients' requests, an ethical principle for the counsellor is to convey the information sensitively to the patients, and in language they understand, so – on the basis of informed consent – they may come to independent decisions (according to the 'Richtlinien und Stellungnahmen des Berufsverbandes Medizinische Genetik e.V. und der Gesellschaft für Humangentik e.V.'). This could be: going on with ICSI or another treatment or learning to accept their infertility and look for alternatives in life. Every counselling situation is unique and requires different/individual approaches. With regard to sex, age, race, religion, genetic status, social circumstances etc. the resulting different ethical conflicts lead to individual opinions and decisions. According to the 'Code of Ethical Principles for Genetics Professionals' (a work by the Council of Regional Networks CORN Ethics Committee) these decisions should be respected by the counsellor within a frame of ethical norms implemented by professional associations.

Let us now return to the couple with a genetic risk. This increased risk for abnormalities in offspring leads to severe ethical, psychological and therapeutic problems not only for the couple. It is an ethical dilemma for the counsellor as well. The main intention of the counsellor should be to help the couple to find a way to cope with their infertility. But what about the ethical and moral ideas of the physician? Does he or she have to preserve the future foetus from harm? By the way – who does this in fertile couples? Does the wish of the couple have priority over the child or is there even a moral obligation over against a future foetus which does not yet exist?

Due to these questions it will be very important that an interdisciplinary team of different professionals from gynaecology, genetics, psychotherapy, ethics and of course the sterile couples themselves work closer together for the benefit of sterile couples and their possible (future) children.

References

Mau, U.A., Bäckert, I.T., Kaiser, P., Kiesel, L. (1997), 'Chromosomal findings in ISO couples referred for genetic counselling prior to intracytoplasmic sperm injection', *Hum Reprod*, Vol. 12, No. 5, pp. 930-7.

Part Five
IVF-TREATMENT: CHANCES AND RISKS

1 Success of in vitro fertilisation

Brian A. Lieberman

Success of in vitro fertilisation (IVF) in this text is defined as the number of live births per treatment cycle commenced. A live birth is the delivery of one or more live babies (twins and triplets are thus counted as one live birth) and who survive at least for one month. A treatment cycle commences with the administration of drugs to stimulate the ovaries and includes those cycles where treatment is cancelled or abandoned before embryo replacement. In discussing success rates it is essential to define the denominator as the rates quoted will be higher if the denominator is the rate per egg recovery or embryo replaced.

The data used in this text are derived from the Human Fertilisation and Embryology Authority (HFEA 1996). All centres providing treatment by IVF or with donated gametes in the UK are required by law to submit information about every treatment cycle commenced. The HFEA data bank is thus both reliable and extensive.

The outcome of IVF is determined primarily by the age of the woman, her previous reproductive history and the duration of the infertility. The outcome is not influenced significantly by the diagnosis of the female factors thought to be responsible for the infertility (Templeton et al. 1996).

The relationship between increasing female age and the live birth rate per cycle commenced is shown in table 1. Younger women have an increased chance of a live birth.

Table 1.

Age (years)	Live birth rate/cycle (per cent)
25	19.9
30	16.9
35	13.9
40	8.2
45	2.5

The relationship between the live birth rate per cycle commenced and the duration of infertility is shown in table 2. The shorter the duration of infertility the higher the chance of a live birth.

Table 2.

Duration of infertility (years)	Live birth rate/cycle (per cent)
0	13.3
1-3	15.3
4-6	14.4
7-9	12.9
10-12	12.4
>12	8.6

The relationship between a woman's previous reproductive performance and the live birth rate per treatment cycle is shown in table 3. Women who have previously been pregnant are more likely to have a live birth after IVF treatment than those never previously pregnant. A previous IVF live birth is a significant positive predictor of a further success.

Table 3.

Number of previous pregnancies	Live birth rate/cycle (per cent)
None	12.5
Spontaneous pregnancies:	
No live births	13.7
One or more live births	15.3
IVF pregnancies:	
No live births	16.6
One or more live births	23.2

There is no statistically significant difference in the outcome of IVF treatment according to the female cause of the infertility provided if the woman is treated with her own eggs. This is not unexpected as IVF bypasses spontaneous ovulation, fertilisation in vivo and gamete/embryo transport. The live birth rate is 13.6 per cent in women with a tubal disorder, 14.2 per cent with endometriosis and 13.4 per cent in unexplained infertility when the age of the woman and the duration of infertility are adjusted statistically.

The live birth rate and the multiple birth rate per cycle are increased when more than one embryo is replaced. The perinatal mortality rate per 1000 births increases with the number of embryos replaced (HFEA 1996). The rates are shown in table 4. The increase in the pregnancy rate is associated with a significant increase in the incidence of multiple pregnancies.

Table 4.

Embryos replaced	Live birth rate (per cent of cycles)	Multiple birth rate (per cent of live births)	Perinatal deaths (per 1000 births)
One	6.0	3.5	7.2
Two	16.4	21.8	25.1
Three	19.9	33.0	33.2

It is important to note that further analysis of the HFEA data shows that the live birth rate per cycle commenced is the same (20.6 per cent and 20.9 per cent) if two or three embryos are replaced provided three or more embryos were available for replacement. The live birth rate is 10.8 per cent if only two embryos were available for replacement. The rate of stillbirth, neonatal death, cerebral palsy and learning disability is increased in twins and triplets.

References

Human Fertilisation and Embryology Authority (1996), *5th Annual Report*, Copies obtainable on request with a SAE to HFEA, Paxton House, 30 Artillery Lane, London. E1 7LS.

Templeton, A., Morris, J.K., Parslow, W. (1996), 'Factors that Affect the Outcome of In-vitro Fertilisation Treatment', *Lancet*, Vol. 348, pp. 1402-6.

2 Success rates in IVF

Urban Wiesing

In discussions about in vitro fertilisation (IVF) the latest success rates of IVF often play an important role. My task will be to reflect upon some questions closely related to that issue. I want to examine the different meanings of 'success', I want to ask the question what does 'success' mean for medicine and what does 'success' mean for the patients. I want to ask how medicine presents its 'success', and last but not least I want to examine the ethical implications of these issues.

As an introduction I will start with a look at the German guidelines for IVF made by a so-called 'Central Commission of the Federal Board of Physicians for the Maintainance of Ethical Principles in Reproductive Medicine, Research on Human Embryos and Genetherapy'.[1] This commission was initiated by the Federal Board of Physicians (Bundesärztekammer) in the 1980s. Their guidelines were published in 1985, and they are now part of the 'Berufsordnung', the professional law of physicians in Germany; that means: they are highly official. The commission stated in 1985: IVF 'is medically and ethically acceptable in appropiate cases, if certain conditions regarding approval and performance are met'.[2] The same commission stated a few pages later that the success rate of IVF 'of currently 10 to 15 per cent needs to be improved urgently'.[3] Let me repeat: The commission believes that IVF is morally sound, but the success rates of 10 to 15 per cent must be improved.

In order to be able to a comment on this statement I have to give some further information: The success rate of IVF in 1985 was far away from 10 to 15 per cent. The cumulated success rate of German IVF-centers, documented in the official journal of the German physicians, in the 'Deutsches Ärzteblatt', was lower than 3.4 per cent from 1981 to 1985 (Semm 1985), and the cumulated success rate up to 1986 was lower than 6 per cent (Fertilität 1987). The documented success rate in the UK in 1985 and 1986 was 8.6 per cent (Voluntary Licensing Authority 1986-1991). Additionally it has to be mentioned that the Federal Board of Physicians argues emphatically for IVF with the Hippocratic obligation to help the sufferer, not with the patient's autonomy.

However, despite the unrealistic notion of the success rates, both statements are remarkable especially in combination. How is it possible that a therapy is medically sound when the success rates must be improved 'urgently'? Is the Hippocratic tradition in medical ethics a convincing argument, when a therapy has to be improved 'urgently'? Which idea of medicine had this commission in mind? I cannot explain what the commission had in mind, to me both statements are not compatible especially when the Hippocratic obligation is stressed 'to help the sufferer'. A treatment with success rates that must be improved 'urgently' is medically not acceptable as long as the success rates have not improved.

The combination of both statements is only acceptable if IVF is not seen as a therapy but as an experiment. But in this case completely different ethical grounds will be needed: the measure is not carried out only to help the sufferer but in fact also to attain scientific knowledge and skills which could be of benefit to future patients. In this case IVF must be offered as such, and it has to be performed according the revised Declaration of Helsinki. That means: it must be limited from the point of view of time, it has to be restricted to trails and to centers with the capacity and skills to do research, the patients have to be informed about the experimental status. But what did happen? Neither did the Commission declare IVF as an experimental therapy nor did it think of these consequences. It did not even ask this question. The worst thing which can happen to a question is not that it can not be answered but that it is not even asked.

Historically seen there has never been a paper scruting of all the indications as to whether IVF is a successful therapy compared with the spontaneous pregnancy rate of untreated couples. Therefore, it is not surprising that in 1990 an investigation of members of the World Health Organisation answered the question as to whether IVF can be regarded as a tested therapy with a decided 'no' (Wagner and Clair 1989). For them the efficiency and unwanted effects of IVF have not been investigated sufficiently.

I believe that the power of judgment of the German commission was severely handicapped by the euphoric expectations regarding IVF and by a naive technological optimism. Optimism in a double sense: Firstly, that the success rates would improve automatically and very soon. But they did not. Secondly, that a successful technology would automatically be helpful for the patient. But it is not. Therefore, historically seen both presuppositions were never met. I have mentioned the guidelines of the Central Commission because they have the most official character and they are very typical. I want to explain this by analysing what medicine considered to be a 'success'.

What did medicine consider to be a 'success' in an IVF-treatment?

Medicine has distinguished between many different steps in IVF-treatment and has given many different results as 'success' rates, for example: Pregnancy rates and birth rates are reported in terms of pregnancies per attempt, pregnancies per fertilisation, pregnancies per transfer. The same is possible with birth rates. And in the scientific articles each of these steps was reported. High 'success' rates were presented which were related only to steps within the procedure. That means: For reproductive medicine a successful single step in IVF was a 'success' and was announced as a 'success'. And with these single steps a 'success' for the patient was calculated. And it was calculated beyond any methodological honesty, but with optimism.

In the literature, especially in the early years, incredibly high success rates can be found or, to put it clearly, were predicted. For example in 1986 Guzick, Wilkes and Jones published an article about 'Cumulative pregnancy rates for in vitro fertilization' in the most respected journal *Fertility and Sterility* (Guzick et al. 1986). They predicted a success rate of 85 per cent after 12 treatment cycles and came to the result: '[...] IVF can lead to successful pregnancy for a large proportion of couples' (p.663). It must be mentioned that in Germany in 1986 the success rate per cycle was about 5 per cent, and no evidence was given that the success rates could be cumulated. As well nobody knew how a woman could survive the torture of 12 treatment cycles mentally and physically. I quoted this article as an example, I could give many more.

That means: The 'success' was not proven, but predicted with presuppositions that were never met. But the success rate of 85 per cent is kept in the mind of the physicians and patients.

How did medicine present the 'success' of IVF?

For the scientists engaged the history of IVF was always a history of 'success'. If you read an article about IVF you will find many numbers and high percentage rates. And in most articles the lowest number is the only relevant one for the patient. The presentation within the scientific community always focusses on other rates, that means: on higher rates than the relevant one. And in the last national overviews about the success rates of German IVF centers the baby-take-home-rate is not even mentioned (Rjosk et al. 1995). It is only possible to calculate this rate on the basis of the published results and other scientificly proven data. And then the success rate is below 10 per cent: The average pregnancy rate is 17.1 per cent per retrieval, the abortion rate is 27.7 per cent, that means the birth-rate per retrieval is 12.3 per cent. It has to be considered, that about 15 per cent of the stimulations are terminated, that means the success rate drops to 10.5 per cent. Unfortunatly 20 per cent of the German

IVF centers refused to provide any success rates.[4] It must be supposed that theses centers are the less successful ones. That means: the average chance of a woman to get a baby via IVF in a German IVF-center is according to the latest national overview below 10 per cent per cycle. And even more surprising: this rate is not mentioned in the article.

Reproductive medicine often defends the low success rate with an argument that must be reviewed critically. Sometimes the argument is stressed that the low success rate of IVF is the same rate as in non-artificial pregnancies. That means: nature should become the criterion for the question whether IVF is acceptable or not. According to the idea: what is as successful as nature is acceptable. But this argument is terribly wrong and once again the idea of medicine is lost. Nature – or the 'normality in nature' – can never give the criterion for acceptable medicine because all diseases are a kind of nature and the central obligation of medicine is to help in case of suffering and that means to act against nature. Medicine as a profession is only conceivable if it is not impossible to be more successful than nature. Otherwise it would make no sense to act as a physician. The ethical foundation of medicine is to help the sufferer, and not to be like nature itself or to restore the 'normality' of nature. To refer to non-artifical pregnancy rates makes no sense ethically.

What did the patients know about the meaning of the different 'success' rates?

The relevant information for the patient, the so-called 'baby-take-home-rate', was always lower than the high 'success' rates of single steps within IVF. But the patients were confronted with a lot of numbers, all of them higher than the relevant success rate. Therefore the patients often develop unrealistically high expectations regarding reproductive therapies. In leading journals worldwide, even in German televison renowned clinicians complained that the results of IVF had been improved by statistical manipulation and that the patients systematically overestimate the chances of success. 'Infertile patients often develop unrealistically high expectations regarding specific therapies. Here the ambiguous statistics must be mentioned' (Blackwell et al., 1987, p.737, see also Soules 1985). The authors name the responsible persons: 'The medical community is partly responsible for these inflated expectations' (Blackwell et al., 1987, p.737).

Is 'success' of reproductive medicine in every case helpful for the patient?

The central question with high impact on the ethical debate arises: Is 'success' of reproductive medicine always a 'success' for the patient, is it helpful for the patient? The answer is: No, in a double sense. Firstly, 'success' in a single step in IVF does not mean that the patient will have a baby. Only one success rate is relevant for the patient: The baby-take-home-rate, and that is usually the lowest rate. And secondly, a baby is not in every case helpful for the patient, because childlessness is a more complex suffering than only a lack of child (Hölzle and Wiesing 1991, Hölzle 1990). I refer to the huge literature about the psychological aspects of infertility. That means that 'success' in reproductive medicine is not always helpful for the patient. The physicians engaged forgot that it is not the same to present high numbers or to help the sufferer. But this is an alienation of medicine from its genuine task – to help the sufferer, and this alienation has a moral impact. For me the most dramatic points seems to be, that the 'success' of medicine is not necessary helpful to the patient, but in most cases of IVF even an additional burden for the patient.

A commission of the 'Academy for Ethics in Medicine' observed in 1990 that 'there are very many «losers» in IVF and only a few «winners»' (Akademie für Ethik in der Medizin, 1990, p.113). This statement should have aroused attention. The question arises: How could it happen – assuming an authentic intention to help from all concerned – that medicine became alienated from its genuine moral task – namely to help the patient? The answer to this question is certainly complex. I believe that one of the reasons lies in the momentum of technology and in the fact that medical ethical tradition was sacrificed to the impending danger of missing a technological development. The technology had such a deep influence on the thinking of the physicians that the fundamental, the basic moral principle of medicine got lost. The short history of IVF gives the impression that traditional and valid norms of medical ethics have been forgotten in view of something tremendously new. And I am afraid that the same might happen when reproductive technology can be combined with genetics. I am afraid that valid ethical norms will be under enormous pressure if it is perceived that a technological development might be missed. I am afraid that experimental therapies will not be offered as such and not be performed according to the revised Declaration of Helsinki. I think that in the light of new technologies medicine has to reconsider what its genuine moral obligation is. And that means: a medical success should be helpful for the patient.

Notes

1 'Zentrale Kommission der Bundesärztekammer zur Wahrung ethischer Grundsätze in der Reproduktionsmedizin, Forschung an menschlichen Embryonen und Gentherapie'.

2 ‘Sie [die IVF] ist in geeigneten Fällen medizinisch und ethisch vertretbar, wenn bestimmte Zulassungs- und Durchführungsbedingungen eingehalten werden’ (Vorstand der Bundesärztekammer, 1988, p.16).

3 ‘deren derzeitige Erfolgsquote von nur 10 bis 15 Prozent dringend der Verbesserung bedarf’ (Vorstand der Bundesärztekammer, 1988, p.36).

4 Even the authors are complaining about the fact that sufficient information about the German IVF centers cannot be provided: ‘a scandal’ (Rjosk et al., 1995, p.52).

References

Akademie für Ethik in der Medizin (1990), ‘Embryonen-Forschung – zulassen oder verbieten?’, *Ethik in der Medizin*, Vol. 2, pp. 107-15.

Blackwell, R.E., Carr, B.R., Chang, R.J., DeCherney, A.H., Haney, A.F., Keye, W.R., Rebar, R.W., Rock, J.A., Rosenvaks, Z., Seibel, M.M. and Soules, M.R. (1985), ‘Are We Exploiting the Infertile Couple?’, *Fertility and Sterility*, Vol. 48, pp. 735-9.

Fertilität (1987), ‘Die In-vitro-Fertilisation (IVF) und der intratubare Gametentransfer (GIFT) in der Bundesrepublik Deutschland (1981-1986)’, *Fertilität*, Vol. 3, pp. 73-81.

Guzick, D.S., Wilkes, C. and Jones, H.W. (1986), ‘Cumulative Pregnancy Rates for In Vitro Fertilization’, *Fertility and Sterility*, Vol. 46, pp. 663-7.

Hölzle, C. (1990), *Die psychische Bewältigung der In-vitro-Fertilisation*, Münster.

Hölzle, C. and Wiesing, U. (1991), *In-vitro-Fertilisation – ein umstrittenes Experiment. Fakten – Leiden – Diagnosen – Ethik*, Springer: Berlin/ Heidelberg/ New York, especially chap. 3.

Rjosk, H.K., Haeske-Seeberg, H., Seeberg, B. and Kreuzer, E. (1995), ‘IVF und GIFT – Ergebnisse in Deutschland 1993’, *Fertilität*, Vol.11, pp. 48-54.

Semm, K. (1985), ‘Seit 1982 102 Entbindungen mit 131 Kindern’, *Deutsches Ärzteblatt,* Vol. 82, pp. 1683-4.

Soules, M.R. (1985), ‘The In Vitro Fertilization Pregnancy Rate: Let's be Honest with One Another’, *Fertility and Sterility*, Vol. 43, pp. 511-3.

Voluntary Licensing Authority (VLA) (1986) The First Report; (1987) The Second Report; (1988) The Third Report; (1989) The Fourth Report. Since the 5th Report: Interim Licensing Authority (ILA) (1990) The Fifth Report; (1991) The Sixth Report. Sumfield & Day: Eastbourne.

Vorstand der Bundesärztekammer, Wissenschaftlicher Beirat der Bundesärztekammer, Zentrale Kommission der Bundesärztekammer zur Wahrung ethischer Grundsätze in der Reproduktionsmedizin, Forschung an menschlichen Embryonen und Gentherapie (eds) (1988), *Weissbuch. Anfang und*

Ende menschlichen Lebens – Medizinischer Fortschritt und ärztliche Ethik, Deutscher Ärzte Verlag: Köln.
Wagner, M.G. and Clair, P.A.St. (1989), 'Are In-vitro-Fertilisation and Embryo Transfer of Benefit to All?', *The Lancet*, pp. 1027-30.

3 IVF, its success rates and their ethical significance

Alberto Bondolfi

The following comments may be seen as a general reflection on the indirect ethical and normative implications of data on in vitro fertilisation (IVF) and its success rates.

One first ethical consideration has to do with the fundamental significance of taking success rates into account when legitimising IVF procedures. The consideration of such data does, in fact, only make sense if the position is adopted that IVF per se is not to be condemned or approved, no matter what the consequences of acting or refraining from acting may be. In other words, taking IVF success rates into account only makes sense from a *teleological* point of view. From a *strictly deontologial* point of view, considerations or observations of this nature should remain irrelevant. Of course, in moderate strains of deontological ethics, the consequences of an action do play a certain role, thus rendering it advisable even in this context not to ignore success rates.

The more the quantitative success rates of IVF increase, the more this medical achievement abandons its status as a 'clinical trial' in favour of 'therapy', even though sterility is not effectively overcome. In society, IVF is increasingly being viewed as plausible and capable of being legally regulated in a 'liberal' manner, i.e. 'not prohibitionistically'. Success rates indirectly legitimise individual reproductive technologies, success being a necessary, if hardly sufficient argument taken in isolation (*conditio necessaria, sed non sufficiens*).

On the other hand, the optimisation of success rates is an argument which gives rise to additional moral problems. In fact, the stricter the defined indication for IVF is, the greater its success, yet at the same time the louder the demands from women with an insufficient indication become. They feel discriminated against being excluded from IVF programmes. Of course, strictly speaking, there is no 'right to IVF', since people do not normally have a right to a medical treatment which is not firmly indicated. It is thus not really correct to speak of discrimination in cases where IVF is rejected as a possible treatment. When refusing treatment, the physicians caring for these women should, however, make an effort to name clearly the reasons for exclusion from their IVF programme, backed up by arguments, as well as to suggest possible alternatives.

A further moral problem arises from the complex link between therapy and research in this field. There can be no doubt that the goal of improving IVF success rates through specific studies must in itself be seen as legitimate, even desirable. Yet how is research with the aforementioned goal to be evaluated ethically if it can only be attained through consumptive embryo research? From a teleological point of view, the manner of evaluating the relationship between this legitimate goal and its envisaged means remains controversial. Defining the status of the non-implanted embryo automatically affects moral evaluation of the proposed research, which counts on consuming such embryos.

Moreover, experimental IVF interventions assume a therapeutic significance which is not only purely individual, the efforts behind them being aimed at the well-being of the woman concerned, but also comprehensive, collectively aiming to surmount female sterility.

In my opinion, individual females undergoing IVF treatment should permit research to be carried out on their own supernumerary embryos. These women would like to profit from the success of this technique and, in submitting to this form of therapy, are already resigned to the fact that indivudal embryos will be lost in the process. Here too, the likelihood of a positive response is to be categorised as relevant, at least indirectly.

From the point of view of the general public – and this point of view is crucial for the process of legal institutionalisation – the argument that there is a direct link between research with embryos and the success of the technique certainly plays a role, albeit not a *crucial* one. The relationship between the well-being of an individual woman, the claims thus arising and the general female public is extremely complex. The laws of a democratic state must attempt to do justice to both levels of this conflict. Studies into the optimisation of IVF must be ethically evaluated within this context. The ethics committees must consider this point in their investigations.

4 Multiple pregnancy

Brian A. Lieberman

The incidence of multiple births is increased after ovarian stimulation used either alone or in conjunction with in vitro fertilisation (IVF) or donor insemination (DI). National data in the United Kingdom is not collected for induction of ovulation but the outcome of all treatment cycles by IVF and DI is published by the Human Fertilisation and Embryology Authority (HFEA). The IVF singleton and multiple pregnancy rates by the number of embryos replaced is shown in Table 1. This data confirms the increased incidence of multiple pregnancies with multiple embryo replacements.

Table 1.

Embryos replaced	No. of cycles	Singleton		Twins		Triplets		Total
		n	%	n	%	n	%	
One	2309	171	95.5	7	4.0	1	0.5	179
Two	6449	1001	77.2	288	22.2	8	0.6	1297
Three	11455	1892	67.9	714	25.5	191	6.8*	2797
Total	20212	3064	75.2	1009	24.8	200	5.0	4073

*Includes 3 sets of quads
Source: Data derived from HFEA 5th Annual Report (1996)

The outcome of single and multiple pregnancies following IVF (fresh and frozen embryos) is shown in Table 2. The probability of a baby being stillborn or dying within the first 4 weeks of life is significantly increased in twin and triplet births (HFEA 1996), increasing from 14.1 per thousand with a single baby, to 58.3 with twins and 90.9 with triplets. It is necessary to record that in the same year the PMR with single but spontaneously conceived babies was 8.0 per thousand.

Table 2.

	Clinical pregs.	Live births	Miscarriage	TOP	Ectopics	Unkown	Babies born	Perinatal deaths /‰ births
Single	3064	2376	448	16	125	65	2380	14.1
Twin	1009	929	114	4	7	103	1747	58.3
Triplet	197	170	41	12	0	3	459	90.9
Quads	3	2	1	1	0	780	6	–
Totals	4273	3477	604	33	132	78	4592	29.7

TOP: termination of pregnancy.

The incidence of cerebral palsy is increased in multiple births (Pharoah and Cooke 1996), rising from 2.3 per thousand infant survivors in singletons, to 12.6 in twins and 44.8 in triplets.

The cost of care and education for surviving twins and triplets is increased compared to singleton births.

References

Human Fertilisation and Embryology Authority (1996), *5th Annual Report*, Copies obtainable on request with a SAE to HFEA, Paxton House, 30 Artillery Lane, London E1 7LS.

Pharoah and Cooke (1996), 'Cerebral Palsy and Multiple Births' *Arch Dis Child*, Vol. 75, F174-F177.

5 Multifetal pregnancies: reduction or prevention?

Guido de Wert

Introduction

One of the results of the development of medically assisted reproduction – more particularly in vitro fertilisation (IVF), gamete intra Fallopian transfer (GIFT), and controlled hyperstimulation – is the increase of multifetal pregnancies and multiple births. Several well-publicised cases have promoted public awareness of the risks involved in these pregnancies and births. I will concentrate on ethical issues related to the management of the risks of multifetal pregnancies in the context of IVF.

Multifetal pregnancies: 'the failure of success'

The usual practice in IVF is to transfer more than one embryo, as this increases the chance that at least one will implant. As a consequence, often more than one embryo implants and develops. According to the international literature, approximately 25 per cent of IVF-pregnancies are multifetal pregnancies.

Especially the larger multifetal pregnancies (triplets and higher-order pregnancies) pose serious health risks for both women and their children (Royal Commission 1993). For women, multifetal pregnancy increases the risk of anemia, miscarriage, toxaemia, high blood pressure, kidney trouble, complicated delivery, and post-birth haemorrhage. Risks for the fetuses include miscarriage, accidents during delivery, and premature birth. Prematurity brings with it another risk: (very) low birth weight, which may have serious and long-lasting consequences. These children usually have breathing problems, and are more likely to have cerebral palsy, poor eyesight, short attention span, poor coordination and motor skills, and poor learning skills as they grow up. Approximately 25 per cent of very low birth weight children have serious disabilities, while a significant number of them have problems requiring special education services. Apart from these health risks, multiple births may also strain the psychosocial well-being of the families involved, especially of the mothers (Garel and Blondel 1992). In view of these problems, larger multifetal pregnancies are considered to be a potentially serious complication of IVF.

The solution: prevention

In order to avoid the risks involved in larger multifetal pregnancies, two strategies have been developed. The first strategy is multifetal pregnancy reduction (MFPR), which involves the killing of one or more fetuses while retaining the desired number of fetuses. How to refer to this procedure is controversial. Terms like selective abortion, selective feticide, selective birth, MFPR, etc., are just some of the possibilities. One may well argue that at least some of these terms reflect some sort of 'Sprachpolitik' (some sort of 'factional language'). I will refer to this procedure as MFPR, the term that has become widely accepted in the literature. The second strategy involves preventing larger multifetal pregnancies.

Multifetal pregnancy reduction

Over the past decade, MFPR has emerged as a staple of infertility therapy. Since the mid-1980s, there has been a strong expansion in the number of procedures that have been performed. MFPR has been welcomed as an important technological advance, which substantially reduces the risk of delivering severely premature infants, who will either die or may have serious disabilites. Nevertheless, the procedure is highly controversial. What, then, are the major moral objections – and are these objections convincing?

A *first* objection holds that MFPR is at odds with the independant ('intrinsic') moral status of the fetus. As we all know, there is no consensus on the foundation and degree of 'worthiness' of human unborn life. For those who consider a 'traditional' abortion to be the moral equivalent of homicide, a MFPR will be equally unacceptable. Those who deny that the fetus has any independant moral status, will in principle consider an abortion as well as MFPR to be morally neutral, 'jenseits von Gut und Böse'. A third, 'middle of the road', position acknowledges that the fetus has an independant moral status, which means that abortion is a morally serious (or at least: not neutral) act. This position, however, does not imply that an abortion is always morally wrong: abortions can be justified for ethically valid reasons. Since this position attempts to draw a line between morally valid and invalid reasons for abortion, it follows that a compatible position on MFPR would search for moral boundaries between permissible and impermissible cases (Evans et al. 1989).

Even though the ethics of traditional abortion is relevant for the ethics of MFPR, the literature points to some differences between these procedures. Right from the start – and now I come to the *second* objection – commentators have stressed the possible risks of MFPR for the remaining fetuses. Three types of risks have been identified: MFPR might cause anomalies in the remaining fetuses (a), it might frequently induce a miscarriage (b), and it might result in premature labour, involving high mortality and/or morbidity (c).

MFPR-practice during the last decade has provided important empirical data on these risks. The risk that the procedure will cause anomalies in the remaining fetus(es) appears to be zero, at least when the procedure is performed by an experienced phycisian, and in the first trimester of pregnancy.

For obvious reasons, much attention has been given (and is still being given) to the risk of pregnancy loss after MFPR. After all, this risk is morally relevant for both 'fetalists' – defined by Rowland as those commentators who have a primary focus on the (protection of the) fetus – and feminists (who primarily focus on the impact of modern reproductive technologies on women) (Raymond 1987). From a fetalist perspective, the possible risk of pregnancy loss further substantiates the claim that a MFPR is at odds with the value of unborn human life. From a feminist perspective, this risk is relevant because pregnancy loss may cause severe emotional stress for the couple, especially for the woman. In view of their/her infertility, the pregnancy lost may have been their only or last opportunity to have children. What, then, is the available data? According to a recent publication, presenting the international, collaborative experience, the risk of pregnancy loss after MFPR increases substantially with the starting and finishing number of fetuses in multifetal pregnancies (Evans et al. 1996). Pregnancy loss rates exceed 20 per cent for patients starting with sextuplets or more, falling to 7.6 per cent for triplets reduced primarily to twins. An important question is, of course, whether these pregnancy losses are all a result of the MFPR, or whether some of these losses represent 'background losses' that whould have occurred regardless of whether the MFPR was performed. The data available suggest that the *spontaneous* loss rate in multiple pregnancies may be quite high, and that a significant proportion of the pregnancy losses that follow a MFPR is not caused by the procedure itself (Berkowitz et al. 1996). At this time, it is impossible to give more precise risk estimations.

A *third* objection to MFPR concerns the possible psychological risks for the survivors: How will these children cope when they learn that some of their (fetal) sibs have been killed in utero in order to improve the outcome of the pregnancy? Will they not suffer from feelings of 'survivor guilt'? In view of this risk, women who have undergone MFPR worry about how best to explain their decision to the surviving child(ren). Some of the women are determined not to inform the surviving child(ren).

Evans et al. (1989) have proposed the principle of *proportionality* as a guiding principle for the ethics of MFPR. They define this principle as 'the duty, when taking actions involving risks of harm, to balance risks and benefits so that actions have the greatest chance to result in the least harm and the most benefit to persons involved'. They rightfully stress that in case of (larger) multiple pregnancies, there are three options, *each of which could result in serious harm*. First, the ('whole') pregnancy could be terminated, causing death to all fetuses and possibly not succeeded by any future pregnancy. A second possibility is to do nothing ('wait and see'), and to risk a very premature delivery. The third alternative is MFPR, involving the risks mentioned before.

Evans et al. define the principle of proportionality in terms of the impact of the various options on the interests of the (future) *persons* involved: the pregnant woman/the couple, and the future (surviving) children. They acknowledge, however, that the fetus, although not considered to be a person, deserves at least some respect, in view of its potential to become a person. This additional moral principle is important. After all, we should acknowledge that MFPR, even if considered to be proportional according to Evans' definition, has its moral price: the (direct) killing of one or more fetuses.
How, then, to ethically evaluate MFPR?

Medical reasons: MFPR is widely accepted when performed for medical reasons. The obstetric and perinatal outcome of multifetal pregnancies is strongly correlated to the number of fetuses. In sixtuplets (and larger multiple pregnancies), the chance that any fetus will survive is low (to zero), while the health of the woman is severely endangered. MFPR can be morally justified as a procedure to reduce the health risks for the woman and to increase the chance that at least some fetuses will survive. ('Radical' fetalists, who consider any direct killing of fetuses to be intolerable, whatever the consequences, will, of course, not accept this 'pro life' justification.) Quadruplet and quintuplet pregnancies impose substantial maternal risks too. Even though the fetuses have a good chance of surviving, perinatal morbidity is substantial. In view of both of these risks, a reduction of these pregnancies seems acceptable. Whether reducing a *triplet* pregnancy is medically indicated, is controversial (Berkowitz et al. 1996). In view of this lack of conclusive medical data, some critics seriously doubt whether a reduction of triplet pregnancies can be morally justified. Apparrently, these critics consider *non*-medical, psychosocial, considerations to be irrelevant for the ethics of MFPR – a view that is reflected in making the medical ratio of MFPR a defining characteristic of this procedure (another example of 'Sprachpolitik').

Psychosocial reasons: Can psychosocial reasons justify a MFPR? This question, of course, is especially relevant in the context of 'smaller' multifetal pregnancies, in particular triplet pregnancies. (After all, most, if not all, infertile couples feel perfectly happy with twin pregnancies.)

Right from the start, many clinics refused to perform MFPR in triplet and twin pregnancies (except in case of specific maternal risk factors). This restrictive policy was immediately rejected by, for instance, the feminist philosopher Overall (1990) as an unacceptable violation of the principle of respect for *autonomy*:

> If women are entitled to choose to end their pregnancies altogether, then they are also entitled to choose how many fetuses [...] they will carry. If it is unjustified to deny a woman access to an abortion of all fetuses in her uterus, then it is also unjustified to deny her access to the termination of some of those fetuses.

This criticism was, I think, somewhat hasty. After all, clinicians involved in the first clinical trials rightly justified a more restrictive policy on the basis of the unknown medical risks of the procedure for the remaining fetuses, more particularly the risk that a MFPR might induce handicaps. It has only recently been established that the procedure itself does not damage the survivors.

In view of this reassuring finding, the moral justification for rejecting MFPR for psychosocial reasons has become weaker. The international working group on MFPR rightly concludes that parental autonomy should be given a higher priority in the decision process than previously (Evans et al. 1993). A second argument for not, a priori, criticising a psychosocial indication for MFPR is that many parents of triplets report considerable stress, social isolation, and depressive symptoms. Several studies suggest that it is almost impossible for a mother to meet the needs of three infants at once and that the mother-child-relationship is often disturbed (Garel and Blondel 1992).

The reluctance with regard to MFPR in triplet (and possibly twin) pregnancies for psychosocial reasons may be based in part on the concern that this might result in a substantial increase in the numbers of MFPR performed. One should realise, however, that infertile women will not lightly opt for a procedure which still carries a risk of inducing pregnancy loss.

Even though (medically as well as psychosocially indicated) MFPR can be morally justified in individual cases, a 'sense of unease' remains (Eser 1990). This urges us to consider the alternative strategy to prevent the problems involved in larger multifetal pregnancies and multiple births: preventing larger multifetal pregnancies.

Prevention of multifetal pregnancies

The ethical debate on MFPR should not be limited to the question as to whether MFPR can be justified in individual emergency situations. Such reductionist debate mirrors an ethical myopia. An important point concerns, indeed, the *cause* of the problem. Most (larger) multifetal pregnancies which make patients request MFPR have a so-called 'iatrogenic' nature, i.e. they are caused by assisted reproductive technologies. Iatrogenic problems should not be created lightly. While there has been (and in some centres: still is – see below) a tendency to accept MFPR as routine part of a 'two-step process of medically assisted reproduction', a strong consensus has emerged that physicians should take appropriate steps to prevent larger multifetal pregnancies. Various arguments in favour of such prevention have been put forward: non-moral and moral, and, with regard to the latter, deontological as well as consequentialist arguments:

- frequent reductions (further) discredit IVF, i.e. they risk hampering the societal acceptance of IVF;
- in view of the value of unborn life, eliminating one or more fetuses can only be justified as a last resort ('ultimum remedium'), i.e. in case of failed prevention of larger multifetal pregnancies;
- a MFPR is not a panacea for the health risks of multifetal pregnancies for the future children. Even though acceptable perinatal outcomes usually can be achieved, there is still a price to be paid in an increased risk of (severe) prematurity (Evans et al. 1993). There is a strong correlation between the starting number of fetuses and the risk of prematurity after a MFPR, even though this risk is substantially lower than in 'untreated' cases of multifetal pregnancies. The risk of extreme premature delivery (25-28 weeks) in reduced sextuplets is 11.5 per cent. In reduced triplets, still 3.3 per cent of the deliveries occurred at 25-28 weeks, while another 7.5 per cent of the reduced triplets delivered at 29-32 weeks (Evans et al. 1996). The point remains that aggressive infertility treatment does have deleterious effects for the children even if MFPR can be performed.

Preventing multifetal IVF-pregnancies demands limiting the number of embryos transferred in a given cycle. Transferring just one single embryo would, of course, be safest. This strategy, however, is currently not a realistic ('viable') option: the 'baby-take-home' rate of IVF would become unacceptably low. How, then, to balance the maximum benefit (in terms of pregnancy rates) derived from multiple transfers (the importance of maintaining an acceptable pregnancy rate) while minimising the risk of multifetal pregnancy?

A first option is to transfer no more than two embryos. This policy would almost completely eliminate triplet (and higher-order) pregnancies, but, again, pregnancy rates would dramatically decrease. In view of this, some guidelines and regulations (amongst others, the German 'Embryonenschutzgesetz' [Bundesrat 1990], the British 'Human Fertilisation and Embryology Authority' [1993], and the Canadian 'Royal Commission on New Reproductive Technologies' [1993]) state that a maximum of three embryos be replaced. IVF-clinics, however, which interpret this guideline as a licence for *routinely* transferring three embryos, will still face triplet pregnancies in a disquieting high percentage of the cases, namely approximately 9 per cent.

Some clinics are studying the 'pros and cons' of a differentiated, 'flexible', transfer policy, replacing preferably no more than two embryos, while allowing of the transfer of more than two embryos in specific cases ('two, unless...'). (This policy has recently been recommended by the World Medical Association [1995].) According to some studies, the transfer of just two embryos in *younger* patients (less than 35-37 years old), when *morphologically good* embryos are available, does not significantly, or just minimally, lower the pregnancy rate, while it effectively prevents triplet pregnancies (Staessen et al. 1993).

What is 'good transfer practice' in case of a suboptimal IVF prognosis (higher maternal age and/or less good embryo morphology)? In these cases, IVF-clinics, including the clinics acknowledging the importance of reducing the number of triplet (and higher order) pregnancies, offer to transfer more than two embryos. After all, so they claim, the pregnancy rate as well as the *multiple* pregnancy rate in these women is substantially lower. The data available up until now shows that the effectiveness of this policy in terms of the prevention of triplet pregnancies varies remarkably. In one clinic, no triplet pregnancy occurred in 1995 (personal communication dr C. Jansen, Voorburg). In another clinic, however, the selective transfer of three embryos resulted in a triplet pregnancy rate of 3-4 per cent, substantially lower than when more than two embryos were transferred as a routine (9 per cent), but still disquieting (personal communication dr C. Staessen, Brussels). This finding illustrates the importance of scrutinising the criteria for transferring more than two embryos.

Against the stream ....: While guidelines and regulations in many countries urge that larger multifetal IVF-pregnancies should be prevented as far as is reasonably possible, more or less restrictive embryo transfer guidelines have recently been criticised. Gleicher et al. (1995) state that these guidelines were not preceded by an investigation of patient attitudes towards multiple births. The results of their questionnaire among infertile patients suggest:

- that most couples express a strong desire for multiple births, as long as these can be limited to triplets;
- that increasing length of infertility is positively correlated with a willingness to risk the conception of multiples *beyond* triplets;

- that increasing female age increases the readiness to consider MFPR as an option (Gleicher et al. 1995).

Gleicher et al. conclude that restrictive embryo transfer guidelines do not concur with the desires of (many) infertile patients, and should therefore be modified.

A similar criticism comes from Simpson and Carson (1996). Their first point concerns the claim that pregnancy rates are similar when, in IVF-patients with a good prognosis, two instead of three or more embryos are transferred. Some studies indicate that, even in this group of patients, lowering the number of embryos to be transferred to two really does decrease the pregnancy rate. More importantly, they question the claim that a restrictive transfer policy is wise or fair even if it does reduce high-order gestations. Their principal objection is that such policies smack of paternalism. IVF-centres, so they argue, should be free to practice IVF in the manner that provides the fully informed couple their *highest* chance of pregnancy.

Is a restrictive transfer policy, indeed, unjustifiably paternalistic? And/or is it unwise and unfair? No. First, it appears that the couples who are most enthusiastic about having multiplets are those who have not had the experience of nurturing children. It is very well possible that many of these infertile couples either are unaware of or deny the medical and psychosocial problems posed by larger multiple pregnancies and multiple births. One should, therefore, question the autonomy of infertile patients who seem willing to accept higher risks of large(r) multiple pregnancies.

Second, it is highly questionable to restrict the normative debate on more restrictive transfer policies to a debate on the respective pros and cons of paternalism and anti-paternalism. Such problem-reduction mistakenly assumes that the only moral issue involved concerns the possible clash between respecting a patient's autonomy on the one hand and promoting her well-being on the other hand. A second moral issue concerns the serious health risks of larger multifetal pregnancies for the future children. Gleicher et al. (1995) completely disregard the *professional responsibility* of IVF-doctors to take into account the interests of future IVF-children. In defence of their ('as you like it'-) position, Gleicher et al. might point at the willingness of at least some couples to consider MFPR in large(r) multifetal pregnancies, thereby reducing the health risks for the surviving fetuses. Interestingly, Simpson and Carson recommend transfering large numbers of embryos only *on the condition* that the couple (woman) accepts the option of MFPR in case of a large multifetal pregnancy. According to these authors, *not* undergoing MFPR is not a real option, because this would involve an unacceptable high risk of having premature infants with severe disabilities. Apparently, Simpson and Carson consider MFPR to be merely an adjunct to aggressive infertility treatment, with no major moral or medical implications. Let me stress again that MFPR is *not* a panacea for the health risks of larger multifetal pregnancies for the future children: there is still a price to be paid in an increased risk of (extreme) prematurity.

Concluding remarks

Larger multifetal pregnancies pose serious risks for both the mother and future children. Even though MFPR may be morally justified in individual emergency situations, the procedure should not be lightly accepted as routine part of a 'two step process' of medically assisted reproduction. A first, deontological, argument for preventing larger multifetal pregnancies, and accepting MFPR only as a last resort, concerns the moral status of the fetus. In view of the lack of philosophical and societal consensus about the status of the fetus, however, a second, *consequentialist*, argument in favour of such prevention may get broader support: aggressive embryo transfer practices can not be justified as 'good clinical practice' in view of (a) the principle of nonmaleficence ('do no harm') – which includes the responsibility to *minimise risk* of harm to future IVF-children – and (b) the fact that MFPR is not a panacea for the health risks of larger multifetal pregnancies for these children. A restrictive transfer policy not only prevents the instrumentalisation of the fetus, inherent in 'banalising' MFPR, it also most effectively protects the health interests of future IVF-children.

References

Berkowitz, R.L., Lynch, L., Stone, J. and Alvarez, M. (1996), 'The Current Status of Multifetal Pregnancy Reduction', *Am J Obstet Gynecol*, Vol. 174, pp. 1265-72.

Bundesrat der Bundesrepublik Deutschland (1990), 'Gesetz zum Schutz von Embryonen', *Gesetzbeschlüsse des Deutschen Bundestages*, Drucksache 745/90, Verlag Dr H. Heger: Bonn.

Eser, A. (1990), *Neuartige Bedrohungen ungeborenen Lebens*, C.F. Müller Juristischer Verlag: Heidelberg.

Evans, M.I., Fletcher, J.F. and Rodeck, C. (1989), 'Ethical Problems in Multiple Gestations: Selective Termination', in Evans, M.I., Dixler, A.O., Fletcher, J.C. and Schulman, J.D. (eds), *Fetal Diagnosis and Therapy: Science, Ethics and the Law*, J.B. Lippincott Company: Philadelphia, pp. 266-76.

Evans, M.I., Dommergues, M., Wapner, R.J. et al. (1993), 'Efficacy of Transabdominal Multifetal Pregnancy Reduction: Collaborative Experience

Among the World's Largest Centers', *Obstet Gynecol*, Vol. 82, No. 1, pp. 61-6.

Evans, M.I., Dommergues, M., Wapner, R.J. et al. (1996), 'International, Collaborative Experience of 1789 Patients Having Multifetal Pregnancy Reduction: A Plateauing of Risks and Outcomes', *J Soc Gynecol Invest*, Vol. 3, pp. 23-6.

Garel, M. and Blondel, B. (1992), 'Assessment at 1 Year of the Psychological Consequences of Having Triplets', *Hum Reprod*, Vol. 7, pp. 729-32.

Gleicher, N., Campbell, D.P., Chan, C.L. et al. (1995), 'The Desire for Multiple Births in Couples with Infertility Problems Contradicts Present Practice Patterns', *Hum Reprod*, Vol. 10, pp. 1079-84.

Human Fertilisation and Embryology Authority (1993), *Code of Practice*, London.

Overall, C. (1990), 'Selective Termination of Pregnancy and Women's Reproductive Autonomy', *Hastings Center Report*, May/June 1990, pp. 6-11.

Raymond, J.G. (1987), 'Fetalists and Feminists: They Are Not the Same', in Spallone, P. and Steinberg, D.L. (eds), *Made to Order: The Myth of Reproductive and Genetic Progress*, Pergamon Press: Oxford, pp. 58-65.

Royal Commission of the New Reproductive Technologies (1993), *Proceed with Care*, Vol. 1, Ottawa.

Simpson, J.L. and Carson, S.A. (1996), 'Multifetal Reduction in High-order Gestations: A Non-elective Procedure?', *J Soc Gynecol Invest*, Vol. 3, pp. 1-2.

Staessen, C. et al. (1993), 'Avoidance of Triplet Pregnancies by Elective Transfer of Two Good Quality Embryos', *Hum Reprod*, Vol. 8, pp. 1650-3.

World Medical Association (1995), *Bulletin of Medical Ethics*, October 1995, p. 11.

6 Multifetal pregnancies: Considerations in couples with a genetic problem

Ulrike Mau

The number of women conceiving 3 or more foetuses has increased dramatically as a result of successful infertility therapy with ovulation-inducing agents and assisted reproductive technology. Guido de Wert (1997) has discussed in detail the ethics of multifetal pregnancy reduction and the widely accepted 'principle of proportionality'.

As a geneticist I would like to point to a special situation: a genetic problem (e.g. balanced translocation of chromosomes) in one parent. This is very often combined with a reasonable – sometimes high – risk of abnormalities, malformations and/or mental retardation in offspring or abortions/ stillbirths. Usually these couples are also treated with in vitro fertilisation (IVF) or intracytoplasmic sperm injection (ICSI) on the basis of informed consent. In cases of such a parental chromosomal abnormality, some authorities tend to transfer more embryos than usual because of a higher risk of abortion. They accept an increased risk of multifetal pregnancies, although there is a high risk of foetal chromosomal anomalies. As a matter of fact these affected foetuses are destined for selective reduction, which means in Germany termination of the pregnancy after chorionic villus sampling (CVS) or amniocentesis.

This deliberate production of multifetal pregnancies and subsequent selective reduction is ethically hard to justify. That is why several IVF-clinics decided to limit the embryo-transfer to two. In these special cases of parental chromosomal anomaly preimplantation diagnosis might be a possible way to improve the situation. Balancing risks and benefits, this possibility might result in the least harm and the most benefit to the persons involved.

There is one more general point I would like to mention. We have to be very careful in the management, how we talk and what impression we transmit to the couple! A lot of couples treated with assisted reproductive technology have a feeling of 'pregnancy on probation', because a number of prenatal tests are recommended before the foetus is accepted as 'good'. All professionals involved should try not to intensify this feeling. ICSI is still not beyond its experimental phase. Because of the limited amount of experiences prenatal tests are excessively recommended. But these tests should be offered to these couples exclusively in the setting of a comprehensive genetic counselling, where all advantages, disadvantages, risks, and limits of the different methods are discussed.

References

de Wert, G (1997), 'Multifetal Pregnancies: Reduction or Prevention?', this volume, Part Five.

7 The effects of IVF on the women involved

Barbara Maier

Introduction

Ten to fifteen per cent of couples in the European countries remain childless unintentionally. In the future the problem of infertility will increase – probably more due to changing social structures than to physical conditions of women and men. More and more of them ask for medical assistance. Often – under various conditions – help is available, but more than half of the people seeking medical assistance remain childless in spite of intensive treatments.

Procedures as in vitro fertilisation (IVF) and intracytoplasmic sperm injection (ICSI) are often hard to bear for the women and men involved, hard to bear in many respects: physically, psychologically, socially, financially, etc. Why then undergo such procedures? The promoting factor is the very strong desire for a child of one's own. Reproductive medicine refers to the suffering of infertile people as legitimation to act under certain conditions. But what kind of pain is this? Suffering is a complex concept, an experience on many levels. Is reproductive medicine sufficiently aware of that? Do we take into consideration possible implications of IVF-treatment and provide strategies to cope with them? I am convinced that the medical performance dominates at the expense of psychological and social implications.

In addition, the discussion on the psychological impact of IVF/ICSI-procedures is often misunderstood as one at the expense of infertile patients seeking help in reproductive medicine. No further discrimination of unintentionally childless women and men by no further discussion is sometimes claimed by people concerned as well as by physicians specialising in reproductive medicine.

The effects of IVF/ICSI on the women involved

The effects of IVF/ICSI on the women involved depend in kind and intensity

1 on the woman's physical and psychological conditions, her relation to her partner, her social situation, on her knowledge about the procedure.
2 on the psycho-social support (from the partner, family, friends and eventually from experts like the psychologist).
3 on the attitude of the physician towards the patient and the application of reproductive technology.
4 on the kind of reproductive technology, and the atmosphere in which it is performed, the level of its social acceptance, on promotion in massmedia and the persuasive effects resulting from it.
5 on the awareness of success-failure rates. No doubt, it is a very positive experience to take one's own baby home. But even this may have negative implications: e.g. in the case of multiple pregnancies, premature birth etc.
6 Last but not least – there are influences not only on the individual but also on the image of women as pointed out by feminist contributions on reproductive medicine. The feminist judgments about IVF are ambivalent: empowering as well as disempowering dimensions are described.

The effects of IVF/ICSI-procedures may appear on various levels: the physical, the psychological (often underestimated but intensively expressed by people concerned) and the social level. Until now nothing has been said about the quality of influence – whether it is positive or negative. Both effects on people are to be observed. In our studies we were oriented to emerging problems – acknowledging the very positive effects when IVF procedures result in a baby, but also when infertile people having undergone unsuccessful IVF-procedures (where 'success' is defined as producing a child) succeed in breaking off therapy and facing the fact of probably remaining childless. For the latter IVF although without success was a completing factor in their strive to become pregnant. They, in their opinion, had done all they could – so that in the future they would not have to blame themselves.

I would like to concentrate on problematic influences of IVF on women involved in the homologous system (Maier 1992, Maier et al. 1993, Ebetsberger et al. 1995), because I do not have experience with the heterologous, which is banned in Austria.

Experiencing infertility and being diagnosed infertile

The disposition of having (or not having) a child seems to be unquestionably given in Western civilisation. Contraceptive means as well as reproductive technologies reinforce the freedom of the individual (couple) to choose the right time for having a baby (and with it to avoid getting pregnant at the 'wrong' time). We are unconsciously convinced of being fertile whenever we want to be (during our fertile life-period).

Being diagnosed infertile therefore means being disqualified in a very essential dimension of our life. Often infertile couples (having tried to become pregnant for a number of years) suspect that they remain infertile; but being medically diagnosed as such they are confronted with a medically defined and seemingly objectified problem. Often this is as shocking as the loss of a very beloved person. Infertile people are confronted with this event and often again with 'loss-experiences', such as described by Mahlstedt (1985), namely the loss of body image, the loss of self-esteem, the loss of status or prestige, of self-confidence or of an adequate sense of competence or control, the loss of security and last but not least a loss of a dream (these people may never experience the effects of parenthood personally, socially, etc.). Being a parent is a part of one's vision of an idealised self as an adult.

Diagnosing also means identifying the infertile part of a couple, the partner who causes the stigmatisation of infertility. (Often both contribute to the infertility problem.) Identifying one means a challenge for the relationship, causing specific interactions on both sides. The readiness of the infertile partner to submit to nearly all medical interventions to save the partnership, and not lose the love and respect of the fertile one; but often also the readiness of the female fertile to undergo, as a quite healthy individual, the IVF-procedures which are performed for ICSI-treatment because of male infertility in order to get pregnant. Women are often inclined to do so. They to a large extent define themselves by mothership, identify themselves as 'real' women only when having been pregnant, delivered and raised children.

Every physician who critically reflects on his or her work knows how often diagnoses are incomplete, relative and anything but definite. This becomes apparent with such unclear diagnoses as idiopathic infertility (which means we really do not know what the cause of the infertility is) but also when we are diagnosing the other way round: no tubal blockage. What do we know: the tubes are open. What we do not know: the micro-structure, the motility etc. As a consequence of diagnosing, a many of infertile people become patients for an illness which fertile people do not understand.

'Psycho-logic' of IVF

The 'logic', the structure and the dynamics of IVF/ICSI which influence the infertile people concerned: To the infertile couples IVF means that something they could not do on their own should be done with medico-technical help. Because they themselves do not have the power to reproduce, their own procreative task has to be passed on to reproductive medicine. IVF means the trust in a technically induced process, which to a large extent does not lie in the hands of the couple involved and often cannot be influenced by them. IVF to them means being dependent on reproductive technologies and so facing their own insufficiency.

There is a 'logic' of fertility. There is a 'logic' of infertility. Sometimes it makes sense remaining infertile; especially when living in a very stressful situation. When undergoing IVF procedures the sense of infertility might often be more concealed than revealed.

Success in IVF-procedures: In spite of well-known low success-rates (20-25 per cent; ICSI 30 per cent), people undergoing IVF have high, unrealistic expectations of becoming pregnant. These are probably induced by the high pressure of suffering from being childless. The change from intensive hope to frustration after unsuccessful IVF-procedures challenges the emotional balance of the woman, the man, and of the couple's relationship.

IVF means stress: physical, psychological, social, financial stress: It pervades nearly all aspects of life. Some of the patients describe the paradoxon of stress-reduction during the procedures. Ch. Hölzle and U. Wiesing (1991) have given explanations for that. The time patients cannot do anything, cannot influence the results, means stress to them because of being confined to inactivity. Whereas acting (even if acting is submission to the procedures, to injections for stimulation, egg-retrieval, embryo-transfer) in this respect means reduction of stress.

To what extent and in which dimension do IVF-procedures also deform the woman, the man, and their interrelationship? For some of them (particularly women) a possibly pre-existing negative attitude toward their own body may be aggravated and intensified. This is particularly the case for functionally sterile patients, seldom for women with tubal blockage! Some of them – with a life-long history in experiencing their own body as disappointing and disobedient in fulfilling their intensive desire for a child – perform IVF (as C. Brähler [1986] has pointed out). The fight against one's own body, which is experienced as a defective machine, serves to overcome the intensive offense (being childless). Helpless anger because of bodily insufficiency is worked out by submitting the body to treatment. The body turns into a foreign body which is to be punished. This means bad consequences for body-consciousness and experience. The body which refuses to produce *the* (female) identity-creating event by becoming pregnant and having a child, may suffer from the procedures, but is kept distant from the woman's self. Such psychosomatic splitting may result in psychosomatic disorders and diseases. Identity problems, problems in sexuality and problems in relationships are possible consequences. In our own studies we found such development four times as often in IVF-women than in the control-group.

The logic of IVF has another problematic characteristic: As a performance (Dennerstein and Morse 1986), IVF allows infertile people 'not to face/trigger a crisis'. There is no sense of coming to grips with this problem of infertility and eventually indeed remaining childless. The chance for mourning diminishes over the time, the search for alternatives is forgotten – and this for perhaps many years. Therein lies *the* cause for the chronic depressive conditions of IVF – (finally) frustrated women.

Points of views of women involved: I have again and again asked our IVF-patients (I consciously call them then patients) the same question: Is IVF the solution for the problems of infertile couples? It is, when successful, with some restrictions. It is not when unsuccessful. Success is defined as procedures resulting in a child. There have been a lot of differentiated answers, for example, that IVF is a post-treatment after several operations which have led to tubal blockage. Infertility viewed in this way is some sort of illness which should be treated by IVF. Another patient pointed to ambivalent dimensions of IVF. 'Once, I had accepted remaining childless ... then I have learned about IVF – and all the troubles started again. Yet my whole life is oriented around this unfulfilled desire for a child and the increasing hope that this desire will be met through IVF-procedures.'

Another answer was: 'Because I must have a child at any cost, I don't think about IVF and my experiences with it. I have to concentrate all my energy on IVF – not on asking myself about the consequences it will have for me and my relationship to my partner'. In this respect IVF serves as a means to avoid confronting the real problems, with possible alternatives such as eventually remaining childless etc. If there is only one option for my life, namely my own child and if this option does not materialise, I will face an existential crisis when I finally realise that it is not possible.

IVF and the longing for a child: Could IVF eventually lead to an addiction-like longing for a child? And if it could, is this because of reproductive medicine itself and its conditions, the application of methods on the basis of questionable indications or because of the pre-disposition of the people concerned? IVF-cycles without success might provoke another attempt and this carries on and on. Instead of facing the sterility-crisis which would be the pre-condition to escape an increasingly strong desire for a child, this very desire begins to dominate their whole lives and overshadows the option to live contently without children. In this situation women are prepared to try again and again – not allowing themselves to stop IVF-procedures although thereby increasingly burning out. For some of them IVF-cycles performed uncritically and too often without psychological support may initiate addiction-like involvement. What does 'addiction' mean in this area? Repeating the IVF-cycles allows those involved to avoid facing the sterility-crisis. Instead they continue with the IVF-cycles, not giving up hope during follicular stimulation, follicular puncture and embryo-transfer and then being forced to endure the long waiting period until there is certainty about having become pregnant or – more frequently – again having menstruation. Disappointment can only be fought back by the next attempt. Some of the women try for years. These years of their life become years of waiting for something which will probably never materialise. Are women who try so hard to become pregnant by nature predisposed to such an obsession-like development or do the methods of reproductive medicine themselves contribute to the women's total preoccupation with the demands of technologies?

People concerned with IVF-procedures often do not speak about them, retreat from families with children and often concentrate only on their longing for a child. Reproductive medicine as a pure medical answer to the complex problems of infertile couples cannot claim to represent the only and sufficient problem-solving strategy for them. On the contrary – it sometimes contributes to increasing difficulties for them – as described above.

After IVF: The question was: How to become pregnant?
The answer: By IVF, ICSI, etc. But what if it does not work?

Patients *after* unsuccessful IVF are a majority which should be taken care of. Psychological support after unsuccessful procedures should be available to them.

Reproductive medicine is often justified by reference to the suffering of infertile people. But when stimulation, insemination, IVF, ICSI are not successful, experts are no longer available to take care of the often increased problems of childless women and men. Own studies on that issue demonstrate that many couples lose other options in their lives, it becomes difficult to relate to others. Disillusion and burnout from unsuccessful treatment often leads to depression, psychosomatic disorders, and even a kind of addiction. Frequently the problems after treatment seem to be even worse than before. These people will most likely go on suffering in the future from the unfulfilled desire for a child, a desire probably intensified by the troubles and pains of IVF.

Some theses about IVF-treatment from a critical point of view

1 Although technological improvement brings with it the temptation to solve problems by technical means, we should not neglect the crucial question: Does reproductive medicine indeed refer to the central aspects of suffering and does it pay enough attention to them in the therapeutic efforts? If so, the treatment must as consequence be interdisciplinary.
2 Primum nil nocere. This should also guide us in IVF-treatment.
3 Before IVF we should provide sufficient counselling, during the procedures and after them psychological support to improve the couples' ability to deal with finally remaining childless.
4 Limitation of IVF-cycles by autonomous patients and physicians corresponding to the needs of patients on various levels.
5 Reassessing the indications should be the task of critical evaluation in every centre which does IVF.
6 The definition of goals is essential from the beginning:
   - Pregnancy *or* acceptance of remaining childless
   - Discussion of alternatives like adoption, foster-parenthood, personal self-realisation-possibilities. This would be the task of psychological support. Not only by psychologists but also by support groups.

In addition, success under the psychosocial perspective is to be redefined. Success should not only be oriented to pregnancies or baby-take-home-rates, but also be seen in successful coping with remaining finally childless. A quotation from U. Auhagen-Stephanos (1992) sums up the task: 'The essential task is to break off the general sterility of life and to allow couples to start once againg living in all its plenty and richness.'

References

Auhagen-Stephanos, U. (1992), *Wenn die Seele nein sagt. Vom Mythos der Unfruchtbarkeit*, Rowohlt: Hamburg.

Brähler, C. (1986), 'Fertilitätsstörung – Kränkung und Herausforderung', in Brähler, E.: *Körpererleben. Ein subjektiver Ausdruck von Leib und Seele*, Berlin.

Dennerstein, L. and Morse, C. (1986), 'Psychological Aspects of IVF', in *In Vitro Fertilisation and Other Alternative Methods of Conception: Advances in Fertility and Sterility Series*, Vol. 2. The Proceedings of the 12th World Congress on Fertility and Sterility, Oct. 1986, Singapore.

Ebetsberger, B. et.al. (1995), 'Die Rolle der Psychologin in der Behandlung bei Paaren mit unerfülltem Kinderwunsch im Beziehungsgefüge zwischen

Institution und Paardynamik', *Psychologie in der Medizin*, Vol.6, No. 4, pp. 21-6.

Hölzle, C. and Wiesing, U. (1991), *In-vitro-Fertilisation – ein umstrittenes Experiment. Fakten. Leiden. Diagnosen. Ethik*, Springer: Berlin/Heidelberg.

Mahlstedt, P. (1985), 'The Psychological Component of Infertility', *Fertility and Sterility*, Vol. 43, No. 3, pp. 335-46.

Maier, B. (1992): 'Versuch einer kritischen Aufarbeitung frustraner IVF-Behandlung in psychosomatisch-ganzheitlicher Sicht', 49. Kongreß der Deutschen Gesellschaft für Gynäkologie und Geburtshilfe, Berlin.

Maier, B. et al. (1993), 'IVF und die Sehn-SUCHT nach einem Kind', Österreichischer IVF Kongreß, Bregenz, Oct.1993, Abstract in *Journal für Fertilität und Reproduktion*, Vol. 3, 1993.

8 In vitro fertilisation and freedom of action

Elisabeth Hildt

Owing to new developments in reproductive medicine our room for manoeuvre in almost all aspects of human reproduction has considerably increased. Not only can we choose whether or not to have a child, we are also just beginning to find methods which help us to have a child which meets at least some of our expectations. Whereas previously infertile couples had no choice – they had to accept their reproductive fate and integrate their childlessness into their concept of life, nowadays the situation is very different. Infertile couples who otherwise could not have had children can now often have a child with the help of reproductive technology involving in vitro fertilisation (IVF). In principle, IVF also enables us to influence the characteristics of the children we may have. By using sperm or ovum donors for IVF, by sex selection, by preimplantation diagnosis (PID), or perhaps in some years' time even by directly modifying some of the genes, we can affect the genetic composition of our descendants.

In social contexts, however, a great number of problematic issues go along with these enormous advances in reproductive medicine and the greater room for manoeuvre they provide. In a giveaway newspaper distributed on the Berkeley campus I read the following advertisement:

> Couple needs sperm donor. Child will have home full of love, music, mathematics, fun, intellect, security, relatives etc. Donor's anonymity will be protected and his kindness rewarded. Please reply with mailing address or Fax number, availability through summer and a description of familial health and personal talents and interests to ...

In another advertisement, a childless couple was looking for a young, attractive and healthy ovum donor with clearly specified height, body weight, and colour of hair and eyes.

In reading this I wondered whether these couples will ever be completely happy with the baby they will have after such an ovum or sperm donation and whether their baby will be able to satisfy their high quality expectations. What at first sight seems to offer more choice, more freedom of action, soon proves to be a great illusion – not least because the genetic reductionism underlying these advertisements is unwarranted. The baby surely will not have 50 per cent of the donor's characteristics, it will only have 50 per cent of his or her genes. In view of the genetic recombination during meiosis it is not possible to plan details of a baby's characteristics in this way. Although the couples can choose *their* sperm or ovum donor according to their wishes, it seems to me that the existence of more alternatives to act, the mere existence of choice in this situation does not necessarily go along with an increase in the couple's freedom of action.

In view of the great advances in reproductive medicine, I would like to ask: Does IVF and the additional room for manouevre it provides for producing the desired baby merely increase a couple's freedom or are there not also many constraints which negatively influence freedom of action? A lot of different answers have been given to the question: Under which circumstances is an action a free one? In the following, I want to refer to some of these different positions and ask to what extent, according to these positions, IVF positively or negatively influences an infertile couple's freedom.

Often, freedom of action is described as 'the freedom to do what one wants to do'. With regard to IVF this definition is unproblematic. It is evident that infertile couples undergoing an IVF treatment *want* to be treated in an IVF programme. Nevertheless, this definition touches an aspect of IVF which has often been considered problematic: the limited opportunity for the couple to influence and control the process of the IVF treatment. The origin of a pregnancy cannot be attributed to their own sexual activity, but rather is the responsibility of a medical doctor. The couple is bound to passively comply with the needs of the medical treatment, they can do nothing but sit and wait. This loss of control over a key bodily process not only leads to a strong feeling of helplessness, but also to a certain alienation towards their own bodies (Hölzle and Wiesing 1991). However, I think one also has to consider here that without the treatment, the infertile couples would not be able to control the situation either. Without the treatment, they would experience the helplessness and loss of control inherent in the infertility experience itself.

Another formulation which plays an important role in the discussion of freedom is 'the principle of alternate possibilities'. It states that persons are morally responsible for what they have done only if they could have done otherwise (Frankfurt 1969). With regard to IVF this formulation is trivial: Although social and internal compulsions may play a role in their decision to begin with an IVF programme, it is clear that in principle the couples could have done otherwise.

Robert Audi (Audi 1993) gives a more detailed definition of 'the principle of alternate possibilities'. He draws a distinction between an action that is compelled – and thus unfree – but not unavoidable, and an action that is unavoidable.[1] While mere compulsion does not necessarily absolve the agent of moral responsibility, in the case of an unavoidable action, according to Audi, the agent is not responsible. In order to give a definition of 'unavoidability', Audi offers the formulation 'Could have done otherwise' (Audi, 1993, p.202):

> 'Roughly, S could not have done otherwise than A at t if and only if S is compelled to A at t and it is not the case either (i) that S could reasonably have been expected to avoid (or try to avoid) the situation in which A occurred, or (ii) that a morally sound person in the relevant situation could reasonably have been expected to do otherwise.'

In short, Audi argues that being responsible for an action does not entail performing it freely, though it does entail that there was at least some time at which the agent could have done otherwise. For a couple seeking reproductive help an IVF is obviously not an unavoidable action in this sense. However, it is also clear that there is a certain degree of compulsion – social norms, social expectations, as well as internal compulsions – influencing the couple. In practice, it is difficult to measure the degree of compelling force, especially for internal compulsions which seem to play an important role in IVF. Particular, the internal compulsion to continue the infertility treatment, the obsession to do almost anything in order to have the desired baby is often so strong that it prevents the couple from discontinuing the treatment. There is a considerable danger that the couple, especially the woman, will enter a vicious circle which drives the couple to go on and on with the infertility treatment, to carry out more and more IVF cycles. The more deeply the couple is involved in the infertility treatment, the more difficult it is to escape this vicious circle (Maier et al. 1993, Koropatnick et al. 1993).

According to Audi, in spite of these internal compulsions, the couple has to be considered responsible for this situation, not least because some years, some months or weeks ago they had decided to begin with the infertility treatment. This clearly shows one of the problems of reproductive technologies: When infertile couples decide to undergo an infertility treatment, they are often not well-informed of possible difficulties, implications and drawbacks of this kind of therapy. Very often they are not really aware of the social and psychological compulsions influencing their decision to start the treatment. Thus, it is absolutely necessary to intensify IVF counselling at the beginning of the therapy, *before* the couples start an infertility treatment. They have to be informed not only of the exact medical procedures and statistical success rates of the treatment, but also of the social and psychological aspects of infertility and infertility treatment. For the couples, this would be an important prerequisite for a free decision whether or not to undergo a certain therapy. Later on, when the couple is already caught in the vicious circle, it is very difficult to quit the treatment because at this point free action is severely restricted by internal compulsions.

According to Gary Watson (Watson 1982), an action is free when what determines an agent's all-things-considered judgements also determines his or her actions. In order to form these judgements, the agent assigns values to alternative states of affairs and ranks them according to worth. In a free action, the agent does what he or she most values. In contrast, in an unfree action, an agent's desires, irrational wishes or unreflected judgements move him or her to action. These irrational aspects may be more or less conscious and they may be based on acculturated attitudes or social norms.

IVF has been challenged for exactly these reasons. Feminist critics in particular point out that in view of social expectations and the social stigmatisation of infertility, the decision to undergo an infertility treatment cannot be considered to be a free one. Due to the enormous pressure of social norms, the women involved cannot really choose other options such as childlessness or adoption. In addition, in view of the low efficiency of the procedure, the high physical and psychological strains and the high risks, IVF seems to be an irrational choice (Koch 1990, Hölzle and Wiesing 1991).

In an interview study with women undergoing an IVF treatment, Lene Koch noticed that in the women's decision to start IVF or to continue the treatment, information with regard to the low success rates and high risks of the procedure did not matter (Koch 1990). In spite of knowing the 'objective facts', i.e. the low statistical success rates, it seemed that each woman tended to irrationally believe that she will be the one to succeed. At first sight, this subjective 'magical belief' in success seems to be the (only) reason why women start IVF treatment despite the improbability of taking a baby home. Not only to feminist critics do these beliefs seem highly irrational.

However, Lene Koch points out that women's seemingly irrational tendency to undergo IVF can be considered perfectly rational and consistent if one assumes that these infertile women act within a different worldview, governed by its own specific rationality. Lene Koch writes (Koch, 1990, p.235):

> Since IVF is the last step in the long line of infertility treatments, it must be tried, before the woman can establish a socially accepted identity as involuntary childless. Where most feminist critics judge IVF on its dubious capacity to produce a child, to the infertile woman IVF is also an element in the procedure to accept infertility. Thus, the desire to try IVF is severed

from the efficiency of the technology, because it is judged by the yardstick of another rationality.

Based on this assumption, what at first sight seemed to be a clearly irrational decision may be perfectly rational from another point of view. In the end, with regard to the question of what constitutes a free action, rationality seems to be a criterion which is not easy to apply. Due to our limited knowledge of an agent's motives for action it is often very hard to characterise an action someone else has done as being based on a rational or irrational decision.

This touches another aspect connected with the advances in reproductive medicine and the increased room for manoeuvre they provide. Because more and more new medical interventions for infertility are offered on the reproductive market, infertile couples increasingly place their hopes in these new procedures. Instead of accepting their infertility, couples again and again begin with new procedures in the hope of having the desired baby. In this way, the process of accepting infertility is slowed down or even prevented. Thus, it may be important to restrict the extent and duration of an infertility treatment in order to allow the couple to start the grief process that is necessary to emotional healing (Koch 1990, Koropatnick et al. 1993, Maier et al. 1993).

Although the above-mentioned compulsions clearly show the problematic nature of IVF, in the end, the increase in a couple's freedom to procreate brought about by IVF is not overridden by the various restrictions of freedom inherent in the IVF treatment itself. However, the positions above dealt with freedom only insofar as the agent is affected by compulsions. An important aspect neglected by these positions concerns the question: What are the limits on the freedom of the individual?

For Alan Gewirth (Gewirth 1978, Steigleder 1992, Beyleveld 1997), these limits are given by the 'Principle of Generic Consistency' (PGC) which says (Gewirth, 1978, p.135): 'Act in accord with the generic rights of your recipients as well as of yourself.' The generic rights are comprised of the rights to freedom and the rights to well-being. According to Gewirth, to interfere with someone's freedom is to interfere with his control of his behaviour, whereas to interfere with someone's well-being is to interfere with the objects or goods at which his behaviour is aimed (Gewirth, 1978, p.251). Gewirth interprets well-being so that it consists in having the general abilities and conditions required for maintaining and obtaining goods.[2]

With regard to an agent's freedom, Gewirth states (Gewirth, 1978, p.271):

> An agent should be free to perform any action, to engage in any transaction, if and only if his recipients are left free, through their voluntary consent, to participate or not participate in that transaction and if and only if he does not inflict basic or specific harm on them.

In the case of IVF, for an agent exercising his or her freedom to procreate, there are several groups of recipients: (a) the husband or wife, (b) the embryos and (c) the child or children resulting from an IVF.

As far as the procreative liberty of husband or wife is concerned, it is necessary that both parties give their written consent to the procedure. In order to avoid disagreement, all possible uses of embryos (implantation, research, destruction) should be approved in advance by both (Shuster 1990).

Human embryos obviously are not able to give their consent. However, it is not clear whether human embryos can actually be considered to be recipients of an action: In contrast to normal recipients they are not prospective (purposive) agents – they are only potential agents. Here, much depends on the position held with regard to the 'Argument from potential'. According to Gewirth, although a potential agent is not the same as a prospective agent, due to the Principle of Proportionality a human embryo does have generic rights to a certain degree. The Principle of Proportionality states that the degree to which someone approaches having the generic features and abilities of action determines the degree to which he or she has or approaches having the generic rights (Gewirth, 1978, p.141). According to Gewirth, the Principle of Proportionality together with the Principle of Generic Consistency require that although an embryo has no right to freedom, it has a right to 'well-being as is required for developing its potentialities for growth toward purpose-fulfillment' (Gewirth, 1978, p.142). Thus, with IVF the embryo's generic rights should be taken into consideration so that it can develop into a prospective purposive agent. This point of view clearly questions all those positions which consider human embryos as mere objects that anyone can use as he or she sees fit.

In contrast, the children conceived via IVF are obviously recipients of the infertility treatment which brought them into existence. The children are or will soon be full-fledged prospective purposive agents. Their rights should be considered from the beginning of the IVF treatment on. These rights may include the right to identity, the right to exist without quality control and the right to createdness.

In summary, freedom of action can be considered to be a criterion appropriate for a critical evaluation of many of the manifold aspects and implicatons of IVF. The criterion of freedom of action serves to assess IVF not only in respect to the agent himself or herself but also to the recipients, i.e. other adult persons, the human embryos, or the IVF children involved.

Notes

1 In contrast, free actions are to be understood as uncompelled.
2 Freedom and well-being are clearly related, however: 'In one respect, freedom is such a general concept that many and perhaps all elements of well-

being may also be viewed as aspects of freedom. The basis of this coalescence is that freedom, especially in its negative form of «freedom from», may be conceived universally as the absence of certain conditions, especially adverse ones. The structure of this view is thus that if some W is a part of well-being, then to have W is to be free from non-W or from deprivation of W.' (Gewirth 1978, p. 250/251)

References

Audi, R. (1993), *Action, Intention, and Reason*, Cornell University Press: Ithaca.

Beyleveld, D. (1997), 'The Moral and Legal Status of the Human Embryo', this volume, Part Seven.

Frankfurt, H. (1969), 'Alternate Possibilities and Moral Responsibility', *Journal of Philosophy*, Vol. 66, pp. 829-39.

Gewirth, A. (1978), *Reason and Morality*, University of Chicago Press: Chicago.

Hölzle, C. and Wiesing, U. (1991), *In-vitro-Fertilisation – ein umstrittenes Experiment*, Springer: Berlin.

Koch, L. (1990), 'IVF – An Irrational Choice?', *Issues in Reproductive and Genetic Engineering*, Vol. 3, pp. 235-42.

Koropatnick, S., Daniluk, J. and Pattinson, H.A. (1993), 'Infertility: A Non-event Transition', *Fertility and Sterility*, Vol. 59, pp. 163-71.

Maier, B., Spitzer, D., Lundwall, K. and Staudach, A. (1993), 'Ganzheitlich psychosomatische Therapievorstellungen bei der In-vitro-Fertilisierung', *Fertilität*, Vol. 9, pp. 189-92.

Shuster, E. (1990), 'Seven Embryos in Search of Legitimacy', *Fertility and Sterility*, Vol. 53, pp. 975-7.

Steigleder, K. (1992), *Die Begründung des moralischen Sollens. Studien zur Möglichkeit einer normativen Ethik*, Attempto: Tübingen.

Watson, G. (1982). 'Free Agency', in Watson, G. (ed.), *Free Will*, New York, pp. 96-110.

9 Freedom through science?

Günter Virt

In principle, I agree with the discerning statement made by Elisabeth Hildt (1997) in respect of the question as to whether in vitro fertilisation (IVF) provides us with a greater potential for freedom. In this context, I would like to be more specific from the point of view of science and the role it plays in our society while identifying a number of issues which reflect the price that has to be paid for such a greater potential for freedom.

In view of a widespread unquestioning belief in science, consideration must be given to the fact that the pressure thus exerted may also produce the opposite effect. That is to say, it reduces the potential for freedom insofar as people feel that the options created by reproductive medicine have to be utilised to the full even though they have either no advantages or even drawbacks in individual cases. 'Society and the majority of individuals are notoriously incapable of withstanding the temptation of what is technically feasible' (Bayertz, 1990, p.16). In addition science itself is strongly influenced by economic issues, leading to pressure and to effects on freedom.

Within the realm of scientific research, there is a striking structural deficit of onesidedness: numerous efforts are made to improve the new options available to reproductive medicine to successfully treat sterility whereas little is done to explore its aetiology. At present, the environmental burden to reproduction is an important scientific issue; the evident lack of research in this area is frightening and calls for compensation. Furthermore it seems, that psychosomatic reasons and effects have received less attention than is necessary. The fact that too little research is done into these problems is not only a restriction to science, but also has an immediate impact on medical practice.

If one is able to avoid the root causes of sterility instead of increasingly depending on reproductive medicine, this certainly means *more freedom*. The opposite is true if spontaneity – which, after all, also has to do with freedom – is replaced by a dependency on sophisticated medical technology, which is a multiple burden, not just time-consuming and costly.

With the exception of strong medical indications physicians themselves must always weigh the prospects for the success of an IVF treatment against the prospects without treatment or of alternative treatment by methods that tackle the psychosomatic problems, when they help overcome the suffering of childlessness. If the physician him- or herself is pressurised by an unquestioning belief in science and fails to really fathom all other alternatives to IVF, he or she violates the principle of beneficence.

Free patients and free doctors must not jointly give in to pressure and look for salvation in a kind of medicine that is fraught with illusions and seems to be able to fulfill wishes even though the medical indications may not warrant such a decision. In individual cases, it may be the more rational and more successful approach to come to a free decision to forego the fulfillment of a wish. Occasionally a compulsion to repeat is reported. Medicine not only is a science but also an art. Thus, great care is required to ensure that under the dictate of an unquestioning belief in science, the desire to help does not turn us into the objects of requests or demands beyond all reasonable weighing of benefits and risks. Free decisions are rational decisions which not only consider immediate consequences, but also late sequelae and the freedom of all those involved in the decision.

The total number of decisions, taken together, influences social attitudes in the future. In what way does IVF change the understanding of procreation, parenthood and also medical aims and how will this understanding affect the freedom of the next generations?

The freedom of decision is not the only aspect of freedom. The full-fledged form of freedom is decidedness. The freedom of decision is characterised by the adage 'the wider the choice, the greater the trouble': IVF is a further option which may make sense in very specific circumstances. However, freedom of decision means that a human being finds happiness and peace with him- or herself and his or her moral demands. And this should be the main ethical criteria in the reflection of freedom.

References

Bayertz, K. (1990), *Gentherapie am Menschen.*

Hildt, E. (1997), 'In Vitro Fertilisation and Freedom of Action', this volume, part 5.

Part Six
HUMAN EMBRYOS IN IVF

1 Human embryos in medical practice

Ian D. Cooke

Medical practice involving human embryos involves the assisted reproductive technologies. Initially a woman's own eggs and her partner's own sperm were used to create embryos. The first experiments developed the technique of natural cycle in vitro fertilisation (IVF) where the woman's own natural single dominant follicle yielded only a single egg. Because of poor success rates gonadotrophin stimulation was used to overcome the natural control mechanisms and create multiple follicles yielding multiple eggs, perhaps 10-15 in each cycle. Variable control of the natural mid-cycle trigger to ovulation led to its interference in optimum harvesting of embryos so this mid-cycle luteinising hormone surge was switched off by a gonadotrophin releasing hormone agonist leading to greater follicle development and the harvesting of even 20-30 eggs. Donor gametes may be used leading to a further three combinations, donor eggs and own sperm, own eggs and donor sperm or both donor sperm and eggs. Donors may be unknown which is usual for sperm, although Sweden, Denmark and New Zealand have introduced legislation to reveal donor identity. Donated eggs have more frequently arisen from known donors, altruism being a common feature of egg donation and in some ethnic groups poorly represented in a particular country, there may be no alternative but to have a known donor. In France 'relational' egg donors are widely used where the potential recipient brings along a donor but the donor's eggs are used for someone else so that the recipient receives an unknown donor's eggs.

Donated embryos could come from embryos surplus to the requirements of other infertile patients or could be created specifically from individually donated sperm or eggs which may or may not have been matched on physical characteristics to the relevant member of the recipient couple.

Finally, embryos may be transferred to a surrogate mother or the commissioning male may use the surrogate's own eggs. These various combinations led to confusion in the definition of mother from the genetic, carrying or social 'mother'. This matter was resolved in the UK by the Human Fertilisation and Embryology Act (HFE Act 1990) which stipulates that the woman who gives birth to the baby is the mother. If the baby is subsequently handed over to a commissioning couple, then formal adoption procedures must be undertaken.

The creation of embryos in IVF depends very much on the predictions for fertility after investigation of a couple. The most important single contributor to prognosis is female age which declines optimally from the age of 31, significantly from the age of 35 and precipitously from the age of 39. The prospects are significantly determined by the female's ovarian response to gonadotrophin stimulation and this can be predicted by assessing the pituitary/ovarian negative feedback mechanism by measuring plasma follicle stimulating hormone concentration on day 2 of the menstrual period. Recently, poor semen samples which formerly failed in IVF can now yield up to 24 per cent live birth rate per treatment cycle by injecting an individual sperm into a single egg (intracytoplasmic sperm injection – ICSI). Recent research is directed to retrieving sperm from the epididymis or testicle following obstruction, such as previous vasectomy or infection, with a good probability of success (percutaneous epididymal sperm aspiration – PESA or testicular sperm extraction from testicular biopsy – TESE). The latter technique has even been used in those cases where spermatogenesis is abnormal and hormone indicators have previously suggested a hopeless prognosis. New work (using immature sperm without the tail yet developed – spermatids) has been described in the literature but further clinical use of this technique is currently proscribed in the UK. These recent developments change the whole perspective on male infertility impacting on public expectation.

The probability of creating human embryos must be distinguished from the live birth rate as only about 20 per cent of embryos proceed ultimately to delivery of a live born infant. Recent data suggest that this is due to major or minor chromosomal abnormalities consequent upon errors in fertilisation. This may be as high as 80 per cent in embryos that look suboptimal but may even be 20-30 per cent of embryos which look ideal.

It is clear that the prognosis at IVF depends on the number of eggs retrieved and the number of embryos created which is dependent upon the quality of both eggs and sperm, the outcome not being predictable, even with the best assessment of the embryos down the microscope. With the availability of any number of embryos, choices must be made as to which embryos will be transferred about 36 hours after their creation and subsequent maintenance in culture and transferred back to the uterus. In the UK, legislation forbids the transfer of more than three embryos back to the uterus in IVF and recent data suggest that with a good quality IVF programme, there is virtually no difference in live birth rate according to whether two or three embryos are returned but this does have a significant impact on the multiple pregnancy rate, in particular the triplet rate. Although not widely publicised, the triplet rate (nationally 3 per cent) is highly variable from clinic to clinic and should be seen as a disaster in medical and sociological terms and not a cause for celebration. All multiple pregnancies, particularly the higher orders, are associated with an increase in perinatal mortality and morbidity rate, prematurity being associated with significant handicap. This has led to the development of fetal reduction, the process of destroying individual embryos in utero in response to the identification of higher orders. Most practitioners will not reduce below two but there is a significant risk of spontaneous abortion of the whole pregnancy after such an attempt. Fetal reduction is frequently done clandestinely (although it is legal in the UK) and some countries such as Israel, where there is no limit to the number of embryos that may be transferred, experience of fetal reduction has been extensively reported in the literature.

Embryo cryopreservation is practicable, whereas at present egg freezing does not yield a viable product. Perhaps 20 per cent of frozen embryos are lost in the freeze/thaw process. Cryopreservation is not universally available and many clinics will decline to freeze embryos surplus to a single transfer if there are not three or more good to reasonable quality embryos, on the basis that transfer of a single thawed embryo subsequently has such a poor pregnancy rate as not to be worthwhile.

There are various motivations for freezing. The couple may wish to have embryos transferred subsequently and if they fail to conceive, following the first transfer without having to go through the invasive procedures of the original egg retrieval. Use of those embryos may be deferred only for some months. If the initial embryo transfer is successful and live birth ensues then such stored embryos may be kept 2-3 years until the first child(ren) grow up. The birth of the multiple pregnancy and the experience of childrearing may discourage parents from returning to use their frozen embryos. Embryos may be donated to other infertile couples but embryos will have different potential for development to maturity, those of couples achieving a live birth will have a much better prognosis than those that fail to develop normally, and this should be considered. It seems, however, that embryo donation for this altruistic reason is uncommon if not rare, couples being much less prepared to give away embryos than gametes prior to fertilisation. Embryos could also be donated for research and a small number do, but this process must be discussed and consent obtained prospectively.

Although it is technically feasible to keep embryos appropriately frozen in liquid nitrogen for many years, the HFE Act 1990 stipulated that they should only be frozen for five years. Of course the five years soon passed and on 1 August 1996 the deadline for destruction of frozen embryos that had been stored for five years arrived. The media responded with enthusiasm and much public attention was focussed on the date and the issue. The Human Fertilisation and Embryology Authority (HFEA) changed its regulations shortly before the deadline so that embryos could be retained frozen provided that written informed consent could be obtained for continued storage. This consent needs to be re-obtained at seven and nine years with a presumption that it was very unlikely that consent would be given for more than 10 years although the deadline could be set aside in exceptional circumstances. It was interesting to note that quite a number of individuals contacted clinics within days of the deadline passing in spite of their previously having been contacted and notified of the date and one wonders about the psychodynamics in these cases. Of course, loss of contact with the clinic for many reasons, even including the death or divorce of a couple, can lead to a failure to observe the above requirements. Posthumous use of embryos would only be allowed legally if this specific situation had been covered in the initial consent and only after appropriate counselling for the concerned individual(s).

Medical and social screening of individuals prior to creating embryos takes place and the issue of 'the welfare of the (potential) child' has been seriously addressed by the HFEA's Code of Practice 1991 et seq. There are different reasons for creating embryos, primarily for infertility but also because of previous genetic abnormalities. Usually this involves use of donor sperm to treat dominant or recessive conditions for which there is no genetic probe existing and where the genetic advice is to substitute one gamete. This could be egg donation. Sperm donation is usually simpler.

The creation of embryos also creates risks for a contributing couple. In IVF there is a small risk associated with egg collection, particularly bleeding, or remotely possible damage to bowel, but there is a risk of about 1 per cent of severe hyperstimulation, the ovarian hyperstimulation syndrome (OHSS), which could be potentially lethal and is a matter for particular thought when women act as egg donors. There is considerable stress, physical and emotional, in egg recovery, again an element for consideration in egg donation. Sperm recovery, particularly through surgical procedures may also carry small risks but usually local and of minor importance.

There are however a number of other issues. Apart from issues of confidentiality, future anonymity and its impact on the developing child and subsequent adult, there is also an important issue on inheritance by the child of the genetic defects that may be involved in the parental infertility. This has received most attention when using poor quality sperm in ICSI. Evidence is beginning to accumulate that such men have microdeletions of genetic material not yet readily identifiable routinely by genetic probes, some of which are likely to be available in the short-term future. The impact of perpetuating the infertility in the next generation has not yet been seriously addressed. Young men with testicular cancer are increasingly having sperm frozen immediately before treatment or sperm retrieved following treatment, the latter perhaps having the risk not only of a genetic defect that could contribute to the development of future cancer, but also the effects of chemotheraphy or radiotherapy could have caused genetic damage. In the female such damage is more likely to compromise ovarian function which will lead to the use of donated gametes but similar questions may arise, particularly in treatment of leukaemia. Already it is evident that such women treated with bone marrow transplants who have donated eggs have poorly grown infants and are at high risk of major pregnancy complications.

The transfer of donated embryos to women over the age of 50 has been discouraged in the UK. A recipient with a successful outcome at the age of 63 has been reported. There was a high frequency of major complications in these pregnancies in spite of meticulous pre-pregnancy screening; maternal mortality, which is related to age, rises significantly in natural conception. The number of elderly mothers is not yet large enough for this to be evident.

Legislation in the UK has been directed to extracorporeal creation of embryos i.e. IVF but has excluded methods of in vivo creation of embryos such as ovulation induction or gamete intra Fallopian transfer (GIFT). Legislation covers the facility including laboratories and pays particular attention to storage. Any regulatory control process needs to address administrative, medical, scientific and societal concerns. In the UK standardised national data and individual licensed clinic data are published annually. Although this purported to help patients, it is not geographically realistic for all patients to travel great distances, but the media have turned this information into a 'league table' which has had a major impact on clinic functioning. In view of this developing perception, this medically, scientifically and ethically contentious area is being turned into a market place for competition with commerical overtones – to the dismay of many participating doctors and scientists.

Control of these important facilities, always newsworthy, can become an instrument of social policy such as access by single persons or male or female homosexual couples. There is great discussion about clinic responses where one partner is HIV positive and an acrimonious debate currently taking place in the UK relates to the removal of payment of donors and encouragement exclusively of altruistic donors. The issue of embryo research proposed by the biologists and opposed by fundamentalists is an area that has hardly been developed. Preimplantation diagnosis has been static for the past five years, its potential not having been realised because of heterogeneity of individual cells within an embryo, limited number of probes being available and the incipient societal debate about cloning and 'designer babies'. It is hoped that a fruitful dialogue between medical science and society will allow the appropriate fulfillment of the potential of this remarkable technology.

References

Human Fertilisation and Embryology Act (1990), Chapter 37, Her Majesty's Stationery Office, PO Box 276, London SW8 5DT.

Human Fertilisation and Embryology Authority (1991), *Code of Practice*, Paxton House, 30 Artillery Lane, London E1 7LS.

2 Are there inconsistencies in our ethical understanding of the human embryo?

Eve-Marie Engels

I will take Ian Cooke's paper (Cooke 1997) as a starting point for some general (1) and some specific (2) reflections on questions in connection with in vitro fertilisation (IVF) and its consequences.

(1) We all should be aware that we are standing at a *turning point* in our attitude towards nature in general and towards human nature in particular, and we should make up our mind in which direction we want to go. On the one hand we are embedded in certain traditions and deeply rooted convictions, intuitions and feelings about what it means to be a human being in contrast to other animals. On the other hand modern biological theories, like evolutionary theory, microbiology and genetics show us the affinities and similarities between all living beings and thus bridge the gap between animals and us. This could be a good starting point for increasing our respect for other creatures. But it seems to me that the conclusions that we are drawing from this affinity just go in one direction: we want to gain more and more power over nature including the human body, thereby subjecting nature to our interests and needs. We are more and more capable of overcoming 'the natural control mechanisms', to use Ian Cooke's words. We are able to outsmart nature in many ways, but we do not yet know how to deal with the effects of our power over nature. Moreover, nature may strike back, as the discussions among scientists on the possibly negative effects of intracytoplasmic sperm injection (ICSI) show (Vines 1996). Thus biological and medical technologies are highly *ambivalent*. They do not only include positive chances for improving the well-being of humanity but also the potential danger of being misused for scientific, economic, ideological and political purposes.

(2) I am going to concentrate on some possible inconsistencies in the moral intuitions and ethical standards of our societies. Obviously during the last twenty years IVF has become a socially accepted method to treat infertility.

Instead of handling the problem of infertility by adopting already existing children or by reflecting more thoroughly on the legitimacy of the claim to a child of one's own our societies have preferred not only to accept but also to *choose* this alternative, as the demand for IVF in spite of its low success rate (about 20 per cent) shows. As we all know the development of IVF was only possible on the basis of research on embryos. Embryo research however is far less generally accepted than IVF, as the societal debates and the legal situation in some countries show. This may be due to an inconsistency, a *double standard*, in our view of the human embryo. If we ascribe dignity to human embryos and if we are convinced that they deserve our protection and should not be the mere instruments and objects of our research we should not make use of reproductive technologies that presuppose this kind of research. Since IVF is a widely accepted method the prohibition of embryo research may have other reasons than the belief in the embryo's dignity, namely fear of the potential abuse of this research and its results.

The same considerations hold for the view of the embryo in the context of *prenatal diagnosis* on the one hand and *preimplantation diagnosis* on the other hand. The acceptance of prenatal diagnosis that may result in an abortion in cases of embryonic abnormality is not consistent with the rejection of preimplantation diagnosis if this rejection is justified by referring to the embryo's dignity or the dignity of handicapped people. Abortion after a prenatal diagnosis may violate dignity even more because the embryo is already in a much more advanced state of development than the fertilised egg in vitro. Here again the rejection of a technology may be due to fears of potential abuse. Ian Cooke addresses the questions of cloning and 'designer babies' in his last paragraph. I however think that those who oppose to embryo research, preimplantation diagnosis, etc. are not necessarily 'fundamentalists'. Newspaper reports and public discussions in late February 1997 about the successful *cloning* of sheep by Scottish scientists and the plans of a British physician to open a practice in Saudi Arabia for providing '*designer babies*', namely sons, not only prove that these fears are realistic but they also show how urgent a public ethical debate is. The contradictory statements of the German ministry of law and of German scientists on the question of whether the German Embryo Protection Act forbids cloning of human beings show once more the necessity of starting an ethical and legal debate *before* scientists set the course.

One of the *tasks of bioethics* is to detect the standards in our moral, ethical and theoretical views and to analyse the reasons for accepting certain practices and for rejecting others. Inventions can only be threatening if they violate our goals and norms. So *firstly* we have to make sure what we really want in the long run and if there is a consensus about this. *Secondly* scientists have to operate in a way that is transparent for others. There has to be an ongoing public discussion on our norms and values that we want to prefer in the long run. The oncologist van Rensselaer Potter who coined the term 'bioethics', defined bioethics as a 'bridge to the future' and a 'science of survival'. We can only build a solid bridge to the future by keeping in mind the experience of the past. Comparing past and present scientific claims and their prospective application can help us to base our appraisal of science on a realistic basis by avoiding prejudices as well as uncritical enthusiasm.

References

Cooke, I. (1997), 'Human Embryos in Medical Practice', this volume, Part Six.

Vines, G. (1996), 'The Genes of the Fathers ...', *New Scientist*, 17 August 1996, p. 18.

3 Supernumerary embryos: some social issues

Anne McLaren

Why supernumerary embryos?

If a couple undergoing the costly and traumatic experience of in vitro fertilisation (IVF) is to be given the best chance of achieving their much wanted pregnancy, it is likely that the number of eggs recovered and exposed to sperm will exceed the number of embryos that should be replaced in the woman's uterus. Where a regulatory system is in place, an upper limit of three embryos to be replaced is usually set. Centres with a high success rate often replace only two, especially where the woman is young and does not herself have a fertility problem.

But not all the eggs exposed to sperm will be fertilised, and not all fertilised eggs will undergo normal cleavage, so women undergoing IVF usually receive hormone treatment to increase the number of eggs recovered. The latest UK figures give a pregnancy rate per cycle of 18.1 per cent for hormone-stimulated IVF, but only 3.2 per cent for unstimulated IVF. The ovulatory response to hormone stimulation is quite variable, and since unfertilised eggs cannot yet safely be cryopreserved for future use, all the eggs recovered are usually exposed to sperm. If the number of eggs exposed to sperm has to be limited to the number of embryos that can be replaced the chances of pregnancy are greatly diminished.

Multiple pregnancies

But why limit the number of embryos replaced? As the number of embryos replaced increases, so does the risk of twins, triplets and even higher multiples. Even with a limit of three, 26 per cent of IVF pregnancies in the UK in 1993 were multiples compared with 1 per cent for spontaneous conceptions.

Multiple pregnancy represents the biggest medical, psychological and social problem involved in IVF today. It carries risks to the health and life of both the woman and her babies. During pregnancy the woman suffers an increased risk of raised blood pressure, pre-eclampsia and miscarriage. The babies tend to be born prematurely: the average gestation period for singletons, twins, triplets and quads is 40 weeks, 37, 34 and 32.5 weeks respectively. They are small at birth: the average birth weight for singletons is 3.5 kg, for twins 2.5 kg, and for triplets 1.8 kg. Mortality is higher at birth (5 times for triplets). Low birth weight babies are more likely to have neurological and other defects (triplet pregnancies produce a child with cerebral palsy 47 times more often than a singleton pregnancy) and have a higher than normal risk of health problems in later life. In addition, the emotional, practical and financial costs of bringing up triplets or even twins is great: surveys have shown that the parents' physical and sometimes mental health may be affected, and their relationship may suffer.

Options

If at the time of embryo replacement there are supernumerary embryos, couples have four options. The embryos can be donated for the treatment of another infertile couple; they can be donated for research; they can be stored for a second IVF attempt or a second pregnancy, provided that the Centre has a freezing (cryopreservation) facility; or they can be allowed to die.

Donation for treatment ('embryo adoption')

Informed consent should be obtained from the providers of both egg and sperm and full anonymity should be maintained. This usually means that the donated embryos will be frozen for a period: even if there was a potential recipient available with an appropriately synchronised cycle, the risk that the donor and recipient couples would become aware of each other's identity would be too great. The donors might be upset if they found out that the recipients' pregnancy had been successful while their own had failed. Unless both recipient partners are unable to produce their own gametes, this 'embryo adoption' (in which the baby will not be genetically related to either parent) must always be an inferior option to using the gametes of at least one of the partners.

Donation for research

Many countries allow the use of donated supernumerary ('spare') embryos for non-therapeutic research, provided that informed consent of both partners has been obtained. Each research project should be approved or licensed by an appropriate regulatory or statutory authority. Certain types of human embryo research are generally regarded as ethically unacceptable (e.g. genetic manipulation, chimera formation, transfer to a non-human animal uterus), and the project should meet certain criteria (e.g. scientific validity, need for human embryos, acceptable objectives, no transfer to uterus, time limit for in vitro culture – usually not beyond 14 days post fertilisation). Acceptable objectives include improvements in infertility treatments, especially IVF, and sometimes also investigations into the causes of infertility, diagnosis of genetic or chromosomal defects, new approaches to contraception, and increased understanding of early human development.

The advances in IVF treatment due to licensed research on supernumerary embryos include improvements in culture media and culture conditions as a result of increased understanding of early human embryo metabolism, successful protocols for embryo freezing and thawing, and safe and effective biopsy procedures for preimplantation genetic diagnosis.

Although there are now more than 20 IVF centres offering preimplantation diagnosis for life-threatening genetic diseases, the procedure is still controversial. The ethical issues that it raises are shared by all approaches to prenatal genetic diagnosis (e.g. amniocentesis, chorionic villus sampling), namely the possibility of increased prejudice against those born with genetic defects and their parents, the problem of which conditions are serious enough to warrant diagnosis and the view that any selection aimed at avoiding the birth of affected babies is ethically unacceptable. The advantage of preimplantation diagnosis over other forms of prenatal diagnosis from the parents' point of view is that it eliminates the emotionally traumatic decision as to whether to terminate the pregnancy if the fetus proves to be affected; its disadvantage is the financial and other costs, and the lack of certainty that a pregnancy will result, since it involves IVF.

Embryo storage

Although thousands of babies have now been born from frozen embryos, with no evidence of any increase in abnormality rate at birth or subsequently, not all the embryos survive freezing, and the pregnancy rate after replacement in most IVF centres is not as high as for fresh embryos. Nonetheless, the storage of supernumerary embryos from a single egg recovery cycle greatly increases the chances of an eventual pregnancy, and many couples have returned for a second or even a third IVF baby from a single batch of frozen embryos.

Animal studies indicate that once embryos are cooled to the temperature of liquid nitrogen, no further deterioration with time occurs. However, in 1990 when the UK Parliament passed the Human Fertilisation and Embryology Act, embryo freezing had only recently been introduced, less information about the health and well-being of the resulting babies was available and public opinion was concerned at the prospect of human embryos being stored for long periods of time. A limit of five years was therefore imposed, and many other countries have adopted a similar limit.

As the first UK embryos to be frozen under licence neared the end of their five-year term, it became apparent that many couples still had embryos stored, which they hoped to use for further IVF pregnancies when their personal circumstances and financial situation allowed. There were also embryos stored from the gametes of young female cancer patients who had received chemotherapy: these women might not wish to start a family for ten years or more. There was therefore pressure to extend the period of storage, and a further Act was passed, allowing storage for ten years, or in exceptional circumstances for more than ten years, up to the woman's 55th birthday.

A condition for any embryo storage in the UK is that both gamete providers must give their informed consent, specifying not only the period of storage but also what should be done with the embryos if they die or become incapable of varying or revoking their consent. Similar consent is required even if the provider of sperm is a donor. For those embryos that reached the end of their five-year limit, both gamete providers were required to give their consent for either a further period of storage or donation for treatment or research. Unfortunately some couples, and in particular some sperm donors, could not be traced to renew their consent, so those embryos could not be maintained in storage but had to be thawed and allowed to die.

Storage of frozen embryos without the informed consent of both gamete providers is not ethically acceptable. If one provider withdraws their consent, for example if the couple separate, storage should not be continued. Unless there is some legislation or Code of Practice in operation that lays down what should happen to the embryos in the event of death or divorce, complex social and legal issues are likely to arise.

4 Social issues surrounding supernumerary embryos

Carmen Kaminsky

The variety of options with regard to the fate of cryopreserved human embryos, especially in consideration of fatal incidents and accidents happening to their genetic parents, have led to ethical and legal disputes inflaming social issues surrounding supernumerary in vitro fertilisation (IVF) embryos. To prevent disputes over frozen embryos, it has been suggested that IVF-partners should form a consensus prior to their undergoing IVF procedures. Prior to consensus-formation between IVF-partners, however, it is necessary to clarify and solve (at least strategically) social issues surrounding decisions about the fate of supernumerary cryopreserved IVF embryos. After all, the question if and under what conditions individuals are allowed to decide the fate of their embryos is itself a social (and ethical) issue.

Social issues surrounding decisions about the fate of cryopreserved IVF embryos have three fundamental aspects: (a) issues concerning the dissolution of biological and traditional social conceptions of what it means to be member of a family; (b) issues concerning the rights and duties of a society as a whole with respect to the interests and well-being of its children; (c) issues concerning diverse emotional and rational attitudes towards the moral status of unborn human life and research on human embryos.

The scientific knowledge underlying contemporary reproductive technology presents a Janus-face towards both biological and traditional social views of the family. This scientific knowledge both supports and challenges these two differing views of social structure and ways of life, including family as well as other sub-groups. The same technologies that can establish biological relationship better than ever in human history also have the potential to deeply question its guiding function. Yet, although the issue of biological relationship might be greatly confused by modern reproductive technologies, it is not – at least not merely – based upon these technologies. Restrictions such as those concerning the intra- or intergenerational adoption of human embryos can therefore be based on forseeable changes in notions of the family only if the conceivable possibilities (*kinds* of individual cases) are put in relation to expectable incidents (*numbers* of similar cases) in order to gain an idea of probable social consequences. Another matter for discussion is whether probable social consequences of classes of cases are to be accepted or prevented. Corresponding principles and grounds will differ according to the interest of a society in the stability of its organisational structures, including its interest in the stability of a given legislative body (e.g. tax-law and legacy).

Even if, however, the organisational structures of a given society are not affected by certain decisions about the fate of supernumerary human embryos, it recognises a duty to take care of the interests and well-being of its actual and future children. Decisions to donate embryos to others for adoption therefore need to be framed by a society's decision about the burdens imposed on the future children concerned. Psychic burdens that might come about, for example, through severely postponed gestational development, especially in non-genetic relations, however, cannot be the topic of specific research, as this would predecide social and ethical acceptability. The sensitivity of a society therefore needs to be maintained as an argumentative dimension.

In view of the impossibility of a consensus on the definition of the moral status of the human embryo, the proposal to have biologically related individuals freely decide how to define the moral status of their embryo might be plausible, yet it seems to be socially completely inacceptable. Possible frameworks for individual consensus-formation with regard to the fate and destiny of supernumerary embryos are therefore highly dependent on socially preferred analogies between those embryos and other entities. Reference to abortion policies as a framework and guideline for letting-die decisions concerning supernumerary in vitro embryos might be acceptable; however, while the analogy with abortion policies may avoid social problems that might arise when individuals want to allow their embryos to perish, it cannot avoid social issues of research on or adoption of supernumerary embryos.

Social issues of research on and adoption of in vitro embryos can neither be solved nor avoided by contracts between individuals. With regard to the adoption of in vitro embryos, the sensitivity of a society about the psychic burdens imposed on children should be relevant for designing frameworks for decision-making. Social policy in this respect should additionally depend on the expected number of incidents. The acceptability of letting-die decisions will be dependent on whether the majority of a society accepts abortion policies as an analogy. Donation of frozen embryos for research obviously poses the greatest challenge to social decision-making. As long as there is no social consensus concerning the frames of individual decision-making, human embryos should not be kept frozen.

5 The status of human embryos in Irish medical practice

Deirdre Madden

In this text I would like to briefly summarise the position in Ireland regarding human embryos which, although in many ways similar to the German situation, is significantly different from other European countries.

At present we do have in vitro fertilisation (IVF) in Ireland which is governed not by legal regulation but by ethical guidelines of the Medical Council which governs the internal standards of the medical profession. These guidelines stipulate, amongst other things, that all embryos created by IVF must be returned to the woman's body and that no more than three are to be transferred to the uterus. This in effect prohibits the freezing of embryos, embryo research, and the 'official' discard of surplus embryos in Ireland. Faced with such guidelines the current practice is to transfer three embryos to the uterus and any others to the cervix where of course they will not be likely to implant. This in turn, if the first IVF attempt was unsuccessful, necessitates the couple going through the drug regime for ovarian stimulation and the egg retreival procedure again at a high emotional, physical and financial cost.

Although I am told that some couples prefer the embryos to be put into the cervix rather than simply discarded in any other way, because it is more in keeping with their dignity, nevertheless I think most couples, despite their religious views, would choose freezing if it were available. I would just like to remind you of the rates quoted by Yvon Englert of 98 per cent of couples in his study choosing freezing (Englert 1997). I think the present situation in Ireland could be termed 'an Irish solution to an Irish problem'.

The problem of the surplus embryo is mainly ethical rather than legal in nature. We must in Ireland and elsewhere decide, as a matter of policy, the status of the embryo and the legal protection it is thereby entitled to. It is not as simple as categorising it as property or persons although these are the legal terms we are familiar with. The ethical argument turns on whether the characteristics attributed to the human embryo entitle it to respect. At the very least it appears to be common case that the embryo should be accorded respect due to its potentiality for human life although these terms are open to different interpretations.

In Ireland these issues are somewhat complicated by the long-running debates concerning abortion and the constitutional protection accorded to the right to life of the unborn. Our Constitution acknowledges the right to life of the unborn and, with due regard to the equal right to life of the mother, guarantees to respect, safeguard and vindicate that right as far as practicable. This therefore is a recognition of the legal rights of the unborn and not just moral rights. So it is important to decide what is meant by the unborn. If the 'unborn' means 'with the potential to be born', 'capable of being born', or 'on the way to being born' as has been suggested by some writers in Ireland then, in my opinion, the pre-implanatation embryo does not qualify for this constitutional protection as it does not come within any of these expressions. At this point in time the embryo may not even be human or individual and cannot have any potential unless it is transferred to the uterus, implants in the uterine wall, and develops the primitive streak. This has relevance for IVF and the status of embryos due to the objections felt by many people in Ireland to embryo freezing. Their arguments, I think, are based on the opinion that IVF is unnatural and harmful to embryos. Freezing, in their opinion, is even more invasive of human dignity and disrespectful. This is based on the idea that a human life is in existence from the moment of conception. This suffers from the difficulty that it is necessary to be more specific in what is meant by conception. Most people do not have the necessary medical information to understand the different stages in the development of the embryo and why these stages should be distinguished.

A few brief points may be made to counteract these objections:

1 Associating the preimplantation embryo with the fetus or 'unborn child' fails to take account of the differences in terms of physiology and development between the two, such as lack of sentience and individuality in the preimplantation embryo. These differences require us to have independent analysis and debate without applying our views on abortion automatically to IVF, the creation of embryos and the issue of what to do with surplus embryos.

2 I fully agree with the idea of respect for the embryo at all stages of its development, though perhaps on a proportional basis. Surely we, in Ireland, could show more respect for human life if we chose to protect the embryos from destruction by requiring them to be donated to other infertile couples or volunteers (although this may interfere with the couple's procreational autonomy) or to be frozen for future use. In any event they should not

simply be put into the cervix as this is really indirectly discarding them. If the Pro-life groups are of the view that the embryo at the preimplantation stage is a human being then surely present practice in Ireland could be regarded as a form of indirect abortion. So far it has not been legally challenged as being unconstitutional whereas if freezing is introduced some groups have threatened to take an injunction to prevent it.

3 I think that the best solution for Ireland from an ethical, medical and legal perspective would possibly be to give the option of freezing at the pro-nucleur stage as is done in some other countries. This appears to have very good chances of success and it may avoid some of the difficulties already outlined. However some people may still argue that once the sperm penetrates the egg a human life has begun. This is matter for an ethical and theological debate rather than a legal one.

In Ireland we are fortunate in one sense, that we are starting with a blank page in terms of legal regulation. We can therefore learn from the experiences and mistakes made in other countries. Consensus on these issues will be very difficult and perhaps unnecessary bearing in mind the differences between the various societies in Europe. However I also feel that morally and legally speaking the rights of the human embryo should not depend on the country in which the medical procedure is taking place. It is surely a more universal question.

I hope that when these questions come up for debate in Ireland that we can have an informed and educated debate and that any changes to current practice will ultimately benefit all involved – the couple, the medical profession and the children who may be born and who will have no voice in this debate.

References

Englert, Y. (1997), 'The Fate of Supernumerary Embryos: What Do Patients Think About It?', this volume, part 6.

6 The fate of supernumerary embryos: what do patients think about it?

Yvon Englert

Introduction

The fate of supernumerary embryos is largely discussed in ethical, political or juridical circles, mainly because the status that will be given to the human embryo in vitro will greatly influence many fields of human reproduction including access to abortion. It is thus not surprising that very few of these debates are focused on those primarily concerned, namely the infertile couples who decided to enter in vitro fertilisation (IVF) treatment and thus are really confronted with this problematic.

The present study firstly describes the ethical basis on which the medical team developed its clinical procedure for all embryos produced in vitro that are not immediately replaced.

The first position is that embryo status in vitro is to be seen differently depending on whether or not the embryo is included in a parental project. Cryopreservation allows the preservation of the embryos as long as the couple wishes to have a child; donation offers another parental project for the remaining embryos. In these situations, the embryos have to be protected. Inversely, an embryo no longer intended for such a project could be destroyed or used for scientific experimentation. Experimentation policy follows the advice of the ethics committee of the Belgian National Fund for Scientific Research: the proposed research has to offer a strong therapeutic interest, the information cannot be obtained using an animal model, the explicit agreement of the couples and of the local ethics committee has to be obtained, and the embryos must be destroyed after experimentation if the protocol does not involve direct therapeutic aims for them.

The second principle is to manage the stored embryos in a co-responsible manner between the medical team and the couples. This implies several mutual agreements and the acceptance of the risk that it may not be possible to find a consensual approach between the fertility clinic and the couples. The mutual procedure agreed by the local ethics committee is the following: the fertility clinic is committed to keep the embryos for a fixed time that may not be extended and to provide full information to the couple. They fill in the document divided in two parts: in the first part the couple is asked if they want their embryos to be cryopreserved or not. It specifies the limit of the storage period and the conditions to transfer. The second part concerns the destiny of the unused embryos after the end of the storage period. Three possibilities are provided: anonymous donation to other couples, experimentation, and destruction. All possible uses of the embryos must be approved by both partners of the couples: if disagreements arise later during treatment, the embryos must be left in storage until a new decision is commonly taken or until the end of the storage period.

The third principle is that the fertility clinic must always have a potential final destination for every produced or stored embryo. This is why the couples have to notify the clinic of their decision before the first treatment. The document is presented to the couple in one of the pre-IVF treatment consultations by the doctor who carries out the treatment. It is followed by an interview with a psychologist familiar with these questions. The completed and signed document is added to the medical file. These ethical principles are summarised in table 1.

Table 1. Fertility Clinic ethical principles regarding experimentation on embryos in vitro

Experimentation is limited to the following situations:

1 strong therapeutic interest
2 absence of a possible animal model
3 informed consent of both memers of the couple
4 approval of the ethical committee
5 destruction of the embryos after experimentation is mandatory when no direct therapeutic aim.

Couples' views

Two hundred couples were interviewed on their views on supernumerary embryos during the psychological consultation before entering IVF treatment. They were also asked to give their opinion on the other reproductive choices (checking of limits), and about the status of the in vitro embryo (did they consider the in vitro embryo as already a child?). One hundred and thirty-one out of 200 did not have had any child at home, 18 were going to have an IVF with gamete donation, 108 couples (59 per cent) identified themselves as Roman

Catholics, 80 (40 per cent) as having no religious beliefs, 12 (1 per cent) as having another religion. Patients' views on the respective importance of genetic lineage and education for defining parental bonding have been codified according to three categories: predominance of genetic lineage, predominance of education, equal balance of both.

Ninety-eight per cent of the 200 couples have decided that their supernumerary embryos will be frozen. In case they do not use these frozen embryos for their own treatment, donation is the most frequent choice (39 per cent) (table 2) but embryo destruction is tolerated by almost all the couples (92 per cent): or they ask for destruction (n= 60 couples) or destruction after experimentation (n= 38 couples) but only 16 per cent of the 102 couples choosing donation explained that destruction was unacceptable. The others consider donation as to be preferred to help other couples and not to protect the embryos. Couples considering the embryo as a child choose destruction (50 per cent) as frequently as donation but refuse experimentation on the embryo (84 per cent). Donation is highest among couples who stress education more than genetic lineage in parental bonding (table 3). This is confirmed by the choice of the couples requiring donor gametes from whom 83 per cent chose donation to another couple. No difference was observed regarding embryo destiny in relation to religion or previous parental experiences. It has been observed in this study that when the couple's opinion focused more on genetic aspects than on the education relationship, they generally chose destruction. As blood relations are lifelong, embryo donation cannot of course be accepted in this case. It would mean that these couples would have to spend the rest of their lives with unforgettable feelings of responsibility. They consider that the embryos belong to them. On the contrary, to consider education as the basis of parental bonding helps acceptance that one's donated embryo develops into another couple's child. It presupposes differentiating between parents and genitors. Couples needing a donor's gametes generally make that differentiation. As expected, these couples also choose donation preferentially. As evidence, couple's choices on supernumerary embryos are the reflection of very personal feelings and attitudes. This emphasises the need for careful and focused counselling to maximise their information about facts and implications.

Couples' opinions on the respective importance of genetic lineage and education in defining parental bonding are more significant in their decision to destroy or to donate their supernumerary embryos than their opinions on the in vitro embryo status, which only determines their attitude toward experimentation.

The public debate

The recent authoritarian decision by the UK legislature to destroy embryos highlights the passionate debate on spare embryos left frozen after IVF treatment. But is the question correctly formulated? Is the problem really what to do with spare embryos? Is it not rather who should decide what to do with spare embryos and how to manage the decision procedure in this field?

In our eyes, the spare embryos' management should be discussed with the couple before entering IVF treatment to determine in advance their possible spare embryos' fate. Such an approach implies that the responsibility for the management of stored embryos is shared between the medical team and the couples, which appears to be an ethical improvement in the management of infertility through IVF.

Does it make a sense to define a time for cryopreservation of supernumerary embryos? There is no biologic evidence that cryostorage must be limited for safety reasons at least within time limits discussed in the British law. The debate is thus purely influenced by social and political motives which does not mean there might not be some reasons to define a limit for the cryopreservation period. Increasing the cryopreservation time may mean the more frequent occurrence of two situations still largely ethically debated: the first situation may be the request for post-menopausal pregnancies using cryopreserved embryos. These possible requests may place clinical teams in difficulties when they are not in favour of such practices or when they are illegal, because it contradicts the meaning of freezing i.e. that frozen embryos are preserved to be replaced at the couples's request. One may even sustain the idea that the undefined cryopreservation period induces difficult decisions for the couples, as illustrated in Bretecher's comic strip 'Le destin de Monique' where a woman is still undecided about whether to replace her frozen embryos when she is 80. A second situation results in difficulties in managing cryopreservation of embryos, when couples break up (divorce or death of one of the partners). Its frequency will be proportional to the length of the cryopreservation period. It is often unclear if one partner can decide solely forever over the frozen embryo's fate. We think the decision must be taken by both parents, having decided to cryopreserve their embryos.

Moreover this is a way to avoid having embryos one does not know what to do with, because one feels uncomfortable about deciding without the couples. If the situation has been discussed and the decisions taken in time, there is no reason to start searching for the couples after years. It is the a posteriori management of spare embryos which creates the problem, not the spare embryos by themselves. It can be expected that contact loss is bound to happen years after the treatment. But, if the couple's instructions are stored in the clinic, nobody has to look for each other at the end of the custody period. And if a couple wants to change their embryos' fate, to find the clinic should not be a too difficult task...

Conclusion

Reproductive medicine cannot always be managed in the same way as any other medical activity. Professional medical rules and experiences usually sustain the way treatments are performed. However, this is changing in some areas of medical care either for economic reasons or ethical ones. Reproductive medicine carries extremely heavy symbolic aspects for society linked to individual autonomy, social morality, sexuality and religion, showing similarities with the abortion debate.

The professionals in IVF-teams should be aware that they can be used as 'puppets' in a game that is much more complex than the pratical problems they are facing in their daily practice. They must both include themselves in the political debate and be careful to protect their patients from undue outside intervention. I believe many problems can be avoided if it is clearly said to the patients at the time of cryopreservation that it is their responsibility to formally request replacement for themselves from the clinic before the end of the custody period. In absence of such a request, the clinic will conclude that the couple has no more child project for the spare embryos. In this latter case, destruction of biological material with no future is in my eyes ethically acceptable, when the couples are reluctant to donate their embryos.

Table 2. Couples' attitudes regarding embryo destiny

asking freezing	196 (98 per cent)
refusing freezing	4 (2 per cent)
Attitude regarding unused embryos at the end of the custody period:	
donation to other couples	78 (39 per cent)
destruction	60 (30 per cent)
experimentation	38 (19 per cent)
donation and experimentation	24 (12 per cent)

Table 3. Opinion on filitation and attitude regarding embryo destiny

	Genetic	Genetic and education	Education
Donation to other couples (alone or in combination with experimentation) n=102	15 (33%)	40 (44%)	46 (74%)
			p<0.001
Destruction and experimentation n=98	31 (67%)	50 (56%)	16 (26%)
	46	90	62

References

Bretecher, C. (1983), *Le destin de Monique*, Ed. Bretecher.

Englert, Y. and Revelard, P. (1996), 'Isn't it Rather «Who Decides» Than «What to Do» With Spare Embryos?', *Human Reprod.*, Vol. 12, No. 1, pp. 8-10.

Laruelle, C. and Englert, Y. (1995), 'Psychological Study of In Vitro Fertilization-Embryo Transfer Participants' Attitudes Towards the Destiny of Their Supernumerary Embryos', *Fertil Steril*, Vol. 63, pp. 1047-50.

7 Putting IVF-clients' views on the fate of their embryos into context

Sigrid Graumann

I wonder what contribution a psychological study (Laruelle and Englert 1995, Englert 1997) on the attitudes of couples participating in IVF-programmes towards their supernumerary embryos can make to the ethical debate?

To me this study seems to ease the conscience of the participating physicians rather than truly to contribute to the ethical discourse on 'supernumerary embryos'. The responsibility for the fate of these embryos is imposed upon the participating couples although they are not solely responsible. The conflictual situation is created by physicians, biologists and couples alike. Englert claims that heated discussions about the destruction of cryopreserved embryos, such as those in the English press, could be avoid simply by allowing the participating couples to decide in advance about the destiny of their cryopreserved supernumerary embryos after IVF-treatment. This does not, however, solve the problem, but only avoids the embarassing public debate. The controversial discussion throughout Europe, and especially the somewhat bewildering offer of Italian women to carry the British embryos to term, showed clearly that there is no ethical consensus in European societies about the acceptability of the destruction of such embryos – despite the fact that 92 per cent of the couples interviewed for this study said they accept the destruction of their supernumerary embryos. What other decision could they have made?

For the interviewed couples the normatively most relevant decision was already made, namely to participate in an IVF-programme and thus to accept side-effects such as the creation of supernumerary embryos. In my opinion, precisely this decision to participate is the ethically and psychologically most relevant. One cannot start with the presumption that the couples ever explicitly reflected on this 'side-effect' of IVF-programmes.

Let me summarise: The couples were offered 3 options for dealing with their supernumerary embryos: donation to other couples, donation for research purposes, or destruction. In addition, the couples were interviewed about their opinions on two other issues, with the intention of identifying their attitudes towards these embryos:

1. What status they ascribe to the in-vitro embryo?
2. Which factor seems to them more important for parental bonding to a child: genetic links ('genetic lineage') or upbringing ('education')?

In asking such questions, the researchers assume a situation where the embryo exists in isolation from the woman who wishes to become pregnant. Starting form this artificial situation (for which the couples are partly responsible) the question of the status of the in-vitro embryo becomes rather rhetorical. The question is actually already answered by the construction of the situation, and this in a rather paradoxical way. On the one hand, there is discussion about the 'embryo' which is involved in a 'parental project', or which is offered to another 'parental project' via donation. In this context the embryo is treated like a subject. On the other hand, for destruction or research purposes, the embryo is discussed as an object. The embryo becomes nothing more than 'biological material with no future'. For the couples this means ultimately that they are offered the rather suggestive choice to confer upon the embryos one of these and no other status, depending on the question. With regard to their destruction or use for research purposes they are merely biological material. They gain value, however, when linked to the couples' hope for a child. Continuing this line of thought, after the establishment of a pregnancy the embryo will become – in the mind of the parents – their child with whom they link their hopes, desires and dreams. Is this not the fundamental paradox the couples have to live with to be able to participate in an IVF-programme? Do not the questions in this study blur rather than clarify this contradiction?

I would like to know what thoughts couples would have about enrolling in an IVF-programme if they were confronted with the moral implications of their decision, including any side-effects. This would mean a much more complex study, which would consist of critical reflection on the concrete decision-making process, combined with a process of clarifying their more general personal moral values. Significantly, in such a study the existence of 'supernumerary embryos' would not be taken for granted! Only such a study would offer a contribution to the ethical question about the destiny of supernumerary embryos.

References

Englert, Y. (1997), 'The Fate of Supernumerary Embryos: What Do Patients Think About It?', this volume, Part Six.

Laruelle, C. and Englert, Y. (1995), 'Psychological Study of In Vitro Fertilization-Embryo Transfer Participants' Attitudes Towards the Destiny of Their Supernumerary Embryos', *Fertil. Steril.*, Vol. 63, pp. 1047-50.

Part Seven
THE STATUS OF HUMAN EMBRYOS

1 The moral status of potential persons

Klaus Steigleder

The American philosopher Alan Gewirth has shown that moral norms possess no independent existence of their own. On the contrary, moral norms come into existence through and between agents, although 'behind their backs', as it were. Every agent logically must accept the supreme moral principle that every agent has the strict obligation to act in accord with the generic rights of her recipients as well as of her own (Gewirth, 1978, p.135).

Now, agency as the ability of knowingly and voluntarily pursuing one's ends is a demanding concept. Not every human being is at least dispositionally able to act and therefore not every human being is an agent. Some are not yet agents, others are irretrievably no longer agents and still others can never become agents in a full sense, e.g. due to very severe forms of mental retardation. This gives rise to the question what, if any, the moral status of these human beings is. If we call, for convenience and according to the customs of bioethics, agents 'persons' and human beings who are not agents 'non-persons' we can reformulate this as the well-known question what, if any, the moral status of human non-persons is.

In this paper I will focus on the moral status of human fetuses and embryos. But, as it will become clear, it will be necessary to give a rough outline of the moral status of infants and young children as well. I want to show that because agents must attribute to themselves and to each other dignity they must, in different ways, regard human non-persons as connected to their dignity and therefore must confer, in different ways, moral status upon them. In order to show this we must briefly consider why and in what way agents have to attribute dignity to themselves in the first place.

Dignity as the basis of generic rights

In order to show that every agent logically must accept a supreme moral principle, Gewirth has developed a sequence of dialectically necessary judgements[1] every agent can only deny on pain of self-contradiction. The first judgement of the sequence is (1) 'I do action A for the end E'. This judgement translates the fundamental structure of an action into a judgement of the agent. Gewirth has shown that this judgement necessarily implies – not semantically but from the reflexive perspective of the agent – further judgements and ultimately the judgement which formulates the supreme principle of morality. Here I shall confine myself to mentioning the main steps of the sequence only and to locating dignity's place in this sequence.

The first step shows that agency has an 'evaluative structure' (Gewirth, 1978, pp.48-63).This means two things. First, the agent has to consider each end of her action at the time of her acting as good according to some criterion. Second, she therefore has to consider her freedom to act and the other necessary conditions enabling her to act at all and the ability to act successfully at all as necessary goods. Gewirth has shown that the contents of these conditions can be specified (Gewirth, 1978, pp.53-58). They comprise, in the Gewirth's terminology of basic goods such as life and physical and psychological integrity, nonsubtractive goods such as not to be stolen from and additive goods such as education. The necessary nonsubtractive and additive goods constitute respectively the necessary conditions for maintaining and furthering one's level of purpose fulfillment, whereas the basic goods consist in the necessary conditions for being and remaining an agent at all.

The second step shows that agency is characterised not only by an evaluative structure but also by a 'normative structure' as well (Gewirth, 1978, pp.63-103).[2] This means that the agent must consider a necessary good as something she has a right to. Now, a right is an other-directed normative concept, but up to this point of the sequence no other person or agent came into play directly or explicitly.[3] So how can we proceed from the necessary goods to right claims? The answer is that the agent has to make two factual judgements which function as premises in the sequence of the dialectically necessary judgements. The first judgement is that the necessary goods are no sure or safe possession of the agent. On the contrary, she is vulnerable and therefore can lose them. This premise contributes to the way the agent wants the necessary goods for herself. Here it is important to note that for the agent the necessary goods are not only necessary because of their instrumental function as means for her acting (and acting successfully at all). There is also a necessity in her wanting these goods. In connection with the first factual premise this wanting must be specified as unconditionally not wanting these goods to be interfered with.

This mode of wanting is latently normative as becomes clear, if we take the second factual judgement or premise into consideration. This is the awareness of the agent that the possession of her necessary goods depends on the conduct of the other agents. The agent can be interfered with by other agents, that is by persons who are able to control their conduct and therefore are able to refrain from any such interference. Therefore, in view of other agents, wanting the necessary goods necessarily takes on the form of an other-directed ought-judgement. The agent must regard all other agents as strictly obligated at least not to infere with her necessary goods. This means that, in view of the other agents, a normative claim is formed. The agent claims the necessary goods as something which is due to her and which she has a right to. Underlying this is a certain sort of necessary self-evaluation which can be interpreted in terms of a normative concept of dignity. For the agent has to attribute a status to herself where, in view of the other agents, she is ultimately not the possible object of a calculation or balancing of the interests of others.

Because the agent must attribute dignity and rights to herself for the sufficient reason that she is a prospective agent, she must acknowledge, in a third and last step of the sequence, that all other agents possess the same dignity and the same rights to the necessary goods. This leads to the supreme moral principle mentioned above.

The moral significance of potential agents

My thesis is that human beings who are not yet agents must possess moral significance for agents for the sufficient reason that they possess the potentiality to become agents. The agent has to attribute to herself dignity by virtue of being an agent. Therefore agency necessarily represents for her an evaluatively and normatively outstanding quality. For it confers on her and every other agent a morally outstanding and unsurpassable status. Now if a being has the potentiality to become an agent and the agent is aware of this capacity, then the agent must see a morally relevant connection between such a being and herself and her dignity. At the same time the agent has to make two distinctions, the first underscoring the connection, the second specifying it.

First, the agent must see an evaluatively and normatively relevant difference between a being who is not yet an agent and those beings who, in principle, possess no potentiality to become an agent. As compared to the latter, the former must possess pre-eminence for the agent by virtue of possessing such potentiality. Second, the agent must see a difference between herself and those beings who are not yet agents. They do not possess the same moral status as agents for they do not possess dignity. The basis of dignity is that the agent inevitably *has* purposes she wants to fulfill. As they are not able to act, potential agents as such cannot meet this condition.

Accordingly my argument is not affected by the standard objection against arguments from potentiality that, for example, a potential president is no president and therefore cannot possess the status or the rights of a president. My contention is not that for the agent the potentiality to agency must possess the same relevance as actual agency, but that for her it must possess *some* relevance. It is not possible that agency can in one case possess unsurpassing significance for the agent and in the other case no significance at all. For the agent to judge otherwise would be inconsistent.

It might be objected that it is important to take into consideration *who* the possessor of something is. One might greatly value one's own million dollars, but attribute no value at all to the million dollars of some other person. Accordingly, the agent can attribute outstanding significance to her own agency, while the potentiality to agency of some other being might be without any value for her. There is no inconsistency involved.

In this form the objection is already directed against the universalisation of the claim to dignity and comes down to the contention that the agent may not attribute the relevance of justifying their dignity to the agency of other agents. This contention is untenable if, for the agent, her having purposes she wants to fulfill is a sufficient reason for her claim to dignity. I shall not discuss this here in greater detail (See e.g. Gewirth 1969 or Gewirth, 1978, pp.115-119). Suffice to say that I do not contend that the agent must value all things she finds valuable for herself similarly when these are possessed by others. But the agency-based dignity forms an evaluation of a higher complexity and level. For the agent her agency is, in a normatively strict sense, *status conferring* and the status, that is dignity and the generic rights has a bearing on how the other agents ought to act against her. Therefore the agent must hold that the agency of others confers on them the same status with equal consequences for the conduct of others including herself.

These considerations show that 'relevance' is an ambiguous term reflecting different levels of complexity and evaluation. In connection with dignity 'relevance' means the presence of a moral status which grounds strict obligations. There is a lower level of 'relevance' at which, for the agent, her own agency is more important than the agency of others. For the agent can only do something with her own agency. On this level a comparability exists between one's own money as against the money of others. Thus the objection misses the point because it does not take into consideration which sense of 'relevance' is meant. The potentiality to agency must be status conferring, if agency is status conferring, even if the potentiality to agency does not confer the same status as actual agency.

Specifying the moral status of infants and young children

Potentiality is not the only morally relevant aspect for the determination of the moral status of human beings who are not yet agents. Another aspect is their different levels of proximity to agency. In order to grasp the moral significance and range of this criterion I first want to consider young children who are very close to agency in the full sense. Thus I want to begin with those human beings whose capacities can be described as 'able to act in a limited, rudimentary or initial way'. Due to insufficient cognitive abilities it is not yet possible to speak of voluntary and intentional conduct covering a relatively long period. The possibility for self-determination and self-control, consciousness of proximate relevant circumstances, and grasp of the effects of one's conduct on oneself and on others are still so much reduced that the individuals in question cannot be held really accountable for their conduct. Needless to say that such a general description covers a whole range of different forms from rudimentary and isolated purposes to more differentiated actions which are more and more integrated into groups of actions and action plans.

Normally a child will go through this whole range of forms. As compared with those who are able to act in the full sense there are differences in competence and capacity which are in part considerable. Nevertheless, in the course of this development precisely that structure progessively emerges which justifies the normative claim of dignity, namely to have purposes one wants to fulfill. It is true that those who are only able to act in a rudimentary way cannot logically be required to perform that special kind of self-evaluation through which the claim to dignity comes into existence. But, as the agent must recognise the decisive characteristic which leads to the justification of her dignity in those individuals, *she* is required to confer on them the same dignity as on herself. Thus, those who are only able to act in a rudimentary way somehow participate in the dignity of agents.

The dignity of rudimentary agents does not justify the same range of rights as does the dignity of agents. For, as generic rights are the rights which constitute agency, they are only partly applicable to rudimentary agents. But insofar as they are applicable (e.g. the rights to life, physical and psychological integrity), these rights are possessed by rudimentary agents. Besides, their dignity justifies rights which are special to them, namely rights to special protection and support.

The scope of the extension of dignity to human beings who are not persons in the defined sense reaches beyond human beings who are not yet agents. For, on the one hand, it includes those human beings who are rudimentary agents but due to very severe forms of mental retardation can never become agents in the full sense. This has consequences for the aspect of potentiality. For even the potentiality to develop to the proximity of agency must confer a moral status. On the other hand, dignity must be conferred on those human beings who are irretrievably no longer agents in the full sense but still show some rudiments of agency.

The argument from rudimentary agency does not apply to newborns. To call newborns rudimentary agents would imply stretching the concept beyond its morally significant characteristics. Nevertheless, there seem to be conclusive reasons for agents to attribute dignity to newborns. For us as agents the newborn baby is a bodily other who despite its dependence possesses a significant amount of independence and whose behavior we contrafactually interpret as rudimentary acts. Accordingly, in the newborn child we must anticipate the agent or at least the rudimentary agent he or she presumably will become.

I am aware that in the presented form this last extension of dignity represents more of a sketch of an argumentative strategy than an argument itself. Nevertheless, I think at least so much has been shown that we may safely conclude that birth would be at best the earliest point for the attribution of dignity to a human being. This brings us back to the task of specifying the moral status of human embryos and fetuses.

Specifying the moral status of human embryos and fetuses

As against infants and young children, the potentiality to become an agent is the only characteristic which is directly relevant for the determination of the moral status of human embryos and fetuses.[4] An important consequence of this is that we are inevitably confronted with an unsurmountable unsharpness in the criteria. We are able to specify the moral status of human embryos and fetuses by spelling out its normative implications in general, but often are not able to spell them out *in concreto*. As we know that their moral status is not that of dignity, we know that there may be circumstances in which the rights or interests of agents have precedence over the status of a human embryo or fetus. But it is impossible to determine exactly which rights can still take such precedence and which cannot.

The general normative implication of the moral status of human embryos and fetuses as potential agents is a general prescription to preserve, protect and foster them. This implies the general prohibition of killing and harming them. General prescriptions and prohibitions can be balanced out by other important normative considerations. This is of importance for the moral problem of abortion. From the general prescription of preservation and protection it follows that basically and as far as possible there should be no abortions and that an abortion is a morally serious matter. But in the case of a direct conflict especially with the generic rights of the pregnant woman the general prescription of preservation and protection can be balanced out. It follows that an abortion *can* be morally justified. Due to the unsharpness of criteria it is not possible to determine *exactly* which rights of the woman can balance out the status of the embryo or fetus and which cannot. On the one hand, there are cases where the priority of the rights of the woman is perfectly clear. On the other hand, there can be no serious dispute that certain reasons for an abortion would be frivolous. But between such clear-cut cases there is an insurmountable gray area. Nevertheless, the normative implications of this are clear in itself. There must be room for free decisions which must not be legally restrained.

The problem of abortion occurs in a conflict situation which is in many respects unique. Things are quite different if the conflict is created in a controllable and somewhat institutionalised way as a side effect of a medical procedure. If hormonal treatments of infertility or the placement of three or more embryos into the uterus as part of in vitro fertilisation or related technologies lead to a significant increase of multiple pregnancies this will morally count against these procedures in the first place. For, on the one hand, the multiple pregnancy is connected with a high probability of serious harm for the mother, the fetuses or the future children the fetuses may become. On the other hand, due to the moral status of human embryos and fetuses, 'pregnancy reduction' is not a morally tenable strategy to deal with this problem. For, if there is a general prescription to protect human embryos and fetuses, 'pregnancy reduction' may be a morally tolerable solution in unforeseen tragic situations, but is not tolerable in the context of a knowingly induced, though unintended, problem.

The distinction between human embryos and pre-embryos

There is some variation in the use of the term 'embryo'. Thus it is important to stress that the above argument from potentiality refers to the embryo in the strict sense and not to the so-called 'pre-embryo'. By this term is usually meant the fertilised human egg (zygote) and the further stages of its development during roughly the first two weeks. During this time there is a process of differentiation during which the pre-embryo differentiates into those cells which develop into the embryonic membranes and into the placenta and those cells which form the embryo proper. Stephen Buckle has made the important proposal to distinguish between two kinds of potentiality here (Buckle 1988). The pre-embryo has the 'potentiality *to produce*', for instance, the embryo. The embryo itself has the 'potentiality *to become*' an agent. It was this last kind of potentiality which figured in the argument from potentiality.

Thus, the moral status of the human pre-embryo is different and much weaker than that of the human embryo. It is difficult to see how the status of the pre-embryo as such could justify a categorical prohibition of its use for research. On the other hand, the question is to be considered to what extent and with what consequences we have to attribute to the human pre-embryo symbolic significance. Furthermore, the human pre-embryo as a possible subject of research is not readily available but produced *in vitro*. The moral evaluation of research on human pre-embryos is not independent from a moral evaluation of the preconditions and the context of the 'production' of the pre-embryos. But all this is not the subject of this paper.

Notes

1 Gewirth explains: 'An assertoric statement is of the form «*p*»; a dialectical statement is of the form «S thinks (or says, or accepts) that *p*»; a dialectically necessary statement is of the form «S logically must (on pain of contradiction) think (or say, or accept) that *p*».' (Gewirth, 1978, p.152).
2 In my presentation of this step I will somewhat depart from Gewirth's presentation. For Gewirth's treatment of the connection between dignity and rights see Gewirth, 1982, pp.27-30, and Gewirth 1992.
3 But we may say that they came into play implictly because, for example, the nonsubtractive good of not being stolen from implies a potential thief.
4 To be sure, the criterion of proximity to agency is applicable to fetuses as well. But here it does not yield definitive and uncontroversial normative results.

References

Buckle, S. (1988), 'Arguing from Potential', *Bioethics*, Vol. 2, pp. 227-53.
Gewirth, A. (1969), 'The Non-trivializability of Universalizabilty', *Australasian Journal of Philosophy*, Vol. 47, pp. 123-31.
Gewirth, A. (1978), *Reason and Morality*, University of Chicago Press: Chicago.
Gewirth, A. (1982), *Human Rights. Essays in Justification and Applications*, University of Chicago Press: Chicago.
Gewirth, A. (1992), 'Human Dignity as the Basis of Rights', in Meyer, M.J. and Parent, W.A. (eds), *The Constitution of Rights*, Cornell University Press: Ithaca, N.Y., pp. 10-28.

2 The moral and legal status of the human embryo

Deryck Beyleveld

This paper is in three parts. Part I discusses some general matters concerning the attribution of moral status to the human embryo. Part II outlines the current situation regarding legal protection of the human embryo in the European Union. Part III sketches an approach to the moral status of the human embryo that lays claim to legal force within the European Union as a whole.

The moral status of the human embryo

General considerations

The general moral status attributed to the human embryo depends, essentially, on two things:

1 which characteristics are deemed necessary or sufficient, on the one hand, for beings to be owed any duties of respect or concern for their interests or welfare, or rights in terms of their interests or welfare, on the other; and
2 beliefs about the ontological status of the human embryo – its nature, capacities, and powers.

Characteristics that have been deemed necessary/sufficient for duties of respect or concern to be owed (or rights to be held) include, e.g.,

(a) being a natural event or system;
(b) being a living organism;
(c) being a sentient being (one capable of pain and pleasure);
(d) being a human being (biologically defined);
(e) being a rational being;

(f) being (in Kant's terms) a rational being with a will (or an agent – a being with the capacity and disposition to pursue purposes of its own choosing as reasons for its acting).

Some of these characteristics (being a natural event or system, being a living organism, and being a human being [biologically defined]) are properties that the human embryo unquestionably has. On the other hand, it is extremely doubtful that the human embryo is sentient, and there is no evidence whatsoever that the human embryo is a reflective rational being, let alone an agent. Such properties are, however, features that the human embryo might develop.

Some of the properties in the above list include some of the other properties. For example, if being a living organism is held to be sufficient for moral status, then being a human being must also be held to be sufficient. It does not, however, follow that those who hold that being, e.g., a living organism confers *some* moral status, may not hold that being a human being, or a rational one, confers a *higher* moral status. The most interesting conflicts between positions occur when there is dispute about what is necessary for *some* moral status to be conferred and what is sufficient for *maximal* moral status to be conferred. The two extremes, are constituted, on the one hand, by the view that being a natural event or system is necessary and sufficient for *maximal* moral status to be conferred and, on the other hand, by the view that being an agent is necessary and sufficient for *any* moral status to be conferred.

One popular view (characteristic of Kantian and contractarian theories, as well as the Gewirthian theory I myself espouse, see, e.g., Gewirth 1978, 1996, Beyleveld 1991) is that beings cannot rationally be accorded maximal moral status (as possessors of inalienable claim rights) unless they are agents. An important question for such theories is whether status as an agent is necessary for a being to be accorded any moral protection, or whether such status is only necessary for maximal moral protection, some moral protection accruing from the possession of other characteristics. In this paper, I shall be addressing this question as it impinges on the moral status of the human embryo.

Moral status of the human embryo if agency is required for claim rights

On the assumption that agency is necessary (as well as merely sufficient) for a being to have claim rights, it remains possible to argue that the human embryo is the possessor of rights (of a lesser or different kind) that generate duties of agents towards the human embryo.

In principle, the human embryo could be granted protection either directly or indirectly. There are essentially two considerations that might be appealed to in an attempt to justify granting human embryos protection directly.

1 It might be contended that human embryos are owed protection because they have some of the features necessary for full moral status. Correlative

to this is the idea that as the human embryo develops it gains greater protection through acquiring more and more of the features necessary for agency.

2 It might be contended that human embryos are owed protection because they are potential agents.

Indirectly, the human embryo might gain protection because not to do so threatens the claim rights of beings with full moral status (in line with which various arguments for vicarious protection might be constructed) or through the idea that agents might contract between themselves to grant the human embryo protections that it might not self-sufficiently be entitled to.

Arguments for direct status

The Principle of Proportionality: This kind of argument is employed by Alan Gewirth, who argues that rational agents (those who avoid contradicting that they are agents) necessarily grant claim rights (generic rights) to the necessary conditions of agency and of successful agency in general to all agents. According to Gewirth, creatures who possess some, but not all the necessary features of agency are to be granted some but not all of the rights of agents in proportion to their closeness to being agents (Gewirth, 1978, pp.121-124 and pp.141-144).

This kind of argument requires the possession of specific properties necessary to be an agent to be sufficient for the possession of specific rights, the possession of all the properties necessary to be an agent being sufficient for the possession of the complete complement of rights protection.

While such an idea is not incoherent, it presents difficulties within the framework of the Gewirthian scheme simply because Gewirth's argument, if valid, proceeds by arguing that agents would contradict that they are agents if they do not consider themselves to have the generic rights, thus that they must (on pain of contradicting that they are agents) consider that they have the generic rights because they are agents, and, hence, must grant the generic rights to all agents. For it to be demonstrated, within such a framework, that agents must grant some generic rights to beings that are not full agents, it must be shown that agents must claim specific rights for themselves on the basis of having properties necessary but not sufficient for agency, and the argument is not structured that way. While this does not mean that an adequate argument is unavailable, it has not yet been presented.[1]

Even outside Gewirth's framework, this kind of argument presents problems when used to grant rights to the human embryo. In principle, the idea would be that the human embryo is a stage in the development of a human agent, and during its development acquires properties necessary to being an agent. So, e.g., the point at which twinning is no longer possible might be thought to be significant, because the preclusion of twinning is necessary for individuation, which is necessary for individuated agency. However, although this might have some emotive appeal, its force in an argument is unclear simply because the fact that possession of property X is necessary for property Y and possession of property Y is sufficient for all R rights to be granted, it does not follow that possession of property X is sufficient for some R rights to be granted.

The Principle of Potentiality: The human embryo is not an agent, but it might be claimed that it is a potential agent, and that some rights protection is owed to it by virtue of this potential.

This idea is open to a logical objection. Judith Jarvis Thomson hints at this when she remarks that 'A newly fertilised ovum, a newly implanted clump of cells, is no more a person than an acorn is an oak tree' (Thomson 1977, p.112-113). And the point is better made by Stanley Benn who points out that '[a] potential president of the United States is not on that account Commander-in-Chief [of the U.S. Army and Navy]' (Benn 1973, p.102) which the actual president would be. The point is that a human embryo has wholly different properties from a human agent, from which it is alleged to follow that we need not (indeed cannot) treat it as though it were a human agent.

Nevertheless, it might be argued that for an agent to fail to grant rights to potential agents requires the agent (by the demands of universalisation) to concede that it would have been permissible for the agent himself or herself to have been damaged or destroyed at the embryo stage, and that to do this is something that the agent cannot rationally will. There are, however, at least two problems with this. First, such an argument requires it to be accepted that agents cannot rationally will that they were never agents, which is not self-evident. Secondly, the argument requires the agent to put himself or herself in the position of the potential agent and treat this position as his or her own. But there is a crucial difference between the positions of the potential agent and the actual agent, viz. that the potential agent cannot put itself in the position of the actual agent. For universalisation to work it is necessary for the positions of the potential and actual agent to be relevantly similar. But, since that is just what the argument is trying to show, it cannot assume this without begging the question at issue.

In addition there are problems concerning the concept of potentiality. Is every human embryo a potential agent? Not all human embryos are viable. Even if some embryos develop into fetuses and go to full-term and are born live, they might be so severely handicapped (even anencephalic) that they can never be agents. Thus, it might be argued, even if potentiality is something that is sufficient for some rights, it is not possible to determine when it applies.

However, when dealing, for example, with the question of the rights of certain nonhuman higher mammals, such as chimpanzees, it is possible to appeal to a precautionary principle to grant rights to these creatures. Certain mammals, such as gorillas, chimpanzees, and dolphins have remarkable capacities. So much so that there can be genuine uncertainty whether or not they are agents. The precautionary principle specifies that because the consequences of treating agents as nonagents is morally dire, uncertain agents are to be treated (insofar as possible) as agents. While there can be no reasonable uncertainty about whether human embryos are or are not agents (they clearly are not) the precautionary principle can be applied to uncertainty about their status as *potential* agents, and this consideration, I suggest is capable of alleviating some of the difficulties associated with determination of potentiality.

There is the thought too, though whether it properly reflects proportionality or potentiality is not wholly clear, that being an embryo is a necessary stage for becoming an agent (at least in the case of biological human beings) and something might be made of the idea that being an embryo is thus a necessary condition of agency in being a necessary condition for becoming an agent.[2]

Arguments for indirect status

The brutalisation argument: It might be argued that to show disregard for the life or well-being of the human embryo shows a disregard for the life of human beings generally. By permitting harm to be caused to human embryos, we brutalise ourselves and make ourselves less sensitive to the rights of human agents. Not to be protective towards human embryos is to threaten the rights of human agents. The human embryo is, thus, to be granted rights vicariously as an expression of the rights of human agents.

One difficulty with such an argument is that it rests very much on empirical evidence that is, at best, lacking.

The psychological damage argument: Many human beings have strong protective feelings towards unborn children. There is an evolutionary explanation for this, as it is quite plausible that protective feelings for the young, including the unborn, confer an evolutionary advantage. This being so, to show a disregard for the well-being of the human embryo is to cause great distress, even psychological damage to those who have (natural, and, indeed generally beneficial emotional responses). Most importantly, to cause them this damage is to violate their rights. Again, the human embryo is to be granted rights vicariously.

Once again, however, this argument rests on empirical assumptions that need testing.[3]

The property argument: It might be argued that the human embryo is the property of its genetic parents (or, at least of its mother). As such, if the mother wishes her embryo to be protected, then the embryo is to be granted that protection.

The obvious difficulty with this argument rests in the idea that the embryo can be property (anyone's property). This is a complex issue that has not to my mind received satisfactory treatment anymore than has the question of whether human tissue can be the property of its possessor.[4] However, if the human embryo can be property then this argument has considerable force.

The contractual argument: Rights are of different kinds. The generic rights that Gewirth argues for are rights that agents must grant simply by virtue of being agents. They might, however, between themselves contract for protections not granted generically and might waive the benefits of rights-protection amongst themselves. In effect, they may use their right to freedom to extend or diminish the protection afforded by the generic rights (amongst consenting agents).

This suggests that, even if the human embryo need not be granted rights simply by virtue of being a human embryo, it might be granted rights (equivalent even to generic rights) by agents who wish to impose the correlative duties on themselves.

An obvious difficulty with this suggestion arises in connection with the imposition of duties (via these rights) on persons who are not party to the contract in question. This will happen more or less inevitably if granted at a societal level, simply because no societies exist in which there is absolute consensus. It may, however, be possible to deal with this in accordance with the same sorts of principles that are used to justify similar impositions in democratic polities.

Two suggestions

Most of these arguments are, I think, inconclusive at best. I would, however, like to make two suggestions.

The first is that, whatever the problems of using potentiality to argue that the human embryo should not be destroyed, the fact of potentiality (or its uncertain possibility) does, I think, generate valid reasons for not damaging the embryo and then allowing it to become an agent. If and when the damaged embryo becomes an agent it will have whatever rights are accorded to agents. An intention to bring into existence a damaged agent is, I suggest, exactly on a par with an intention to damage an existing agent.

The second suggestion is that, while an appeal to the principle of proportionality may not be successful in conferring direct protection on the human embryo (or partial agents generally), it would seem to have undeniable force when used in the context of vicarious arguments. Thus, e.g., the more properties of agency that a creature possesses the more likely it is that ill-treatment of that creature will have a brutalisation effect or a psychological damage effect, and so on.

The legal status of the human embryo

The legal status of the human embryo varies considerably from one European Union country to the next. I shall not attempt a detailed survey, but merely indicate the range of variation.[5]

- EU countries range from having no specific laws regulating the treatment of human embryos (leaving the use of human embryos, at one extreme, entirely to the policy of hospitals or various medical bodies), through regulation on the advice of national bioethics councils or professional bodies, to having comprehensive and specific legislation.
- Whereas some countries permit (or at least do not prohibit) research on surplus embryos created for in vitro fertilisation (IVF), others prohibit this (including Germany and Austria); while Sweden only permits such research for the purpose of improving IVF treatment.
- Some countries (including the UK) permit the creation of human embryos specifically for research, whereas others (e.g., Austria, France, Germany, Spain, and Sweden) do not.
- Time limits for the duration of human embryo culture (where permitted) are, however, generally set at 14 days.
- Not all countries permit the freezing of human embryos, and those that do impose different time limits for storage – e.g., 1 year in Austria and 5 years in Spain. Furthermore, in some countries limits set may not be extended, whereas in others (e.g., Sweden and the UK) they may be extended under varying conditions.
- Some countries legislate the disposal of embryos (e.g., France, Spain, and the UK), whereas other do not.
- Some countries specifically permit the creation of human embryo banks (e.g., the UK), whereas others (e.g., Sweden) do not.
- Some countries permit artificial division of human embryos (e.g., Denmark), whereas others (e.g., Germany and Spain) do not.
- Embryo cloning (by nuclear transfer), and the gestation of embryos in a nonhuman environment (including ectogenesis) are, however, generally not permitted.
- It is generally impermissible to attempt to implant embryos after they have been subjected to research procedures (although Denmark does not rule this out if it can be done without transmitting defects).

The reasons for this variation are no doubt complex, and merit study. Certainly, they cannot be accounted for wholly, or even mainly, by whether or not the country in question is mainly Catholic, Protestant, or Secular (although this factor would seem to account for differences in practices between, e.g., the Catholic and Free Universities of Belgium).

Whatever the reasons for it, this absence of consensus is significant from a moral point of view. The scope for EU citizens or scientists to evade prohibitions existing in one country by transferring to another country (or utilising its services) is considerable, and this serves to nullify the effect of legislation which may be driven by moral objections.

In the final section of this paper, I shall sketch an approach to the search for a moral consensus that lays claim to legal force within the EU countries and may thus be a foundation for harmonisation within the EU.

Sketch of an approach to a legal-moral consensus

All countries in the EU are party to the European Convention on Human Rights (ECHR) (and other human rights Conventions). The rights enshrined in these Conventions reflect a consensus about morality that has legally binding force within the EU.[6] It is tempting, therefore, to say that, insofar as the variation in legislation concerning the human embryo reflects moral disagreement in the EU countries, these can be referred to the ECHR (in particular) for adjudication. However, the matter is not that simple. For one thing, the ECHR is thought by many to grant considerable derogatory powers to individual governments in relation to its provisions. For another, it does not explicitly declare how possible conflicts of rights are to be adjudicated. And finally, although the Convention prescribes that

> [t]he enjoyment of the rights and freedoms set forth in this Convention shall be secured without discrimination on any ground such as sex, race, colour, language, religion, political or other opinion, national or social origin, association with a national minority, property, birth or other status

it does not specify whether or not the subjects of these rights are human beings (biologically defined) or human beings more narrowly defined (as persons or agents). Unless these difficulties can be overcome, appeal to the ECHR will be of little practical value.

However, on the issue of derogatory powers, at least, there should be nothing to argue about, simply because Article 14 of the ECHR, in effect, specifies that the rights granted by the ECHR are held simply by virtue of being 'human', howsoever this is to be understood. If this is so, then the rights enshrined in the ECHR cannot be derogated from except for the sake of more important rights of similar status. As far as the issue of the interpretation of being human is concerned, it should be noted that 'may' implies 'can' as much as 'ought' does, and this means that rights cannot meaningfully be granted to those who do not have the power to exercise them. The rights enshrined in the ECHR (as civil and political rights) are, at least focally, rights that require the powers of agency to exercise and are not possessed simply by being human (biologically defined).

This, however, does not deal with the second issue, which concerns how various rights and goals are to be weighed against each other. And it also does not deal with the question as to whether any of the rights that are focally directed at agents may be extended to protection of the human embryo (and other beings with some, but not all, of the necessary conditions of agency).

In order to tackle these problems, I suggest that it can be shown that anyone who recognises *any* human rights must, on pain of contradicting that this acceptance is an acceptance of human rights (in the sense applicable to civil and political rights as well as to social and economic rights), accept a particular moral principle, Alan Gewirth's 'Principle of Generic Consistency' (PGC)[7] as the principle for identifying, interpreting, and ordering human rights. The ECHR (and other human rights instruments) must, therefore, be interpreted in line with the PGC. If this argument is valid then law and morality within the EU must be referred to the PGC as the ultimate principle of validity (both moral and legal), *unless* adherence to the idea that there are human rights is given up.[8]

The principle of generic consistency

The PGC states, 'Act in accordance with rights to the generic conditions of agency of your recipients as well as of yourself'.

According to this principle, all agents have inalienable rights to the generic conditions (or features) of agency (GF). GF fall into two main categories.

(a) Things like life, freedom of action (in the sense of the capacity to guide one's actions by one's own maxims), sufficient mental equilibrium to give active expression to one's desires, and anything else that is necessary for the *possibility of even attempting to act*, interfering with which will have a systematic restrictive or adverse effect on the possibility of even attempting to act (e.g., clothing, health, shelter, food, and the necessary means to these).

(b) Things like accurate information, interference with which will have a systematic adverse effect on one's ability *to succeed* in the pursuit of one's goals.

GF that fit category (a) are termed 'basic', whereas those that fit into (b) fall into two further categories:

(i) Things, like having others be truthful and keeping their promises, that are needed to maintain the capacities for purpose-achievement that one already possesses – which are termed 'nonsubtractive'.

(ii) Things, like educational provision in accordance with one's abilities, that are necessary to improve one's existing capacities for purpose achievement in accordance with ones potential – which are termed 'additive'.

The rights granted by the PGC are

- both negative and positive, negative rights being rights to non-interference with the objects of the rights, positive rights being rights to provision of or to assistance with securing the objects of the rights;
- claim-rights, these being correlative to duties on the part of other agents not to interfere with what the right-holder has a right to *against the will of the right-holder* (or to provide or assist the right-holder with what the right-holder has a right to *if the right-holder so wishes*);
- (as a structure) held equally and reciprocally by all agents: in holding rights against other agents, agents owe equal duties to these other agents.

The rights granted by the PGC cannot be overridden by *any* considerations except (in case of conflict) by more important rights within the structure of rights granted by the PGC, importance to be assessed by a criterion of degrees of necessity according to which rights to the basic GF are more important than rights to the nonsubtractive GF, which are more important than rights to the additive GF (because possession of the basic GF is necessary for possession of the nonsubtractive GF, but not vice versa, etc.).

The argument for the PGC from the acceptance of human rights

This argument runs as follows.

(1) Anyone who grants that someone *(X)* has a right to have or do something *(p)* must grant that *X* has a right to the means *(m)* to having or to doing *p* (and this is true whatever *p* might be). (For *X* not to grant rights to *m* is, at least implicitly, for *X* to retract the grant of a right to have or to do *p*.)
(2) Therefore, *if* there are conditions for the pursuit and achievement of rights, *whatever these rights might be* (generic conditions of rights [GCR]), then anyone who grants rights to anyone must grant these persons rights to the GCR.
(3) If there are GF then they will also be GCR.
(4) There are GF.
(5) Therefore, there are GCR.
(6) A rational person (one who observes canons of deductive and inductive logic and seeks efficient means to pursue his/her purposes) will attach more importance to the basic GCR than to the nonsubtractive GCR than to the additive GCR. Within each of these categories a rational person will attach more importance to those conditions, interference with which has a more proximate and extensive effect in interfering with the possibility of

action/successful action. The GCR are, in this sense, to be ordered in importance according to a criterion of degrees of necessity.

(7) Therefore, anyone who grants that *X* has a right to have or do something (no matter what this might be) rationally must grant that *X* has rights to the GCR in accordance with the criterion of degrees of necessity.

(8) Anyone who holds that there are human rights (rights held simply by virtue of being human) rationally must hold that all human beings have human rights to the GCR in accordance with the criterion of degrees of necessity.

(9) At least insofar as human beings, as the recipients of rights, are capable of exercising rights (as the civil and political rights Conventions suppose), being human is to be interpreted, at least focally, as being an agent.

(10) At least insofar as the grant of human rights has this restriction, the supreme principle of human rights rationally must be taken to be the PGC.

It is, of course, perfectly possible that a Convention on human rights as a Convention might grant rights that the PGC does not grant, grant rights that the PGC prohibits, or simply fail to grant rights that the PGC requires. Nevertheless, the argument to the PGC from the supposition of human rights entails that such a Convention must, as a Convention on human rights, be governed by the PGC, and this fact places severe constraints upon the interpretation of a Convention on human rights conceived as a Convention on human rights.

The general rules of interpretation are as follows.

I. Where a Convention grants rights explicitly that the PGC does not grant then, *provided that the PGC does not prohibit the grant of such rights,* such a grant will be legitimate under the 'indirect' applications[9] of the PGC (provided that the Convention itself is authorised by the PGC).

II. Where a Convention merely fails to grant rights explicitly that the PGC requires, the Convention is to be taken as granting these rights implicitly, on the same ground that requires the Convention to be regarded as operating with the PGC itself (even when it does not declare the PGC explicitly as its governing principle) – viz., that anyone who claims that there are human rights must, on pain of contradicting this claim, assent to and use the PGC as the principle determining these rights (and, similarly, must assent to the rights that derive directly from the PGC). To deny that the PGC is the governing principle of what is alleged to be a Convention on human rights, or to fail to use the PGC as the governing principle of such a Convention, is to contradict that the Convention is a Convention *on human rights*.

III. Where a Convention grants rights explicitly that the PGC requires not to be granted, then – on a strict interpretation – such grant must be considered to be invalid, an error made by the drafters of the Convention. However, a strict interpretation need not always be given. What the PGC requires is, to some extent, dependent on particular circumstances. This is because the PGC grants rights according to a criterion of degrees of necessity for action and successful action, which ranks particular rights in three levels (and also ranks rights within these levels hierarchically), and determines which rights are to be given precedence when rights come into conflict. However, whether or not the rights of individuals will come into conflict will depend on contingent circumstances attending social interaction. Thus, although the PGC is the absolute principle of human rights, the rights it grants are, with one exception,[10] not absolute, but depend upon contingent circumstances attending the interaction of individuals. Now, although the PGC does not, for the most part, grant rights absolutely, there are rights that will only be capable of being overridden by other rights in extreme situations. In most circumstances, these rights will pertain. Because they have this status, such rights might be articulated explicitly in a Convention even though there are circumstances in which the PGC would overrule them. As such, on a weaker interpretation, human rights conventions are not to be rejected because they enshrine rules that do not have absolute validity under the PGC. Provided that such rules for rights have validity under the PGC in most circumstances, they may be treated as 'rules of thumb' for rights. It is only where rights are granted that the PGC generally would not grant, that it becomes necessary to declare the rights to be invalid or, in extreme cases, to reject the Convention.

Conclusion

In applying the PGC, many details remain to be worked out. However, one thing is certain: if the arguments I have just presented are valid, then as long as debate about the moral/legal status of the human embryo is to take place within the context of a recognition of human rights, this debate is to be referred to the kind of consideration indicated in the first part of this paper by reference to the PGC.

Notes

1 For a general discussion of Gewirth's use of his Principle of Proportionality, see the criticism by James F. Hill (1984) and the reply by Gewirth in the same volume at pp.225–227.

2 Insofar as Gewirth appeals to potentiality to grant rights to the unborn, he appears to have something like this in mind (Gewirth, 1978, pp.143–144). Not to be confused with this consideration, it might also be contended that to deny protection to the human embryo is to threaten the human species.

However, this will not provide protection for specific embryos. Furthermore, whatever force it has rests on the idea that it would be morally wrong to bring it about that there will be no future agents, which is not self-evident.

3 For a discussion of various indirect arguments (albeit in the context of the issue of rights of non-human animals), see Peter Carruthers (1992).

4 A wide-ranging, but not to my mind very helpful discussion, is contained in the Report by the Nuffield Council on Bioethics (1995).

5 I am grateful to Lorna Leaston for providing me with a summary of the current regulatory position, from which this résumé is derived.

6 The UK, and some Scandinavian countries adhere to a doctrine of dualism according to which ratified international treaties do not automatically become part of domestic law, but only if and when incorporated by domestic statute (which the UK has not done in relation to the ECHR). I have argued elsewhere that this is an incoherent doctrine in relation to human rights treaties (See Beyleveld 1995). In any case, due to the European Communities Act 1972 and the practice of the European Court of Justice to declare anything illegal that violates the ECHR, it is obvious that the ECHR has been indirectly incorporated into UK law (See Browne-Wilkinson, 1992, pp.399-402).

7 Gewirth does not argue from the acceptance of human rights (which acceptance requires justification), but from an agent's claim to be an agent. Gewirth maintains that an agent contradicts that it is an agent if it does not accept the PGC or violates it in practice. I defend this argument in Beyleveld 1991.

8 For a presentation of this argument, Gewirth's own argument, and some other arguments for accepting the PGC, see Beyleveld 1996.

9 To apply the PGC directly is to deduce what the PGC requires from the PGC, together with the circumstances of the application. However, it may not always be possible to determine what the PGC requires in this way. This is because (a) the circumstances may be so complex that persons can reasonably disagree about what the PGC requires in these cases; or (b) the decision that needs to be made is optional in terms of the PGC (e.g., driving on the left-hand side of the road v. driving on the right-hand side), but is one that must be made because persons cannot be permitted to perform either option indiscriminately. The PGC handles these cases by prescribing (in its direct application) legitimate dispute-resolution procedures. Decisions made according to these procedures are indirect applications of the PGC. The conditions of legitimacy and the binding of these applications are discussed in detail in Beyleveld and Brownsword 1994.

10 This is the right of an innocent person not to be killed against his/her will.

References

Benn, S.I. (1973), 'Abortion, Infanticide, and Respect for Persons', in Feinberg, J. (ed.), *The Problem of Abortion,* Wadsworth: Belmont, California, p. 102.

Beyleveld, D. (1991), *The Dialectical Necessity of Morality: An Analysis and Defense of Alan Gewirth's Argument to the Principle of Generic Consistency*, University of Chicago Press: Chicago.

Beyleveld, D. and Brownsword, R. (1994), *Law as a Moral Judgment*, Sheffield Academic Press: Sheffield.

Beyleveld, D. (1995), 'The Concept of a Human Right and Incorporation of the European Convention on Human Rights', *Public Law*, pp. 577–98.

Beyleveld, D. (1996), 'Legal Theory and Dialectically Contingent Justifications for the Principle of Generic Consistency', *Ratio Juris*, Vol. 9, No. 1, pp. 15–41.

Browne-Wilkinson, L. (1992), 'The Infiltration of a Bill of Rights', *Public Law*, pp. 397–410.

Carruthers, P. (1992), *The Animals Issue: Moral Theory in Practice*, Cambridge University Press: Cambridge.

Gewirth, A. (1978), *Reason and Morality*, University of Chicago Press: Chicago.

Gewirth, A. (1984), 'Reply', in Regis, E., Jr. (ed.), *Gewirth's Ethical Rationalism: Critical Essays With a Reply by Alan Gewirth,* University of Chicago Press: Chicago, pp. 225–7.

Gewirth, A. (1996), *The Community of Rights*, University of Chicago Press: Chicago.

Hill, J.F. (1984), 'Are Marginal Agents «Our Recipients»?', in Regis, E., Jr. (ed.), *Gewirth's Ethical Rationalism: Critical Essays With a Reply by Alan Gewirth,* University of Chicago Press: Chicago, pp. 180-91.

Nuffield Council on Bioethics (1995), *Human Tissue: Ethical and Legal Issues,* Nuffield Council on Bioethics: London.

Thomson, J.J. (1977), 'A Defence of Abortion', in Dworkin, R.M. (ed.), *The Philosophy of Law*, Oxford University Press: London, (reprinted from *Philosophy and Public Affairs* Vol. 1, No. 1, 1971, pp.46-77).

3 The legal status of the human embryo

Hans-Georg Koch

In this short comment I cannot deal with all the details of the imaginative presentation made by Deryck Beyleveld (1997). Instead, I have to restrict myself to some notes and reflections.

To begin with the general question of status: Every opinion about the embryo's status is confronted with certain difficulties in trying to conform to common legal rules. It is difficult, for example, to substantiate why abortion is widely allowed – as it is in some countries –, if the 'early' embryo is granted its own status as a (developing) human being. It is, on the other hand, difficult to refer to criteria like 'rational being with a will' or 'agent' and to apply these criteria to new born children, whose intellect has not yet developed or to apply them to human beings who have largely lost their intellectual capabilities (e.g., by an accident) but who are nevertheless not deprived of the attribute 'human' by the legal system. After all, the cause of these difficulties is the fact that in virtually all legal systems the event of birth is a significant moment with regard to a persons's legal protection – also in countries where even a child 'capable of being born alive' enjoys increased legal protection. Opinions questioning the 'moral importance' of birth in favour of a legal protection which becomes effective already in an early phase of the developing process argue in many ways inconsistently – as can be demonstrated, for example, by their refusal of ectogenesis.

Apparently birth means something like a definite initiation into human society. But this also means that, although it is a natural event that produces this legal step, it is not only a step of nature but also a process of legal attribution and thus a value judgment.

Of course you can dispute to which 'natural event' during the development of the embryo such an attribution should be tied, whether the full moral status should be reached abruptly or – similar to the development's process-character

– whether it should be possible to distinguish between certain gradations. In my opinion, the better arguments seem to support the latter position.

This argument is not necessary to justify abortion – which can be justified, for example, by viewing abortion as a privilege granted to the pregnant woman considering that she is being 'used' by the embryo and that she does not have to tolerate this 'utilisation' under all circumstances. In contrast to this, the crucial question is the extent to which it is permissible to instrumentalise the embryo in the interest of a third person, for example, a physician performing research.

Professor Beyleveld showed that this problem is treated very differently in the various European countries. The Convention on Human Rights and Biomedicine (Council of Europe 1996) does not clarify the situation either, in formulating (Art. 18 (1)): 'Where the law allows research on embryos in vitro, it shall ensure adequate protection of the embryo'. It is not surprising that – in Germany – a general prohibition of the so-called 'verbrauchende Forschung' (research which destroys embryos) is derived from this paragraph (see the statement from the German Federal Government, p.3). Unequivocal – and presumably capable of leading to consensus – is Art. 18 (2): 'The creation of human embryos for research purposes is prohibited'.

In my opinion, it is a problem which requires weighing up. To mention only a few problems, the creation of human embryos for non-reproductive purposes must be clearly rejected. Such an instrumentalisation, so to speak 'ab ovo', would be incompatible with the German Constitution's conception of what it means to be human. The production of chimerae or hybrid beings using human genetic material seems to me to be not only a question of individual human dignity, but also a question of the way the human species sees itself, so to speak of the 'dignity of humankind'. It may be necessary to regulate some reproduction measures like cryoconservation (freezing of embryos) – but in my opinion they do not have to be prohibited. As to the problems resulting from the possibility of 'split' motherhood, other questions about the legal (and moral) status of an embryo may be in the foreground. The most difficult question is the permissibility of scientific research in which surplus in-vitro embryos are destroyed. I do not think that a ban without exception would be necessary if strategies were designed to prevent the creation of 'embryos doomed to die'. This estimation is mainly based on the opinion that in-vitro embryos have a lower status. I think there are good arguments supporting this position, above all the viewpoint of the 'reduced potentiality'. An embryo not yet implanted in the uterus has only a provisional chance of becoming a human being. The discussion about a brain-dead woman's pregnancy which was maintained artificially ('Erlanger Baby') show that we consider a certain period of 'intrauterine interaction' between mother and fetus to be essential for human genesis and that this period is just as important as the genetic development. To my mind, it would therefore be an inappropriate reduction to the 'genetic point of view' to give a full legal (and moral) status to the embryo simply from the moment of fertilisation.

References

Beyleveld, D. (1997), 'The Moral and Legal Status of the Human Embryo', this volume, Part Seven.

Council of Europe (1996), *Convention on Human Rights and Biomedicine*, Directorate of Legal Affairs: Strasbourg.

German Federal Government, Bundestags-Drucksache 13/5435.

4 Legal regulations in Europe

Calum MacKellar

Since the first successful case of in vitro fertilisation (IVF) in 1978 and its extension to genetic diagnosis, a multiplication of technological and medical possibilities often far removed from the initial scientific discovery has been initiated. Not only can the eggs and sperm of a specific married couple be used for fertilisation but a variety of possible new techniques in assisted reproduction resulting from the IVF process are now present. With the assistance of these new reproductive possibilities towards childlessness being generally recognised as progress, they have, nonetheless, created extensive new ethical problems for our societies. Moreover, no discussion concerning embryology is possible without also examining the diverging and controversial status of parenthood and the status of the human embryo. Though comprehensive debates concerning what should be permissible and where an uninfrigeable moral line should be drawn regarding these techniques have begun, most governments in Europe are still trying to find a legislative solution to the complex ethical problems being studied.

Initially most countries developed guidelines contained in 'rules for guidance' with some additional circulars which were not legally binding per se. However, due to the explosive growth of the fertilisation techniques these guidelines have quickly become new legislation throughout most of Europe. When one considers the different legal regulations of IVF in the European Union and other European states, from an international perspective, it also becomes evident that a real mosaic of diverse regulations is present corresponding to the specific legislative directions each country has taken. Every government has walked down the road of bioethical regulation at their own pace and manner with often the most minimal considerations towards international cooperation. Though a precise comparison between the different regulations concerning IVF in the respective countries would be extremely time consuming it is possible to analyse the most important points from the examples of some national legislations:

Required forms of cohabitation: This can vary from no legal requirements concerning marriage or a one-to-one relationship, as in Great Britain, to the condition found in Italy or France where the couple must be heterosexual and either married or have been living in common-law marriage for at least two years.

Consent: There is a general agreement throughout the European countries that written consent must be obtained before any treatment.

Surrogacy: Only a few countries have any legislation concerning the carrying of a child by a woman for the benefit of an infertile woman who will become the future mother. In Great Britain and Denmark, surrogacy is only allowed under the condition that no money is paid for the service. In Norway, on the other hand, the practice is forbidden altogether.

Storage of sperm, eggs and embryos: The storage of sperm, by cryopreservation, is far less regulated, if at all, than for eggs or embryos where more stringent regulations are effective. This can vary from being banned altogether as in Denmark or Switzerland or being possible for up to five or even ten years, in special cases, as in Great Britain.

Identity of sperm and egg donors: A great variety of legislations exist between each set of national regulations. In Germany there is no donor anonymity for sperm donors whereas in Britain donors are anonymous. In France it has been established by law that recipients and donors of unfertilised and fertilised eggs may not be informed of each other's identity. If, however, there is a therapeutic necessity, there is the option for a doctor to give medical information about the donor couple, though without them being identified.

Embryo and sex selection: Most legislations allowing the fertilisation of supernumerary embryos make it possible, when there is a risk of genetic disease, to identify and select unaffected embryos for procreation through preimplantation diagnosis. In some countries, however, this procedure is not possible. In Germany, for example, the Embryo Protection Act specifically prohibits the use of a human embryo for any purpose other than its maintenance and healthy development. Since the cell taken from an embryo for preimplantation diagnosis is totipotent and could, theoretically, also develop into a human being, German legislation has proscribed the technique.

Conditions for in vitro fertilisation: The two possibilities presented are homologous IVF, where the gametes are provided from the hopeful couple and heterologous IVF where the gametes of a donor are used. In Denmark there are no specific rules of law for accepting unfertilised eggs and sperm. In Norway, however, treatment may only be carried out with the couple's own eggs and sperm. Additionally, though most countries do not have a specific age-limit for IVF, it is generally agreed that the technique should be discouraged after a woman's 45th year.

Donation of embryos: Here again a great variety exists in the legislation. In Great Britain embryo adoption is made possible, on condition of written consent from the donors. In Austria, however, the donation of fertilised eggs is forbidden.

Utilisation of embryos: An often lively debate has preceded the legislation concerning the destiny of embryos, especially with respect to research. In Germany together with some other countries, embryos can only be used for implantation into a woman. By contrast, for some countries like Sweden, non-therapeutic research is permitted, but regulated. Experiments on fertilised eggs are only acceptable if performed within 14 days after fertilisation and if the donors of egg and sperm cells have consented. Experiments may not be aimed at developing methods for achieving potential hereditary genetic effects. A fertilised egg which has been subject to experimentation is to be destroyed after the stated time. Finally, for a minority of countries, no formal political or legal decisions have yet been taken, though, in the absence of directly relevant laws, experiments may be accepted through recommendations of an ethical committee or 'code of practice' promulgated by a professional body, without legal force.

The great variety of legal regulations reflects the different moral heritages of each country corresponding to the many aspects of traditions, customs and in some cases the degree of possible relationships between a state and a respective religious and moral persuasion. This is the case, for example, in the Republic of Ireland, where the authority of the Catholic Church is very much respected. In countries like Switzerland, on the other hand, it is the legislative process itself with the possibility of a national referendum, that has enabled its citizens to reflect, discuss and decide for themselves the complex issues at stake. In May 1992 after a referendum on the 'Misuse of reproduction and genetic technologies' the Swiss citizens decided by 1,270,816 votes (73.8 per cent) against 450,676 votes (26.2 per cent) for fertilising only as many eggs outside the woman's body as can be implanted without delay and to prohibit the donation of embryos and the use of surrogate mothers.

The diversity in legislation between the various countries can also reflect the solutions to sociological problems encountered by them to the new medical possibilities related to IVF. It has been observed that the lack of legislation for a specific social problem has often resulted in a legal crisis leading some national parliaments to legislate quickly in often very controversial circumstances. Though the resulting decisions are acknowledged to be incomplete and imperfect, the lack of time, limiting appropriate informed and encompassing discussions which would have been required, is made responsible for the legal imperfections. This was the case in Great Britain, where members of parliament were obliged to legislate, after an emergency late sitting, the possibility for scientists to fertilise eggs from aborted female human foetuses. The resulting prohibition was contested by many scientists as being inappropriate and without a suitable discussion by the general public.

A possible assistance in such difficult situations could be envisaged through a comparison of the different legal regulations in Europe on IVF. It would then be possible to study some of the problems arising in some countries to the advantage of others where such problems have not yet been experienced. Indeed it is always better to learn from other peoples' mistakes than from one's own. The comparison of legal frameworks and their corresponding problems can then be considered as a positive and useful procedure through the assistance and information it could provide to the legislators. Moreover, it would greatly enhance the knowledge of considerations and experiences to be taken into account in any new legislation. International cooperation in this field would contribute, additionally, to a possible European consensus on the most important and sensitive problems facing humanity, as for example the mixing of human gametes with those of other species, while continuing to respect the moral traditions and customs of each country.

Legislative cooperation would additionally discourage 'bioethical tourism' in the field of IVF which is sometimes envisaged as a simple but often morally difficult solution to some sociological problems. Recently, in Great Britain, the press extensively reported the case of Diane Blood, a widow, whose husband died from meningitis. Mrs Blood asked the Human Fertilisation and Embryology Authority of Great Britain for permission to use sperm taken from her husband while he was dying to try to obtain a child. The Embryology Authority, however, turned down the application on the grounds that her husband had not given specific written consent. Mrs Blood then appealed against the Authority, suggesting the possibility of taking her husbands sperm abroad to a country where such insemination would be possible. This was again rejected by the Authority but a review of the decision was decided. Finally, following extensive discussions concerning additional facts submitted by Mrs Blood, her request to undertake the procedure abroad was accepted.

In conclusion, though many legislations throughout Europe may vary considerably, the legal framework in the field of IVF must be accepted as an on-going process requiring the most careful precautions and discussions. Even the manner by which legislation is decided is open to controversy. Should decisions be taken by referenda of whole populations or should a free-vote by their members of parliament be sufficient? Indeed are moral problems best decided by a majority-vote or should one just accept the guidelines proposed by an ethical committee or the dogmatical directives of a religious persuasion? These are difficult questions. The possibility of international cooperation throughout the European Union should, therefore, be considered as one of the most valuable sources of assistance in this important area.

5 A distinct category? About the moral status of human surplus embryos

Egbert Schroten

In applied ethics, the issue of the moral status of human surplus embryos can be phrased in terms of the question: What ought (not) to be done to/with them, and why? Deryck Beyleveld, in his clear and thoroughgoing lecture on the moral and legal status of the human embryo, rightly points out that the answer to this question essentially depends on:

> (1) which characteristics are deemed necessary or sufficient for beings to be owed any duties of respect or concern for their interests or welfare, on the one hand, or rights in terms of their interests or welfare, on the other; and
> (2) on certain beliefs about the ontological status of the human embryo – its nature, capacities and powers. (Beyleveld, 1997, p.247)

Against this background, he makes many useful distinctions. In my short statement, I want to add another distinction which, from a moral point of view, seems to be important as well.

In Western cultural history, the issue of the moral status of the human embryo has been discussed within the context of abortion.[1] Whether there was a social reason (for instance family planning in some circles in the Roman Empire) or a medical reason, there was no question of surplus embryos. An embryo was an embryo in the future mother's womb, and thus taken to be a future child. And in the medical setting there was always in the foreground or in the background, the difficult question of having to choose between the life of the mother and that of the future child. In other words, whatever positions were taken – medical, moral, philosophical, theological – the status of the human embryo was discussed in the context of a parental relationship. Various 'theories' (for instance the *pars viscerum matris* model, in which the fetus is seen as part of the intestines of the future mother) point in this direction.

Although the problem of abortion is still with us, through the various forms of in vitro fertilisation (IVF) we now face a new situation: medically assisted procreation. In this situation there are human embryos in vitro, which means that they are not in the womb. As long as these embryos are (to be) transferred, we could see them, and for that matter treat them, as if they were embryos in the womb and, therefore, future children in spe, i.e. we hope them to be children, eventually. However, the so-called surplus embryos, which are for one reason or another not transferred, are in a peculiar position. In vitro or in cryo-preservation, they are still human embryos but (at least for the time being) not future children in spe.

Does that make a difference? I think, it does. The presupposition is that we cannot reduce a human being to its genetic make up. Of course, the genetic make up is a necessary condition for being a human being (Schroten 1994). But the reason why we, traditionally, care a great deal about human embryos is that they are taken to be future children. The famous classic expression of Tertullian (± 200 A.D.) is symptomatic: *Homo est et qui est futurus* (human is also who will be human).

With IVF, as with other technologies, we are confronted with an extension of our responsibility, which means in practice an extension of the realm of decision-making. Through IVF, we have brought ourselves into the position where we have at our disposal human embryos who are not future children in spe, because for one reason or another (e.g. biological), we decide not to transfer them into the womb. It means that IVF makes it necessary to distinguish between two categories of human embryos: embryos to be transferred and surplus embryos, i.e. embryos not to be transferred. Embryos in the first category (including embryos for donation) should be treated as embryos in the womb, as future children in spe or in terms of Alan Gewirth and Deryck Beyleveld, as future agents in spe. Embryos in the second category, although they are human embryos, are not future agents in spe. However, they are not 'mere' human tissue or 'biological material' either. The point I want to make is that human surplus embryos should be treated as a distinct category.

If we follow what is worked out in Deryck Beyleveld's contribution, it would mean that surplus embryos, not being future agents in spe, should not be accorded maximal moral status. To emphasise the peculiarity of this category and our respect for them in sharing human genetic inheritance, one could argue for their destruction, since research on these embryos would imply using them in a purely instrumental way. Nevertheless, I would argue for the possibility of research on surplus embryos on teleological grounds. If, and only if, it is clear that an important human therapeutic aim cannot be attained by other means, research on these embryos might be allowed under very strict conditions (which is necessary, for instance in view of the possibility of 'industrialisation' of embryo production) (Council of Europe, 1996, Art. 18,2). To avoid misunderstanding, informed consent of the partners is presupposed.

If we accept this way of reasoning, it implies a case by case approach and a *broadly based* multidisciplinary licensing body to assess, monitor and control the research, within a legal framework which clearly indicates the limits within which such a research can be done (for instance a time limit, such as 14 days).

Notes

1 I want to take the opportunity to announce a thesis of one of my PhD students, Jan te Lindert, on this subject, which will be published probably towards the end of 1997.

References

Beyleveld, D. (1997), 'The Moral and Legal Status of the Human Embryo', this volume, Part Seven.

Council of Europe (1996), *Convention on Human Rights and Biomedicine*, Strasbourg.

Schroten, E. (1994), 'What Makes a Person?', *Theology*, Vol. 97, No. 776, pp. 98ff.

6 Research on human embryos

Lorna Leaston

The legal status of the embryo varies considerably from one European country to another. Whilst the reasons for this are both varied and complex, and the proper subject of further research, I want to confine my observations to one notable feature common to a number of European jurisdictions.

It can be observed that many European jurisdictions – but notably not the UK – distinguish in legal terms between (a) the use of 'spare', or supernumerary, embryos for research and (b) the creation of embryos specifically for the purpose of research. Whilst most jurisdictions permit (a), many do not permit (b). Article 18 of the European Convention on Bioethics explicitly prohibits the creation of embryos solely for research purposes, while leaving open the question of research on embryos 'surplus' to requirements.

The significance of this distinction must not be overlooked. Legislation of a member-state prohibiting the creation of embryos solely for research purposes, can rely on this legislation to prevent access to diagnostic methods such as preimplantation diagnosis (PID). In PID an embryo is specifically created, through in vitro fertilisation techniques, for the purpose of testing and analysing its genetic make-up. On the basis of this information, a decision is made about whether or not to implant the embryo. Since the embryo has been created solely for research purposes, PID is often held to be objectionable.

Whilst there are numerous ethical objections to PID (Hildt 1996), I wish to focus solely on this objection, premised as it is upon a belief that there is a fundamental moral distinction between the research use of 'surplus' embryos, and the creation of embryos specifically for research purposes. If the distinction can be demonstrated to be an artificial one, based upon a logical fallacy – as I believe it can – then objections to 'research' of this kind, to be convincing, must be argued from a different premise.

According to the literature, many theorists posit a morally relevant difference between 'surplus' embryos produced as part of a programme designed to result in embryos for implantation, and 'research' embryos created solely for research purposes. The latter is often prohibited, or at least, disapproved of – on the grounds that there is something degrading about producing embryos at will merely for research purposes. The researcher is often held to be guilty of 'exploiting' the embryo; creating it in order to serve ends other than its own end, or good. However, as various commentators have noted, this argument wrongly presupposes the embryo has ends. To have ends, as Dieter Birnbacher notes in his paper (Birnbacher 1997), one must, as a minimum necessary condition, be conscious – which is not the case with the early embryo. Nor, he continues, can the embryo be said to be an end since ends pertain not to human beings, but to end-states which human beings desire to bring about.

There is a further problem. The argument rests on a logical fallacy, namely, that the idea that the mere creation of a human being can be regarded as its 'use'. Since being born is not considered a benefit (although being born healthy is), for parallel reasons the creation of an embryo for the purpose of therapeutic research cannot in itself be considered harmful or detrimental to the embryo. The point at issue is not its deliberate creation, but that of the experimental procedure to which it is subjected.

As such, there is no morally relevant difference between embryos already in existence because they are superfluous to requirements, or those who are intentionally created for research purposes.

Any legal protections to be accorded to the embryo in the form, for instance, of restrictions relating to the way embryos are to be treated as reseach subjects (if necessary at all), must be assigned to the embryo by virtue of its status as a moral agent, or to safeguard the claim-rights of fully-fledged agents who are affected in some way by the procedure. What is not permissible is that such protections are assigned to the embryo on the basis of a criterion relating to the initial intention of those who created them. Whether an embryo was deliberately created for research purposes, or for the purpose of implantation, is of no moral relevance; the legal status of the respective embryos ought, therefore, to be determined independently of considerations relating to the source of such material. Since it is claimed the distinction is a superficial one, the onus of responsibility for proving otherwise must rest with those European jurisdictions (including Netherlands, Spain, Sweden, etc.), which legislate to prohibit the creation of embryos solely for research purposes, whilst permitting research on 'surplus' embryos.

References

Birnbacher, D. (1997), 'Do Modern Reproductive Technologies Violate Human Dignity?', this volume, Part Nine.

Hildt, E. (1996), 'Preimplantation Diagnosis in Germany?' *Biomedical Ethics*, Vol. 1, No. 2, pp. 28-9.

Part Eight
CONNECTING LINES BETWEEN IVF AND PREIMPLANTATION DIAGNOSIS AND GENE THERAPY

1 Connecting lines from a medical point of view

Hansjakob Müller

Preimplantation diagnosis seen in the context of prenatal diagnosis

As a medical geneticist, one first considers preimplantation diagnosis (PID) in the context of the established methods of prenatal diagnosis (PND) (Müller 1990, Miny et al. 1995). The techniques used for this purpose, and the phases before and during pregnancy in which it can be employed, are shown schematically in fig. 1. As a general rule it should be possible to carry out a PND examination as early as possible without endangering the pregnancy or the health of the unborn child, and the result of the examination should be a very reliable. On the basis of these criteria, PID can be considered favourably.

PID has a number of obvious advantages: only non-affected embryos are transferred to the woman's uterus; no abortion is needed in the event of a pathological result, and there is no need to begin what amounts to a pregnancy on probation as is the case if the health of the foetus has to be determined by conventional PND. After a PID examination, a woman can accept her future child from the beginning of the pregnancy. She does not have to hold back her feelings towards it until the 10th or even the 18th week of gestation when it has been established whether it will be healthy or not, i.e whether it will be aborted.

PID has obvious medical drawbacks. It requires a complex and distressing procedure of medically assisted reproduction, namely in vitro fertilisation (IVF) with embryo transfer (ET). On the one hand the prospects of a pregnancy after IVF and ET are limited, while on the other hand there is a risk of multiple pregnancies if a number of embryos are simultaneously transferred back into the mother.

Two distinct methods of genetic preimplantation diagnosis exist: either preconception genetic analysis or analysis of embryo cells. To some degree, these procedures are associated with different medical, genetic and ethical problems.

The cornerstone of progress in this field is constituted by advances in the micromanipulation of oocytes and in embryo biopsy techniques. The nuclei, or respectively the DNA for PID, can be obtained by removal of the polar body (Verlinsky et al. 1990) or by biopsy of the blastomere or trophoectoderm. In a landmark article, Handyside et al. (1989) demonstrated the possibility of sampling a human embryo cell at the four-cell stage and of determining the sex of the embryo before implantation. The first successful outcome of PID was achieved in 1990 with the birth of twin girls whose mother was known to be at risk of transmitting X-linked mental retardation and adrenoleukodystrophy (Handyside et al. 1990). PID has also been carried out for many monogenic disorders (Verlinsky et al. 1990, Harper and Handyside 1994, Black 1994, Verlinsky and Kuliev 1996).

Preconception genetic analysis

Selection of gametes opens up intriguing prospects for the prevention of inherited diseases. Whereas gene typing of individual sperms is not possible, it has been successfully carried out, by an indirect approach, on oocytes.

The genome of the oocyte can be evaluated by removing and analysing the first polar body (Verlinsky et al. 1990). This involves induction of superovulation to retrieve several follicles, the genetic analysis of polar bodies, and transfer of only unaffected fertilised oocytes or embryos to the mother (Verlinsky and Kuliev 1996).

In the absence of crossing-over, the first polar body will be homozygous for all alleles not contained in the oocyte and the second polar body. If crossing-over has occurred, the oocyte will be heterozygous and its genotype cannot be predicted. Therefore, the location of a gene on the chromosomes in relation to their centromere and telomere is important: For telomeric genes the probability of crossing-over approaches 50 per cent, while for genes close to the centromere its frequency may be very low. Despite the crossing-over mechanism, it can be presumed that in a substantial proportion of the polar bodies, the normal or the abnormal allele will be homozygous. In the case of a heterozygous polar body, the determination of the genotype of the oocyte could be attempted by aspiration of the second polar body after fertilisation.

The procedure of polar body removal seems not to decrease the viability of the resulting embryos. The pregnancy rate per transfer in the polar body manipulated cycles was 19.9 per cent, actually much higher than the expected rate for IVF cycles in couples of advanced maternal age (Verlinsky et al. 1996). More than a dozen healthy children have already been born after polar body diagnosis (Verlinsky and Kuliev 1996).

In the case of X-linked diseases, in IVF the number of female embryos available for embryo transfer could be increased by the use of an X-enriched sperm fraction achieved by separation of X- and Y-bearing sperms. Johnson et al. (1993) improved the sexing of human sperms using the difference in the amount of DNA; the natural female-to-male ratio was altered from 1:1 to 4:1. If this type of separation becomes more reliable, it could become a clinically useful option.

Genetic testing of embryo cells

Although preconception genetic diagnosis has a number of clear advantages, embryo biopsy is needed in the following situations: (1) If the paternal allele cannot be analysed. (2) If there is a possibility that the test will not be effective for telomeric loci because of the likelihood of a high cross-over frequency resulting in a heterozygous state of the polar body. (3) If gender determination is needed. Further indications for this procedure are mentioned in the section on indications for PID. Embryo biopsy performed at the four- to eight-cell stage then becomes an indispensable complement to preconception genetic analysis. Using standard IVF techniques to obtain multiple embryos for analysis, embryo biopsy is usually performed 3 days after retrieval (Black 1994) and ET on the same day or one day later depending on the complexity of the genetic tests needed. Embryo cryopreservation is available if more time is needed to arrive at a reliable test result. Thereafter, the unaffected embryos can be transferred in a future cycle. Human blastocyte biopsy was first undertaken by Dokras et al. (1990). The trophoectoderm cells can be biopsied without affecting the inner cell mass from which the embryo is derived. Despite these advantages, this method has hardly ever been used in humans. Pregnancy rates following transfer of blastocytes remain very low (Verlinsky et al. 1993).

A total of 328 embryo transfers following PID resulted in 83 pregnancies, with at least 40 healthy babies born (Harper quoted by Unterhuber 1997). Pregnancy rates after PID do not differ substantially from those achieved after routine IVF (Harper and Handyside 1994). More important, micromanipulation does not appear to affect ongoing normal development.

Technical aspects of genetic testing

IVF has created an opportunity to perform genetic studies on polar bodies, blastomeres or trophoectodermal cells. The same methods for detecting genetic conditions after birth can be used for PID (McLaren 1987) if only a very small number of cells is needed. Direct PID of monogenic diseases became possible after the introduction of the polymerase chain reaction (PCR) for DNA analysis (Saiki et al. 1985) and for chromosomal abnormalities after the introduction of the fluorescence in situ hybridisation (FISH) technique

(Delhanty et al. 1994). It can be applied for the visualisation of specific chromosome aberrations in interphase nuclei (Grifo et al. 1990, Verlinsky et al. 1996). An alternative to the FISH technique is 'primed in situ synthesis' (PRINS) (Koch et al. 1989). In this procedure, chromosome identification is performed by in situ annealing of specific oligonucleotide primers, followed by primer elongation by a Taq DNA polymerase in the presence of labelled nucleotides. This technique may contribute to a significant improvement in gender determination and aneuploidy detection in single human blastomeres (Pellestor et al. 1996).

PID is functioning, but it is not yet routine. The techniques for the reliable detection of most genetic disorders still need intensive research with particular emphasis on safety and diagnostic accuracy. The small number of nuclei available increases the risk of diagnostic error or technical failure. Although it is not unlikely that even a four- to eight-cell embryo contains chromosomal mosaicism, PID does not allow this condition to be detected. Other questions also remain unanswered, such as the possibility of a pathological condition changing to a normal one during the first days of embryonic development (e.g. reduction of trisomy to disomy). Therefore, once pregnancy has been achieved, the results are usually monitored by traditional PND.

Indications for preimplantation diagnosis

This section presents various situations in which PID could be considered.

1. Couples who are infertile and have to conceive by IVF but who do not have a particular inheritable risk of having offspring with a genetic abnormality.

1.1. IVF procedures are carried out under light-microscope observation. Thus embryos are morphologically classified according to their appearance before their transfer. The morphological criteria include the size and shape of the blastomeres, aspects of the cytoplasm and the presence of fragments (cf. Weymarn et al. 1980). The correlation between the chromosomal status and the morphological appearance of the early embryo is still poorly understood. The incidence of chromosome aberration is undoubtedly higher among embryos with a clearly abnormal appearance. A more extensive investigation of these relationships is needed. In my view it is unethical to transfer an abnormal embryo, likewise, it is unethical not to carry out a thorough genetic investigation of those embryos that are not transferred because they do not have a normal appearance.

1.2. In the context of an IVF, the same indications will probably apply to PID as are now generally accepted for PND. Here, above all, maternal age ranks high on the list. It is a well-known fact that the incidence of de novo numerical chromosome aberrations increases with maternal age.

If FISH or PRINS techniques on single cells allowed the more common chromosome aberrations to be detected and could produce consistent results, the avoidance of transferring aneuploid embryos would be of special benefit to elderly women with no genetic risk except their age who undergo infertility treatment through IVF. In this connection it should be borne in mind that some couples, because of a prolonged investigation of their infertility, have already reached an advanced age for reproduction. The success rate of IVF and ET would be improved by transfering only chromosomally normal embryos.

1.3. Intracytoplasmic sperm injection (ICSI) (Markert 1989) represents a new option for a couple to have children when the man is not fertile. In ICSI, in contrast to conventional IVF, only one sperm is needed to fertilise an ovum. It is injected directly into it. Sperms can be obtained from the ejaculate or by microsurgical sperm aspiration (MESA), or by testicular sperm extraction (TESE) if they cannot be ejaculated. ICSI is also used when sperms are themselves unable to penetrate the ovum.

So far, pregnancy rates after IVF are in a similar range, irrespective of whether achieved with or without ICSI. However, there is still uncertainty with regard to possible risks for the health of children conceived by ICSI, even if there are so far no indications of potential dangers to health during the first years of life. Such risks could be related to the mechanical perforation of the zona pellucida and the ovum and to the attachment of potentially pathogenic microorganisms to instruments and sperms (Moss 1996). The use of aged or immature sperms may also constitute a source of risk. No conclusions as to the clinical use and safety of MESA and TESE can yet be drawn.

2. Some forms of male infertility are consequences of genetic abnormalities which can also result in additional complications (Müller 1990). An important fact in this connection is, above all, that chromosome anomalies in the partner can be the cause of his childlessness. Carriers of balanced chromosome aberrations (Chandley 1979) are among the men who attend infertility clinics. Such persons can produce genetically unbalanced gametes. If these are used for ICSI, there is a risk that children conceived in this way could also be carriers of a clinically manifest, unbalanced chromosome aberration. Also in its balanced form, the aberration can be passed on to the next generation (Buckett et al. 1996). There are indications that in women too, chromosome aberrations could be more important as a cause of infertility and repeated IVF failure than was formerly assumed.

Single gene mutations (Müller et al. 1994) and microdeletions (Reijo et al. 1996) of the Y-chromosome can lead to male infertility. It may also result from a number of clinically more complex monogenic diseases such as Kartagener syndrome or myotonic dystrophy. If infertility is overcome with ICSI, there is a large risk that the same predisposition will be passed on to a subsequent generation. A more thorough ethical evaluation is needed in order to determine whether ICSI can be justified in this situation.

3. Women and couples in a specific genetic risk group who have experienced PND and abortion but still want a healthy child of their own although they cannot accept a further round of conventional PND. In this connection, I remember a woman who had given birth to a child with congenital myotonic dystrophy which died after a short time and who had experienced two pregnancies which were aborted because the foetus was affected. She wanted to have healthy children, but without the stress of conventional PND. PID would offer an alternative.

4. PID for at-risk couples who for ethical reasons will not consider termination of pregnancy (abortion) under any circumstances. PID makes it possible to overcome the most sensitive issue in PND and the avoidance of genetic disease, namely the problem of abortion. It is considered as an option for couples for whom the termination of a pregnancy is not acceptable. The abortion of an affected male foetus could represent a psychological dilemma for a female carrier of an X-linked disorder such as Duchenne's muscular dystrophy. Even if she is not fundamentally opposed to abortion, she could tend to identify the foetus with her affected brother.

5. PID on embryos for couples at risk for Huntington's disease and certain other dominantly inherited disorders (Schulman et al. 1996). PID allows the disease to be prevented in their own offspring without disclosure of the parental phenotype. Only embryos without the mutant gene are transferred to the uterus. The parents would specifically not be given any direct or indirect information on their own genetic situation. The specific foetal risk can, if PID is performed accurately, be reduced to zero. This approach may also be applicable to other late-onset dominant disorders such as Charcot-Marie-Tooth disease.

Lines towards germline gene therapy

IVF would be a prerequisite for the conduct of germline gene therapy (GLGT) in humans. However, it has been proscribed by virtually all committees, organisations or legislative bodies that have concerned themselves with it. With regard to GLGT, differing views are taken of PID. PID can constitute an alternative to GLGT in the case of severe genetic diseases which already manifest themselves in utero or very early in life. On the other hand, PID would also be an important basis for the development of GLGT in humans. It would make little sense to transfer an embryo in which gene therapy had failed or in which the transferred foreign gene had implanted itself in a normal gene and thus damaged the latter.

While no research on GLGT is being carried out in humans, transgenic animals are steadily gaining importance in medicine and animal breeding. Transgenic animals are living creatures in which, by methods of genetic recombination, a foreign gene has been implanted or an own gene has been destroyed ('knocked out') or modified. They are produced as models in order to obtain an insight into complex biological networks or into the nature of certain inherited diseases. They are also used for the toxicological testing of new drugs and other substances, and for the production of human proteins ('gene pharming'). Finally, it is expected that transgenic pigs will provide human-compatible organs for xenotransplantation. The experience gathered with such animal experiments can probably be transferred to humans and is likely to influence the discussion on human germline gene therapy. PID after such therapy – if ever accepted – could well become mandatory.

Biological and medical perspectives

PID, in comparison to PND, gives rise to hardly any new ethical questions except in the case of special new fields of application. These have already been referred to in connection with ICSI and GLGT.

The term 'totipotency' occupies an important position with regard to the ethical assessment of embryo biopsy and the legal admissibility of PID. It is used in different ways, referring either to an embryo cell's capability of contributing to every tissue in the body including the germline, or its capacity to develop on its own into a live-born young. There are a number of unclear points since in this respect differences exist between the various species and it is, understandably, not possible to carry out corresponding experiments with human embryos. The similarity in pattern and timing of early development between mouse and human suggests that the mouse embryo may be a better indicator of human blastomere potential than either the sheep or the rabbit embryo. Single cells taken from 4- and 8-cell stages of mouse embryos are no longer totipotent in the latter sense (Tsumoda and McLaren 1983, Kelly 1977). The objection that the required single cells used for genetic studies would otherwise have a chance of developing into an individual is not a tenable ground for the prohibition of early embryo biopsy.

PID, like PND, must be used to help diagnose severe genetic disorders which manifest themselves early in life, in order to prevent the occurrence during childhood of severe, untreatable illnesses and handicaps. Any kind of genetic examination, however, must be accompanied by appropriate genetic counselling. The persons concerned must be involved in the decision-making process and the ethical discussion. In addition, all PID should take place within the framework of controlled studies in order to eliminate as quickly as possible uncertainties in connection with the clinical use of PID and related technologies such as ICSI.

The duty to provide medical aid to those in need also includes the specific professional requirement to pursue new possibilities precisely in those cases where the chances of prevention or cure are currently non-existent or highly unsatisfactory. Any medical assessment of PID must take this fact into consideration.

Acknowledgement

Anne McLaren, Cambridge, contributed decisively to the relevant parts of this review article with her verbal comments during the meeting 'IVF in the 90s' in Stuttgart and also with her written note on totipotency (McLaren 1997).

Fig.1. Timetable for the use of prenatal examination methods

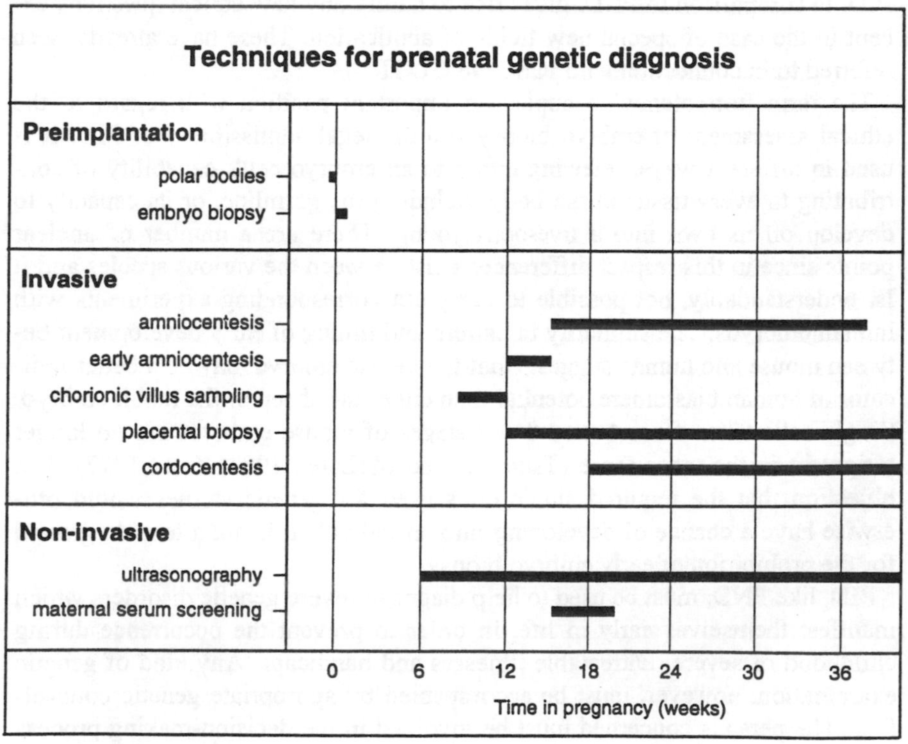

References

Black, S.H. (1994), 'Preimplantation Genetic Diagnosis', *Current Opinions in Pediatrics*, Vol. 6, pp. 712-6.

Buckett, W., Aird, I., Luckas, M., Kingsland, C., Lewis-Jones, I. and Howard (1996), 'Karyotyping Should Be Done Before Treatment', *Brit Med J*, Vol. 313, p. 334.

Chandley, A.C. (1979), 'The Chromosomal Basis of Human Infertility', *Brit Med Bull*, Vol. 35, pp. 181-6.

Delhanty, J.D.A., Griffin, D.K., Handyside, A.H., Harper, J., Atkinson, G.H.G., Pieters, M.E.H.C. and Winston, R.M.L. (1993), 'Detection of Aneuploidy and Chromosomal Mosaicism in Human Embryos During Preimplantation Sex Determination by Fluorescent In Situ Hybridisation (FISH)', *Human Mol Gene*, Vol. 2, pp. 1183-5.

Dokras, A., Sargent, I.K., Ross, C., Gardner, R.L. and Barlow, D.H. (1990), 'Trophoectoderm Biopsy in Human Blastocytes', *Human Reprod*, Vol. 5, pp. 821-5.

Grifo, J.A., Boyle, A., Lavy, G., DeCherney, A.H., Ward, D.C. and Sanyal, M.K. (1990), 'Preembryo Biopsy and Analysis of Blastomeres by In Situ Hybridisation', *Am J Obstet Gynecol*, Vol. 163, pp. 2013-9.

Handyside, A.H., Kontogianni, E.H., Hardy, K. and Winston, R.M.L. (1990), 'Pregnancies from Biopsied Human Embryos Sexed by Y-Specific DNA Amplification (Letter)', *Nature*, Vol. 344, pp. 768-70.

Handyside, A.H., Penketh, R.J.A., Winston, R.M.L., Pattinson, J.K. and Delhanty, J.D.A. (1989), 'Biopsy of Human Preimplantation Embryos and Sexing by DNA Amplification', *Lancet*, Vol. I, pp. 347-9.

Harper, J.C. and Handyside, A.H. (1994), 'The Current Status of Preimplantation Diagnosis', *Curr Obstet Gynecol*, Vol. 4, pp. 143-9.

Johnson, L.A., Welch, G.R., Keyvanfar, K., Dorfmann, A., Fugger, E.F. and Schulman, J.D. (1993), 'Gender Preselection in Humans? Flow Cytometric Separation of X and Y Spermatozoa for the Prevention of X-linked Diseases', *Hum Reprod*, Vol. 8, pp. 1733-9.

Kelly, S.J. (1977), 'Studies of the Developmental Potential of 4- and 8-Cell Stage Mouse Blastomere', *J Exp Zool*, Vol. 200, pp. 365-76.

Kent-First, M.G., Kol, S., Muallem, A., Blazer, S. and Itskovitz-Eldor, J. (1996), 'Infertility in Intracytoplasmic-sperm-injected-derived Sons', *Lancet*, Vol. 348, p. 332.

Koch, J.E., Kolvraa, S., Petersen, K.B., Gregersen, N. and Bolund, L. (1989), 'Oligonucleotide-priming Methods for the Chromosome Specific Labelling as Alpha Satellite DNA in Situ', *Chromosoma*, Vol. 98, pp. 259-65.

Markert, C.L. (1983), 'Fertilisation of Mammalian Egg by Sperm Injection', *J Exp Zool*, Vol. 228, pp. 195-201.

Mayor, S. (1996), 'Technique for Treating Infertility May Be Risky', *Brit Med J*, Vol. 313, p. 248.
McLaren, A. (1987), 'Can We Diagnose Genetic Disease in Pre-embryos?', *New Scientist*, Vol. 116, pp. 42-7.
McLaren, A. (1997), 'A Note on Totipotency', *Biomedical Ethics*, Vol. 2, No. 1, pp. 7-8.
Miny, P., Tercanli, S., Gänshirt, D. and Holzgreve, W. (1995), 'Pränatale Diagnostik', *Therapeut Umschau*, Vol. 12, pp. 792-800.
Moss, T.R. (1996), 'Illustration of Sperm May Show Attachment of Potentially Pathogenic Micro-organisms', *Brit Med J*, Vol. 313, p. 334.
Müller, Hj. (1980), 'Genetic Aspects of Human Infertility', *Schweiz Rundschau Med*, Vol. 68, pp. 1702-9.
Müller, Hj. (1990), 'Pränatale Diagnostik', *Schweiz Med Wschr*, Vol. 120, pp. 269-74.
Müller, Hj., Rey, J.P. and Scott, R. (1994), 'Genetic Aspects of Human Infertility', in Brunetti, P.M., Perrenoud, A. and Sprumont, P. (eds), *Changements dans le processus de la reproduction humaine*, Editiones Universitaires Fribourg Suisse: Fribourg, pp. 69-75.
Pellestor, F., Girardet, A., Andréo, B., Lefort, G. and Charlieu, J.P. (1996), 'Preimplantation Embryo Chromosome Analysis by Primed in Situ Labeling Method', *Fertility and Sterility*, Vol. 66, pp. 781-6.
Reijo, R., Alagappan, R.K., Patrizio, P. and Page, D.C. (1996), 'Severe Oligozoospermia Resulting from Deletions of Azoospermia Factor Gene on Y Chromosome', *Lancet*, Vol. 347, pp. 1290-4.
Saiki, R.K., Scharf, S., Faloona, F., Mullis, K.B., Horn, G.T., Erlich, H.A. and Arnheim, N. (1985), 'Enzymatic Amplification of β-Globin Genomic Sequences and Restriction Site Analysis for Diagnosis of Sickle Cell Anemia', *Science*, Vol. 230, pp. 1350-4.
Schulman, J.D., Black, S.H., Handyside, A. and Nance, W.E. (1996), 'Preimplantation Genetic Testing for Huntington Disease and Certain Other Dominantly Inherited Disorders', *Clin Genet*, Vol. 49, pp. 57-8.
Tsumoda, Y. and McLaren, A. (1983), 'Effect of Various Procedures on the Viability of Mouse Embryos Containing Half the Normal Number of Blastomeres', *J Reprod Fert*, Vol. 69, pp. 315-22.
Unterhuber, R. (1997), 'German Law Clashes With State of Reproductive Medicine', *Nature Medicine*, Vol. 3, p. 13.
Verlinski, Y., Cieslak, J., Ivakhnenko, V., Lifchez, A., Strom, C. and Kuliev, A. (1996), 'Birth of Healthy Children After Preimplantation Diagnosis of Common Aneuploidies by Polar Fluorescent in Situ Hybridization Analysis', *Fertility and Sterility*, Vol. 66, pp. 126-9.

Verlinsky, Y., Ginsberg, N., Lifchez, A., Valle, J., Moise, J. and Strom, M. (1990), 'Analysis of the First Body. Preconceptual Genetic Diagnosis', *Human Reprod*, Vol. 5, pp. 826-9.

Verlinsky, Y., Handyside, A., Simpson, J.L., Edwards, R., Kuliev, A., Muggleton-Harris, A., Readhead, C., Liebaers, I., Coonen, E. and Plachot, M. (1993), 'Current Progress in Preimplantation Genetic Diagnosis', *J Assist Reprod Genet*, Vol. 10, pp. 353-60.

Verlinsky, Y. and Kuliev, A. (1996), 'Preimplantation Polar Body Diagnosis', *Biochemical and Molecular Medicine*, Vol. 58, pp. 13-7.

Weymarn, v. N., Guggenheim, R. and Müller, Hj. (1980), 'Surface Characteristics of Oocytes from Juvenile Mice as Observed in the Scanning Electron Microscope', *Anat Embryol*, Vol. 161, pp. 19-27.

2 The possible impact of preimplantation diagnosis for infertile couples

Dieter Meschede and Jürgen Horst

Over the past two decades human procreation has become the subject of powerful medical interventions, the two most prominent being assisted reproduction and prenatal diagnosis. Preimplantation diagnosis (PID) may be regarded as the culmination of this development. In order to recognise or exclude genetic disorders it combines in vitro fertilisation (IVF) with the molecular or cytogenetic analysis of a sample from the very early conceptus (Handyside 1993).

To date, PID has been used mainly for the detection of monogenic disorders diagnosable on the basis of a DNA test. Some pilot studies are now under way to investigate the possibility of cytogenetic diagnostics in preimplantation embryos in order to pick up chromosomal disorders such as trisomies or unbalanced translocations (Munné et al. 1993). For the time being, however, cytogenetic PID is still in an experimental stage of development (Reubinoff and Shushan 1996).

Couples may enter a PID program in two different ways – often, the primary concern will be a genetic disorder (e.g. cystic fibrosis, myotonic dystrophy, thalassemia) that the couple's offspring has a significant risk of inheriting. In this setting, IVF is a technical adjunct of PID and is only necessitated by the need for direct access to the early conceptus. A second group of patients possibly making use of PID could be couples who are being treated for a fertility problem. Here, IVF needs to be done anyway, and an embryo biopsy can be performed with relative ease as an additional procedure to safeguard against some genetic defects in the conceptus.

The therapeutic power of IVF has been vastly enhanced by micromanipulative technology that allows the handling of gametes and embryos with great precision. The most important of these techniques is intracytoplasmic sperm injection (ICSI), now the standard procedure for the symptomatic treatment of severe male factor infertility (Tournaye et al. 1995).

It has been argued that the rapidly growing use of ICSI and related techniques facilitates the implementation of PID programs 'via the backdoor' and opens the floodgate for a general genetic screening of embryos conceived in vitro. As a matter of fact, most institutions that currently perform PID build on an active local IVF/ICSI program.

We were interested to learn to what extent infertile patients treated with IVF/ICSI could potentially make use of PID, were this technology available to them (German law currently precludes the use of PID, but the issue is under intensive ethical and legal discussion). Our institute runs a special genetic counselling program for patients considering ICSI and similar procedures (Meschede et al. 1995, 1996). At the time of writing of this text we had completed the evaluation of 329 cases. For each of these couples an individual genetic risk assessment was performed. Any risk of ≥0.5 per cent for a major congenital disorder was considered as 'significant'.

It turned out that, with the current technical state of PID, for none of the 329 couples would there have been an unequivocal medical indication to use this technique. This surprising result is explained by the fact that in the vast majority of cases with a 'significant' risk factor present, this was for a chromosomal or multifactorial disorder for which PID cannot (or cannot safely) be applied at this point.

Three cases with a risk of a monogenic disorder (hemophilia A, fragile X syndrome, Duchenne muscular dystrophy) in their offspring represented borderline indications for PID. Hemophilia A, though technically diagnosable in a preimplantation embryo, can be treated with very satisfactory results, so the justification for a PID procedure is questionable. Due to the peculiarities of the underlying mutation, diagnosis of the fragile X syndrome based on one or a few cells from a preimplantation embryo would in a high percentage of cases probably be unsafe. Finally, the couple at risk for Duchenne muscular dystrophy in their children did not desire specific genetic investigations and would not use any type of prenatal or preimplantation diagnosis should ICSI be successful. In addition, with molecular analyses in the female partner it might have been possible to exclude her as a carrier of the disorder, obviating any need for PID.

In summary, our data do not support the notion that PID will – all ethical, legal, and financial considerations aside – be applied on a large scale to infertile couples presenting for IVF/ICSI treatment. However, this issue needs to be reconsidered should PID turn out to be an effective and safe approach to demonstrate chromosomal abnormalities in early human conceptuses.

References

Handyside, A.H. (1993), 'Diagnosis of Inherited Disease Before Implantation', *Reproductive Medicine Review*, Vol. 2, pp. 51-61.

Meschede, D., De Geyter, C., Nieschlag, E. and Horst, J. (1995), 'Genetic Risk in Micromanipulative Assisted Reproduction', *Human Reproduction*, Vol. 10, pp. 2880-6.

Meschede, D., Lemcke, B., De Geyter, C., De Geyter, M., Wittwer, B., Nieschlag, E. and Horst, J. (1996), 'Genetic Risk Factors Among Infertile Couples Treated with Intracytoplasmatic Sperm Injection', *Human Reproduction*, Vol. 11, Abstract Book 1 (ESHRE 1996 – Meeting of the European Society for Human Reproduction and Embryology, Maastricht), Abstract P137, p. 158.

Munné, S., Lee, A., Rosenwaks, Z., Grifo, J. and Cohen, J. (1993), 'Diagnosis of Major Chromosome Aneuploidies in Human Preimplantation Embryos', *Human Reproduction*, Vol. 8, pp. 2185-91.

Reubinoff, B. and Shushan, A. (1996), 'Preimplantation Diagnosis in Older Patients. To Biopsy or Not to Biopsy?', *Human Reproduction*, Vol. 11, pp. 2071-5.

Tournaye, H., Liu, J., Nagy, Z., Joris, H., Wisanto, A., Bonduelle, M., van der Elst, J., Staessen, C., Smitz, J., Silber, S., Devroey, P., Liebaers, I. and van Steirteghem, A. (1995), 'Intracytoplasmic Sperm Injection (ICSI): The Brussels Experience', *Reproduction, Fertility and Development*, Vol. 7, pp. 269-78.

3 Legal regulation of IVF and preimplantation diagnosis in Germany

Stefan Müller

In vitro fertilisation (IVF) in Germany is regulated by the Embryo Protection Act (Gesetz zum Schutz von Embryonen 1990) and the guidelines of the Federal Physicians Chamber (Richtlinien 1994). The Embryo Protection Act (ESchG) reserves to physicians the sole right to perform IVF (ESchG §9) and also regulates a number of other matters associated with IVF such as embryo and sex selection (ESchG §3), donation of embryos (ESchG §1) and also post-mortem fertilisation (ESchG §4).

The guidelines of the Federal Physicians Chamber dictate the medical indications for an IVF. These are different kinds of infertility. These guidelines have to be transferred into the professional law of each state's physicians chamber. Before this transfer is done the guidelines are only relevant as a description of the state of the art with no legal competence. Some states' Physicians Chambers, such as Hamburg (Berufsordnung 1995), have already transferred the latest version of these guidelines, others, such as Lower Saxony (Richtlinien 1988), have only transferred an older version of these guidelines. Even others, such as Bremen (Berufsordnung 1990), have not transferred any of these guidelines, which means that there are no special medical indications for an IVF. The states' approval to use an IVF is only given when this IVF is used in a sterility-therapy (Richtlinie 1991), but no special medical indications for this therapy are required from a legal point of view. In all the IVF guidelines transferred by the states' Physicians Chambers there is no indication for an IVF for the use of a preimplantation diagnosis (PID). But some Physicians Chambers, such as Hamburg, under their professional regulations, do not allow their members to use PID.

PID of genetic diseases is done with the aim of helping those couples who would prefer selection to occur at this stage rather than during pregnancy. Following IVF or an uterine lavage (which is at this time not working properly in connection with a PID), biopsy and removal of one or two cells from the early 'pre-embryo' provides the material for molecular genetic diagnosis without interfering the development of the embryo. If the diagnosis is positive for a hereditary disease the embryo will be rejected, otherwise the embryo will be transferred to the uterus of the mother. After the embryo has nested into the uterus, the pregnancy of the mother will start. PID has been successful so far for a number of hereditary diseases such as cystic fibrosis, Tay Sachs disease and Lesch-Nyhan syndrome.

In Germany any examination of totipotent cells (i.e. cells up to the eight-cell stadium) is forbidden by the Embryo Protection Act (ESchG §6.1, §8.1). In most cases analysis of cells for a PID is done on totipotent cells. But in the near future it should be possible to analyse non-totipotent cells. Examination of non-totipotent cells for a PID is not forbidden by the Embryo Protection Act.

Also forbidden under the Embryo Protection Act (ESchG §1.2) is the fertilisation of an ovum for any other reason than to cause a pregnancy in the woman to whom the ovum belongs. This seems to be an ethical inconsistency. On the one hand the embryo is totally protected before the pregnancy starts by the Embryo Protection Act, on the other hand an abortion is – under specific circumstances – allowed some weeks later (Strafgesetzbuch 1995). Whether this ethical inconsistency in German legislation can be maintained will be revealed in the near future.

There has to be a public debate on the question: Will German society use the chances provided by PID for genetic counselling in cases of hereditary disease? If the answer is 'yes', then the legal regulations have to be changed to take advantage of the chance and to prevent abuse of this new technology.

References

'Berufsordnung für Ärzte im Lande Bremen' (1990), *Bremer Ärzteblatt*, Vol. 11, pp. 13-20.

'Berufsordnung der Hamburger Ärzte/Ärztinnen' (1995), *HÄB*, Vol. 7, pp. 272-82.

'Die Richtlinien zur Durchführung des intratubaren Gametentransfers, der In-vitro-Fertilisation mit Embryonentransfer und anderer verwandter Methoden erhalten folgende Fassung:' (1994), *Deutsches Ärzteblatt*, Vol. 91, pp. 58-62.

'Gesetz zum Schutz von Embryonen' (Embryonenschutzgesetz) (1990), *BGBl.*, Vol. I, p. 2746.

'Richtlinien zur Durchführung der In-vitro-Fertilisation und des intratubaren Gameten- und Embryotransfers als Behandlungsmethode der menschlichen Sterilität' (1988), Kammerversammlung der Ärztekammer Niedersachsen.

‘Richtlinie für das Verfahren zur Genehmigung von Maßnahmen zur Durchführung künstlicher Befruchtung durch Ärztinnen, Ärzte, Einrichtungen und Krankenhäuser’ (1991), *Amtsblatt der freien Hansestadt Bremen*, Vol. 75, pp. 665-9.
‘Strafgesetzbuch §218a, Schwangeren- und Familienhilfeänderungsgesetz’ (1995), *BGBl.*, Vol. I, p. 1050.

4 Connecting lines from an ethical point of view

Paul Schotsmans

Introduction

The birth of Louisa Brown has brought more or less a revolution in the reflection on the beginning of human life. Preimplantation diagnosis (PID) and human gene therapy are further steps in the application of medical progress on human reproduction. Connecting lines are certainly present: the ethical evaluation of in vitro fertilisation (IVF) can and should indeed be the frame of reference for the ethical approach of PID and human gene therapy.

I will therefore address this challenging topic from a clarification of my own ethical position concerning IVF. As a representative of the Leuven personalist approach, I consider an act, a decision, the use of a technique etc. as morally good, if it promotes the human person in all his or her dimensions and relationships. I consider it therefore to be a crucial task for the ethicist to clarify these dimensions and relationships of the human person. Louis Janssens (1980-81), promotor of the Leuven school,[1] described several dimensions such as subjectivity, corporeality, technological creativity, relationship, solidarity, historicity and transcendence. For the sake of clarity, I essentially stress three foundational dimensions for the promotion of the human person, adequately considered in all his or her dimensions and relationships: uniqueness, intersubjectivity and solidarity (Schotsmans 1992). The promotion of these dimensions represents in my view the realisation of the humanly desirable, as Paul Ricoeur would describe it (Ricoeur 1975). But the most fundamental characteristic of personalism is that we also have to take into account our basic historicity in our unique confrontation with reality, in order to make sound moral judgements. The dynamic character of this approach is therefore illustrated by our moral duty to protect or to realise as many of our pre-moral values as possible, knowing quite well that we cannot possibly realise them all. This is the reason why we should speak more accurately about the realisation of the 'most humanly possible' or 'le meilleur humain possible' (cf. also Ricoeur 1975).

In vitro fertilisation

The dilemmas concerning IVF can be grouped around three poles. The problem of the indication is the first one: do we reserve this technique to couples that are confronted with the impossibility of realising their wish for a child, or do we accept the application of IVF also for lesbians, homosexuals (through surrogate motherhood) or individuals who claim their right to have children? From the perspective of the uniqueness of every human person, even from his or her first beginnings, we have the crucial problem of the moral status of the human embryo. Finally, also, the society as a whole cannot ignore its duty to provide adequate provisions and quality control as an expression of an attitude of solidarity. The fact that several European countries diverge significantly in their legislation makes clear that further reflection on the best way to integrate IVF in a health care system is needed. This is even more important for those European countries where the legislators have failed to provide adequate societal control mechanisms, e.g. as is the case in Belgium.

It is my firm belief that IVF can be integrated from a comprehensive and dynamic personalistic approach (Schotsmans 1993). Our three anthropological orientations function indeed as three perspectives for developing ethical guidelines in order to integrate the technique. The dimension of intersubjectivity would imply limiting the application of the technique to stable, heterosexual and infertile couples. This conclusion diverges from those who reject IVF for the reason that they stress radically the principle of the inseparability of the procreative and unitive dimensions of human sexuality; it diverges also from those who claim an individual right to have children. Our more moderate acceptance of IVF is clinically realised through the integration of psychological counselling as 'locus ethicus' to help couples cope with their infertility problems and with the integration of the peculiar character of the IVF technique.

Much more difficult is, however, the evalution of the moral status of the human embryo. In the light of what is humanly desirable, I stress the need to realise as much as possible an adequate protection of the human embryo. In the light of the dynamic structure of the personalist approach, I can accept that the value of curing infertility or the value of realising an infertile couple's wish for a child can be positively and proportionally balanced against the negative value of the loss of embryos during the application of the technique. In the light of these orientations, the Leuven Hospital Ethics Committee (1993) could accept that IVF cannot be offered without the inevitable loss of embryos, e.g. during the cryopreservation procedures, and eventually, the final decision 'to let them perish', when the couple's wish for a child has been successfully fulfilled.[2] This does not yet imply, however, the acceptance of experimentation on human embryos. To understand this I refer again to the dimension of historicity. At this moment, in the Leuven evaluation, the issue of experimentation is not yet sufficiently clarified. The disproportion of values, i.e. the instrumental use of human embryos, is too high to accept also the development of experimentation procedures.

The societal dimension is expressed through the open communication about procedures, contracts with couples and quality control. This Louvain openness for societal control is unique in a country where no legislation on IVF exists. The recent Convention of the Council of Europe (1996) is a promising international development for more consistency in European legislation, so that IVF tourism can be more and more excluded.

These positions stand now – and to understand this, the notion of historicity is again crucial – under two strong pressures. First, the very important requirement of consistency. Can we accept throwing fertilised human oocytes away (thereby destroying them or – more euphemistically – letting them perish), and say no to preserving them for possible later use, e.g. implantation research, without consistency? Second, the pressure of recent developments in the application of PID. It may be clear that this diagnostic procedure must be judged by evaluating the moral legitimacy of the IVF technique, which I accept (here I see no serious ethical problems), but also by the legitimacy of experimentation on the human embryo.[3] Here again, the personalist approach is challenged by recent developments to clarify how the promotion of the human person, adequately considered in all his or her dimensions and relationships, can be realised.

Connecting lines with PID and human gene therapy

As it counts for IVF, also PID and human gene therapy must be ethically evaluated in the light of their intrinsic values. Many scientific, clinical and ethical problems still limit the wide application of these techniques at the moment. Let us therefore make profit of this situation to develop an ethical framework for their integration.

Scientific and clinical evaluation

We are confronted here with a technique where we do not yet have sufficient data to come to an objective scientific evaluation of the benefits of its application. A premature application could, however, lead to some dangers. Looking back at one of the new methods of IVF, namely the intracytoplasmic sperm injection (ICSI), more and more scientific and clinical warnings come from the medical profession. It would be unscientific and unethical not to take these warnings seriously. In the light of this, I personally would reject the quasi scientific nihilism of some who are practising reproductive technology. ICSI gives us an indication that the medical risks are not yet totally clarified. The same is certainly true for PID and human gene therapy. While techniques are improving and suggest that in the future the identification of certain genetic diseases will be almost 100 per cent effective, the special 'biology' of the pre-implantation human embryo with its mosaicism is such that error is unavoidable. Mosaics (existence of several genetically different cell lines within the same embryo) is a serious problem for PID programmes since analysis of a single (or even 2) cell(s) may give rise to an erroneous result. This fact must, in any case, be included in the information given to the couples (Plachot 1996). As gene therapy moves into the second half of its first clinical decade, somatic cell gene therapy is widely accepted in principle by opinion leaders and public policymakers. There are initial promising results in a handful of gene therapy studies, and both new biotechnology companies and more established pharmaceutical companies are increasingly interested in this field. But we can still, at this moment, only hope that the review process will continue to protect potential recipients of gene therapy from undue risks (Walters and Palmer, 1997, p.152).

I consider it therefore a moral duty to support as much as possible an open societal debate on medical progress in the application of these new techniques. Information of the public and awareness of the peculiar character of this type of research are absolutely necessary. This, however, also makes it clear that I do not think we should ban the development of these techniques. An honest scientific and clinical evaluation will remain always the first step in a sincere ethical reflection.

Clearly, PID and human gene therapy make us aware of our responsibility to future generations. But it remains difficult to clarify how is to be integrateted the well-being of future generations. I must therefore stress once again the need for a careful risk assessment, in agreement with the Report on the Ethical Implications of Biotechnoloy, by the Group of Advisors to the European Commission (1996, p.17):

> Because of its present risk assessment, somatic gene therapy should be restricted to serious diseases for which there is no other effective available treatment... Because of the important controversial and unprecedented questions raised by germ-line therapy, and considering the actual state of the art, germline gene therapy on humans is not at the present time ethically acceptable.

An ethical evaluation

We are searching for connecting lines. Our ethical evaluation must therefore remain general and open for future analysis.

Professional ethics: I shall first refer to professional ethics as the context to integrate clinically and ethically the application of these – and all kinds of – new medical developments. This implies that I shall suggest restricting their use to the therapeutic and clincal context of medical practice. One of the most important motors for an unreflective development of medical technology seems, however, to be a radical interpretation of the principle of self-determination. Any reference to the clinical context must then be banned and replaced by the free and deliberate decision of the individual client in the health care system. This implies that medicine and medical technology will be reduced to a market mechanism, whereby professional guidelines and modes of conduct are no longer valid. As important as every applied reflection in medical ethics is (and will therefore remain) the foundation of a sound professional virtue-ethics in medicine.

An even more important issue will also be to define the borders between the 'clinically acceptable' and what we can call in general the significance of medical technology for enhancement reasons. This may be clear on the individual level of the choice of parents concerning PID. It is even more true for human gene therapy. Walters and Palmer think that genetic technologies will provide one method for improving the human condition (as will also non-genetic approaches). Given the relatively early stage of development in the genetic technologies, they consider it too early to make any reliable prediction of how important these technologies can be or will be in the coming centuries. In their judgement, health-related physical enhancements by genetic means are morally justifiable in principle. Non-health related physical enhancements and intellectual and moral enhancements for persons who already are functioning within the normal range, seem to be more problematic. Possible child abuse and the allocation of these enhancements would make them highly problematic (Walters and Palmer, 1997, p.130-133). I would agree, when it can be clarified how health-related enhancements can be integrated in the professional duty of physicians to help to attempt to provide a better life and a better world to our descendants.

The moral status of the embryo: The nature and the moral status of the human embryo is a vast and difficult subject. Terminological, empirical, normative and metaphysical issues are intertwined in the arguments for and against particular criteria and definitions. For those who, drawing on the sanctity of life and similar doctrines, maintain that human life begins with the conception and that the fertilised oocyte must be respected 'as a person', it makes little difference if 'embryo' is used in a wide or narrow sense. In both cases, abortion and experimental research on embryos can almost never been ethically justified. However, for those who do not share this view and hold that it is difficult to find any non-arbitrary cut-off point, it is more important (a) to be specific about the precise sense of 'embryo', and (b) to make explicit the claims and rights that go with the definition of the concept, as well as under what conditions these rights may be overridden (Hermeren 1996).

Here, I would like to situate myself within the context of my Roman Catholic Community and its debate on the moral status of the human embryo. In 1987, the Sacred Congregation for the Doctrine of the Faith issued the Instruction 'Donum Vitae'. When it deals with the status of the embryo, its conclusions are unambiguous. It refers to: 'unconditioned respect', 'treated as a person from the moment of conception'; 'rights as a person must be recognised'. John Paul II stressed this viewpoint further in his Encyclical Evangelium Vitae (John Paul II, 1995, Nr.63):

> This evaluation of the morality of abortion is to be applied also to the recent forms of *intervention on human embryos* which, although carried out for purposes legitimate in themselves, inevitably involve the killing of these embryos. This is the case with *experimentation on embryos,* which is becoming increasingly widespread in the field of biomedical research and is legally permitted in some countries.

I would think it is right to suggest that the Roman Catholic Community shares a more tutioristic approach, trying to protect the embryo as much as possible. In light of this and/or despite this uncriticised consensus, it must be clear also that the debate on the moral status of the embryo inside the Roman Catholic Community remains open. Recently, some Catholic moral theologians, e.g. R.A. McCormick, P. Verspieren and J. Mahoney, have brought more diversity in the Catholic approach to the human embryo. While the official magisterium still rejects any nuance, R.A. McCormick accepted the distinction between genetic and developmental individualisation. The former is certainly present from the earliest beginnings of life, the latter is not: 'Developmental individualisation is completed only when implantation has been completed, a period of time whose outside time-limits are around fourteen days' (McCormick, 1989, p.345). This implies an open attitude to integrating not only IVF, but also PID and human gene therapy, again, of course, in the context of its clinical application.

It may, however, be clear that the debate about an adequate protection of the human embryo has been and will always remain a point of discussion. From recent statements about absolute (Honnefelder 1996) versus relative protection, there is a long way to go. Crucial for our debate here is, however, that the question of appropriate protection for the human embryo raises the more general question of the embryo's moral status.

Human dignity or 'le meilleur humain désirable': Both the clinical-ethical debate about the integration of IVF, PID and human gene therapy as therapeutic interventions and the debate on the moral status of the human embryo touch our understanding of human dignity, or in more personalist terms, our conception of the most humanly desirable (P. Ricoeur). Simply referring to the anthropological dimensions as perspectives for the ethical integration of the three techniques, is enough to bring a certain distance from some popular and rather simplistic ethical positions in this debate. Indeed, it may help us to reject radically any one-sided approaches, based e.g. on the principle of self-determination, and also the utilitarian approach, whereby consequences and benefits are more important than a thorough study of the understanding of human dignity. Under the influence of so-called 'Principlism' (Beauchamp and Childress 1995), medical ethics has unfortunately moved too strongly in the direction of the analysis of medical decision-making and has forgotten to pay the same attention to the foundation of medicine as a healing profession. Our anthropological options make clear that the clinical context of the physician-patient relationship must remain the basis for the promotion of the human person, adequately considered in his or her dimensions and relationships. The profession of medicine is indeed fully relational, even so that the enrichment of the other as other remains the most important ethical directive.

This is even more clearly illustrated by the application of our approach to reproductive technology, PID and human gene therapy. Human persons are situated, incarnated, corporeal human subjects. The more a medical intervention neglects the physicalness of the human being as an expression of his or her personhood, the more it becomes in my view problematic. Therefore, artificial insemination with the semen of a donor creates more ethical problems than the application of IVF for the infertile couple. So, we can go on in this line of reasoning: it will be almost impossible to integrate clinically and ethically surrogate motherhood.

Human gene therapy is another possible example. The first applications of this technique are forcing us to (re)examine the lines of demarcation against eugenics on the phenotype. I could go on: personalised embryo selection will strengthen the temptation in the ethos of the population to arrive at state policies on eugenics. To have the courage to recognise this, is, in my view, also a matter of consistent ethical reasoning.

To conclude

Is it an illusion to hope that the personalist approach can function in a kind of preventive way as a way to integrate new advancements in medical technology? The rapid changes in reproductive technology, genetic diagnosis and human gene therapy seem to suggest that it is and that ethical evaluation comes always after, if not much too late. This observation does not, however, discharge us from the duty to openly evaluate the values of new technologies. Science, medical technology and practice, medical ethics and law all have their specific agenda. But a real interdisciplinary approach creates the framework for an appropriate ethical reflection. Conscience has to do with 'science', 'knowing', 'understanding'... this may even be all that is ethics about: to keep our minds open, to analyse values, and to strengthen basic attitudes of trust and devotion, although – for me – always in the light of the humanly desirable.

Notes

1 Other users of the Leuven approach are Joseph Selling and Roger Burggraeve.

2 This position is rather unique in the Catholic community: only four Catholic institutions (Nijmegen, Lille, and the two Louvains) announced, shortly after the appearance of the Vatican's Instruction Donum Vitae (1987), that they would continue to provide IVF to otherwise infertile couples.

3 'This is within the moral philosophy of different persuasions, by the *moral legitimacy of the IVF technique* (i.e. human technological intervention in the fertilisation process, a procedure which in a large number of cases provides the basic pre-condition for recovering the embryo which will be analyzed) and the *legitimacy of experimenting on the human embryo*' (Bompiani, 1996, p.6).

References

Beauchamp, T.L. and Childress, J.F. (1995), *Principles of Biomedical Ethics*, Oxford.

Bompiani, A. (1996), 'Ethical Aspects of Preimplantation Diagnosis', *Third Symposium on Bioethics. Medically-Assisted Procreation and the Protection of the Human Embryo*, Strasbourg, 15-18 December 1996, distributed document.

Council of Europe (1996), *Convention for the Protection of Human Rights and Dignity of the Human Being with Regard to the Application of Biology and Medicine: Convention on Human Rights and Biomedicine*, Directorate of Legal Affairs: Strasbourg.

Group of Advisers to the European Commission (1996), *On the Ethical Implications of Biotechnology*, Office for Official Publications of the European Communities: Luxemburg.

Hermeren, G. (1996), 'The Nature and Status of the Embryo: Philosophical Aspects', *Third Symposium on Bioethics. Medically-Assisted Procreation and the Protection of the Human Embryo*, Strasbourg, November 1996, distributed document.

Honnefelder, L. (1996), 'Nature and Status of the Embryo: Philosophical Aspects', *Third Symposium on Bioethics. Medically-assisted Procreation and the Protection of the Human Embryo,* Strasbourg, November 1996, distributed document.

Hospital Ethics Committee (Faculty of Medicine, K.U. Leuven) (1993), 'Renewed and Updated Recommendations on In Vitro Fertilization and Embryo Transfer', in Borghgraef, R. and Schotsmans, P. (eds), *The Technological Advances in Health Sciences and the Moral Theological Implications*, University Press: Leuven, pp. 79-84.

Janssens, L. (1980-81), 'Artificial Insemination. Ethical Considerations', *Louvain Studies*, Vol. 8, pp. 3-39.

John Paul II (1995), *Evangelium Vitae. On the Value and Inviolability of Human Life*, Libreria Editrice Vaticana: Rome.

McCormick, R.A. (1989), 'Therapy or Tampering: The Ethics of Reproductive Technology and the Development of Doctrine', in Idem, *The Critical Calling. Reflections on Moral Dilemmas since Vatican II*, Georgetown University Press: Washington D.C.

Plachot, M. (1996), 'Preimplantation Genetic Diagnosis: Technical Aspects', *Third Symposium on Bioethics. Medically-Assisted Procreation and the Protection of the Human Embryo,* Strasbourg, November 1996, distributed document.

Ricoeur, P. (1975), 'Le problème du fondement de la morale', *Sapienza*, Vol. 28, pp. 3123-337.

Schotsmans, P. (1992), *En de mens schiep de mens. Medische (r)evolutie en ethiek*, Kapellen.

Schotsmans, P. (1993), 'Bioethics and Human Reproduction. An Ethical Approach of In Vitro Fertilization and Embryo Transfer', in Borghgraef, R. and Schotsmans, P. (eds), *The Technological Advances in Health Sciences and the Moral Theological Implications*, University Press: Leuven, pp. 15-26.

Walters, L. and Palmer, J.G. (1997), *The Ethics of Human Gene Therapy*, Oxford University Press: New York.

5 How 'tailor-made' do we want our offspring to be?

Paulus Liening

The issue of the connections between in vitro fertilisation (IVF) and preimplantation diagnosis (PID) cannot be overestimated in its significance for future developments – especially if the success rate of IVF rises: let us assume so in a kind of thought experiment for the next few minutes. Let us also assume that the combination of IVF and PID could be used generally – and not only to help infertile couples. Let us assume furthermore that genetic tests and so the possibilities for PID could become better and better. (The question which cannot be discussed here is whether these assumptions have a realistic background or are mere science fiction.)

Let me make three points. My *first point* concerns the idea of an integrally personalist approach. I feel warm sympathy for Professor Schotsmans' (1997) integrally personalist approach (although this approach shares with all variants of anthropological approaches the difficulty of drawing specific conclusions on bioethical questions), but nevertheless I will give an outline of an extremer position, call it the *agent-provocateur-position* if you like. The basis of my argumentation is the disagreement with one of Paul Schotmans' central premises, namely that there is a need to protect the human embryo as much as possible. But first let me mention a general aspect concerning the limits of an integrally personalist approach. At least complementary to this approach, we have to regard institutions, structures and the 'logic of the civilisation process'. I mention just one aspect: From the view of my own work on questions of resource allocation and priority setting, especially in a situation of ever-growing possibilities on the one side and probably permanently scarce resources on the other side, I must say that not being able to have a child may cause some suffering, but cannot really be set on the same level with (e.g.) the enormous needs in palliative medicine. Also, of course, resources spent in medicine compete with resources spent in the social sector. So we have good reasons to estimate many children growing up in poverty and without sufficient support as in much greater need than a couple with a wish for a child. But I admit that criteria for resource allocation and for distributive justice in general are controversial. Nevertheless we have no choice: we have to find a consensus.

My *second point* concerns the context of IVF/PID and 'the logic of the civilisation process'. I will briefly list some points characterising this context. Generally we can say, that the legibility of the genetic code does not allow us to re-enchant or even to re-sacralise nature. The decoded message can not be interpreted as a command to leave evolution untouched as the highest and most just authority. To take that which is obviously contingent as unchangeable is no longer possible. In my view, there is a not irreversible, but a very strong logic of civilisational development and IVF and PID exist as a consequence of this process. This means that biotechnology is deeply anchored in the urge for security and in 'possessive individualism'. Daily the territory ruled by chance is diminishing. Exaggerating, one could say that anyone who wants preventive medicine has to accept genetic engineering in the long run. It is also not very astonishing that we observe a change of public interest from the question of whether IVF/PID is ethically acceptable to the question of who shall profit from those new technologies. Biotechnology is also deeply anchored in the continuing medicalisation of the welfare state. In the German fairy-tale about the race between the hare and the hedgehog, it is – against all experience-based expectations – the hedgehog who is winning the race: he is always already there. In our context the hedgehog stands for a only too understandable medical casuistic healing ethics – and for a profit-oriented research-interest, too. The logic of the research-system and the involvement of economic interests create a system with its own internal dynamics, a so-called 'super-structure'. Once again exaggerating, one could sum up ironically: On n'arrête pas le progrès.

My *last point* concerns consequences for bioethics. (Please do not interpret this as bioethical fatalism; or – even worse – as a variant of happy postmodern anarchism. If anything at all, it tries to be a 'realistic-constructive resignation'. Indeed, I would prefer not to be a pessimist.) In my view all fundamental arguments are known and have been exchanged. A full consensus cannot be expected to be reached. Disturbing questions like 'How tailor-made do we want our offspring to be?' may lead to the temptation to become fundamentalist out of pragmatic reasons. But this is no way out... What I want to stress is not that bioethics is running out of work. On the contrary, the more bioethical development has an utopian dimension the more the role of bioethics has to be damage limitation. Many new and immensely significant questions are arising – I think there is no necessity (and not even the possibility) to list them all here. So there is a lot of work to do for bioethicists.

References

Schotsmans, P. (1997), 'Connecting Lines From an Ethical Point of View', this volume, Part Eight.

Part Nine
A FUNDAMENTAL APPROACH: TECHNICALISATION OF REPRODUCTION

1 Limits of reproductive technology

Brian A. Lieberman

Summary

The limits of reproductive technology will be considered in terms of the current state of the art, future developments and, where appropriate, obligations on the physician to consider restricting the use of the technique.

Introduction

The birth of Louise Brown in 1979 in Oldham followed treatment by in vitro fertilisation (IVF) (Steptoe and Edwards 1978). Her birth was the consequence of research, including that on embryos, conducted by Steptoe and Edwards. As so often is the case in science, however, their triumph was dependent upon the seminal observations of William Cruikshank who, 200 years ago, first recognised eggs in the oviduct of rabbits four days after mating (Cruikshank 1797) and Walter Heap of Manchester who in 1891 demonstrated that it was possible to transfer successfully embryos between Belgium hares and Angora rabbits (Heap 1891). The last two decades have witnessed further progress in fertility treatments. Refinements of the existing technologies and new developments may increase the live birth rate per treatment cycle commenced.

Effective treatments now exist for the majority of, if not all, forms of female infertility and the introduction of intracytoplasmic sperm injection (ICSI) provides a highly effective means of treating couples in the presence of a severe sperm disorder (Palermo et al. 1992). Effective as the treatments may be, the scientific advances have helped the infertile, but often have failed to correct the underlying disorder and in some instances may have allowed the disorder to be passed onto the next generation.

The biosynthetic human follicle-stimulating hormone (FSH) was licensed for IVF treatment in Europe in 1996. These drugs are by and large only marginally more effective, but significantly more expensive than urinary gonadotrophins (Out et al. 1995). Their use will not reduce the incidence of ovarian hyperstimulation syndrome (OHSS) nor increase significantly the live birth rate compared to the cheaper urinary derived products. The introduction of these drugs is likely to limit the number of women undergoing treatment in the public sector where funding is tightly controlled and will significantly increase the cost to a private patient. It is likely that clinicians will attempt to develop more cost effective alternative protocols of stimulation to contain the cost of IVF.

Patients and other purchasers of fertility treatments wish to buy the most cost effective treatment, but the pressure to produce the most babies per treatment cycle commenced is associated with high rates of multiple pregnancy. The ultimate denominator should be the rate of healthy non handicapped children per treatment cycle commenced, as the costs of hospitalisation, care in the community and special education need also to be taken into consideration.

Ovulation and ovarian stimulation

The development of the anti-oestrogen, clomiphene citrate and the introduction of gonadotrophins derived from the urine of post menopausal women both in the early 1960s provided for the first time an effective means of ovarian stimulation. These drugs were initially prescribed in anovulatory women, but have been used widely since 1970 to produce more than one egg in ovulatory women undergoing treatment by IVF.

Their use has been associated with higher birth rates, but this is associated with both a significant increase in the rate of multiple births and risks to the life and health of the women from the OHSS. The incidence of OHSS ranges from 2-7 per cent and varies in severity. The severe forms (1 to 2 per cent of all women being stimulated) are life threatening and demand early diagnosis and active management.

At present a 'long regime' is used in the majority of centres. This consists of the administration of a gonadotrophin releasing hormone (GnRH) agonist or analogue. These drugs cause the release of natural FSH from the pituitary and if administered continuously will result in a state of pituitary FSH exhaustion (known as pituitary desensitisation or downregulation). It thus becomes possible for the clinician to have total control of the ovulatory process but in so doing large amounts of exogenous FSH are required to stimulate the ovaries. GnRH antagonists (rather than agonists) are currently undergoing clinical trials. These drugs have an advantage over the agonist in that it may be possible to inhibit the luteinising hormone (LH) surge (the signal from the pituitary to the ovary that the egg containing follicles are mature). It will thus become possible to avoid the use of the agonist with a consequent reduction in the amount of FSH necessary to induce ovarian stimulation.

The introduction of biosynthetic gonadotrophin technology will also allow scientists to manipulate the molecule. It will thus become possible to synthesise long-acting preparations and perhaps alternatives to be used at different times during the stimulation to mimic the natural process more closely.

More effective drugs provide clinicians with more powerful means to stimulate ovulation. This facility should not be used to override the body's 'natural' processes. The importance of weight reduction in the treatment of overweight women with polycystic ovaries (a body mass index in excess of 27) is well established. Attempts to induce ovulation in the overweight polycystic ovaries patient should be delayed until the body mass index (BMI) is within the normal range.

It is essential that drug therapy in anovulatory underweight women (BMI <19) should be withheld until they have gained the required amount as pregnancy in underweight women is associated with a higher incidence of growth retarded and premature babies.

Intracytoplasmic sperm injection (ICSI)

This technique was developed in Belgium to treat couples where the male partner has a significant sperm disorder (Palermo et al. 1992). It is highly effective and is probably the most important advance in infertility treatment since the introduction of IVF. Preliminary follow up studies of the children conceived after ICSI show an increase in sex chromosome abnormalities (from 0.02 to 2.0 per cent). Studies are also in progress to determine whether microdeletions of the Y chromosome are transmitted to male offspring. These deletions are known to be associated with azoospermia. The outcome of these studies and also the long term follow up of the children conceived after IVF/ICSI are awaited with keen interest.

The implantation rate of ICSI embryos is similar to, if not greater than, that after conventional IVF reflecting the younger age and absence of fertility disorders in the female partner. It is thus incumbent upon the clinician to advise the couple to consider limiting the number of embryos replaced to less than three.

Both mature sperm cells and spermatids (immature sperm cells with the correct number of chromosomes but lacking a tail) can be used to fertilise the eggs with ICSI (Fishel 1996). The use of spermatids is not permitted in the United Kingdom although it is technically possible to obtain the cells by testicular aspiration. An apparently healthy child has been born following this procedure. In the UK, the Human Fertilisation and Embryology Authority (HFEA) require further proof as to the safety of the procedure and the health of the children before licensing the use of spermatids for routine clinical use. This line of argument is reasonable but at the same time the Authority has not yet licensed a clinical research project in humans to address this question.

Treatment with spermatids remains illegal in the UK pending the outcome of research which may be forthcoming from countries with less stringent licensing procedures. Clinical IVF was introduced without these controls and is it unethical to provide such treatment (using spermatids) to those who require such treatment provided they are fully informed as to the experimental nature of the procedure?

Egg (oocyte) cryopreservation

The birth of a healthy baby after egg freezing and thawing, and subsequent IVF was first reported by Chen in 1986. It has not yet been possible to repeat this sequence of events and the cryopreservation of eggs for routine clinical purposes is not yet a practical proposition. The ability to successfully freeze and thaw eggs is not only of major clinical importance in view of the paucity of egg donors for the treatment of women suffering from premature ovarian failure and to prevent the birth of children with genetic disorders, but is of ethical importance in those groups of people who have objections to the cryopresevation of embryos and who regard life as beginning at the moment of fertilisation. The technique would also be useful in the management of young women undergoing treatment of cancer which would result in the removal or destruction of their ovaries. Eggs could be removed, frozen and subsequently subjected to IVF at a later stage in their lives when they wish to have children.

Cryopreservation of ovarian tissue

Gosden (1994) has shown that it is possible to restore fertility in oophorectomised sheep by ovarian autografts stored at –196 °C. These experiments open the way to the storage of ovarian tissue with a view to subsequent in vitro maturation of the eggs. This would be of great benefit to young women undergoing chemo- or radiotherapy for cancer when the treatment destroys their eggs, and also to help overcome the shortage of donated eggs for the treatment of women with premature ovarian failure or to prevent the transmission of sex-linked disorders.

Embryo cryopreservation

The ability to freeze and thaw embryos is invaluable. Follow-up studies of children born after the replacement of freeze/thawed embryos have not shown an increase in the incidence of major or minor malformations and their social and intellectual development is similar to children conceived normally (Sutcliffe et al. 1995).

The live birth rate per cycle of frozen embryo replacement remains static (Horne et al. 1996). To improve this rate it is necessary to examine the population group undergoing treatment, the drugs used to stimulate the ovaries, the IVF and culture techniques and finally the method of cryopreservation, thawing and replacement. It is of ethical importance to address these matters as it is only with a robust and effective cryopreservation programme that clinicians are able to support the argument in favour of limiting to one or two the number of embryos replaced in a cycle of IVF.

Preimplantation diagnosis

This technique has to date been used with IVF at a limited number of centres to prevent the birth of children with single gene recessive disorders e.g. cystic fibrosis, Lesch-Nyhan syndrome, Duchenne muscular dystrophy (Handyside 1991). Preimplantation diagnosis (PID) could also be used to prevent the birth of individuals who are carriers of an autosomal dominant gene disorder that will in later life cause severe mental retardation (Huntington's chorea). It is also possible that the technique could be applied to those with a family history of breast, ovarian and bowel cancer. PID requires a highly organised team of scientists, clinicians and geneticists to provide the necessary counselling and to undertake the complex clinical and laboratory procedures. It is extremely difficult to establish a precise diagnosis from a single cell (a blastomere) and whilst this is possible, the magnitude of the technical problems is likely to limit the introduction of the technique on a wide scale.

Currently the need for PID is usually determined by the birth of a child with a severe disorder invariably associated with mental retardation, profound handicap and a shortened life expectancy or the family history of a disorder such as Huntington's chorea. The identification of the genetic basis of an ever-increasing number of serious diseases e.g. breast and ovarian cancer and Alzheimer's disease is inevitable and this will lead to an increased demand for PID. It is highly unlikely that a genetic basis for homosexuality, criminality and other forms of behaviour thought by some to be unacceptable will be identified. It would be most unfortunate if the prevention of severe disease is curtailed by the banning of PID because of unwarranted fears of the technique being abused.

The procedure involves IVF, the biopsy of a four or eight cell embryo to obtain a single blastomere and to submit the cell to a variety of techniques depending on the nature of the underlying disorder. It is necessary to determine the sex of the embryo to prevent the birth of another child with a sex-linked disorder or to use gene probes to detect the presence or absence of a particular gene.

The identification of cancer-related genes raises important ethical questions with respect to the use of PID to prevent the development of cancer in mid or late life. Not all individuals at risk will develop the cancer. Will gene probes be used to screen embryos derived from couples only with the appropriate history and undergoing IVF treatment or would some individuals seek such screening for all their potential children? This would require IVF/PID techniques to be applied to an ever increasing population but before this could ever reach the realms of clinical practice a far clearer understanding of the role of tumour-suppressor genes is necessary. Would this be an appropriate use of resources?

The transfer of genetic material

It is now possible to place the nucleus of a cell of an adult live sheep in the egg of a ewe having first removed the genetic material from that egg. This results in the birth of lambs from the 'reconstituted' embryo identical to the donor of the nucleus. The animal experiments are of great interest scientifically and may benefit specialised agricultural and biosynthetic processes, e.g. producing human proteins for pharmaceutical purposes and the breeding of livestock (Wilmut et al. 1997).

The theoretical implications of this animal research are that a nucleus could be taken from a human cell and replaced into a human egg, having first removed the genetic material. The reconstituted embryo could then be placed in a woman and it would thus be possible to produce a human identical to the nuclear donor. There are no indications to use this technology in the treatment of human infertility nor are there indications to clone human beings. However it is theoretically possible that this technology could be used to prevent the birth of a child with mitochondrial disorder. Mitochondrial disorders are inherited via the cytoplasm of the egg. It would thus be possible to use the nuclei of the woman and her partner and the cytoplasm of a healthy egg donor to create the embryo.

This procedure would be illegal in the UK, as it would require a licence from the Human Fertilisation and Embryology Authority. The use of embryos for such purposes may be possible in countries without strict regulations governing research on and the use of human embryos.

References

Chen, C. (1986), 'Pregnancy After Human Oocyte Cryopreservation'. *Lancet*, Vol. 1, pp. 884-6.

Cruikshank, W. (1797), *Transactions of the Royal Society*, pp. 197-214.

Fishel, S., Aslam, I. and Tesarick, J. (1996), 'Spermatid Conception: A Stage Too Early, or a Time Too Soon', *Hum Reprod*, Vol. 11, pp. 1371-5.

Gosden, R.G., Baird, D.T., Wade, J.C. and Webb, R. (1994), 'Restoration of Fertility to Oophorectomized Sheep by Ovarian Autografts Stored at -196 °C', *Hum Reprod*, Vol. 9, pp. 597-603.

Handyside, A.H. (1991), 'Pre-implantation Diagnosis by DNA Amplification', in Chapman, M., Grudzinskas, G., Chard, T. and Maxwell, D. (eds), *The Embryo: Normal and Abnormal Development and Growth*, Springer: London, pp. 81-90.

Heap, W. (1891), 'Preliminary Note on the Transplantation and Growth of Mammalian Ova Within a Uterine Foster Mother', *Proc R Soc*, Vol. 48, pp. 457-8.

Horne, G., Critchlow, J.D., Newman, M.C., Edozien, L., Matson, P.L. and Lieberman, B.A. (1996), 'A Prospective Evaluation of Cryopreservation Strategies in a Two Embryo Transfer Programme', *Hum Reprod*, Vol. 12, No. 3, pp. 542-7.

Out, H.J., Mannaerts, M.J.L., Driessen. S.G.A.J. and Coelingh Bennink, H.J.T. (1995), 'A Prospective, Randomized, Assessor-blind, Multicentre Study Comparing Recombinant and Urinary Follicle Stimulating Hormone (Puregon versus Metrodin) in In-vitro Fertilization', *Hum Reprod*, Vol. 10, No. 10, pp. 2534-40.

Palermo, G., Joris, H., Devroey, P. and Van Stirteghem, A.C. (1992), 'Pregnancies After Intracytoplasmic Injection of a Single Spermatozoon into an Oocyte', *Lancet*, Vol. 340, pp. 17-8.

Steptoe, P.C. and Edwards, R.G. (1978), 'Birth After Reimplantation of a Human Embryo', *Lancet*, Vol. ii, pp. 366.

Sutcliffe, A.G., D'Souza, S.W., Cadman, J., Richards, B., McKinley, I.A. and Lieberman, B.A. (1995), 'Minor Congenital Anomalies, Major Congenital Malformations and Development in Children Conceived from Cryopreserved Embryos', *Hum Reprod*, Vol. 10, pp. 3332-7.

Wilmut, I., Schnieke, A.E., McWhir, J., Kind, A.J. and Campbell, K.H.S. (1997), 'Viable Offspring Derived from Fetal and Adult Mammalian Cells', *Nature*, Vol. 385, pp. 810-3.

2 Do modern reproductive technologies violate human dignity?

Dieter Birnbacher

Introduction: Problems with the use of the concept of human dignity in recent German bioethics

Frequent reference to the concept of human dignity as a normative principle is a distinctive feature of German bioethical discussion. On the one hand, the concept plays a major role in the moral rejection and legal prohibition of some of the new methods of reproduction and of gene manipulation. On the other hand, it is typically invoked, both by ethicists and lawyers, as a kind of ultimate article of faith rather than as a principle open to rational debate. Its typical function is that of a 'conversation stopper' (J. F. Keenan) apparently settling an issue once for all and tolerating no further discussion. The explanation of this phenomenon seems to be sociological rather than philosophical. The more pluralistic the values of a society become, and the more relativistic its thinking about these values, the more strongly the need is felt for a taboo concept defining, in a negative way, its residual moral identity. This may help to explain the characteristic absoluteness and emotionality associated with the concept. At the same time, it signals an inevitable intellectual quandary: It is difficult to *argue* for a taboo. Either a taboo is deeply felt and firmly established in a society, so that it is unnecessary to argue for it; or, as in a pluralistic society as ours, the taboo is no longer shared by all, so that it becomes increasingly difficult for the majority to convince the dissenting minority by argument.

In many respects the use of the concept of human dignity in recent bioethical discussions of reproductice technologies is problematic. One example is the way that the concept has been used in an inflationed way overstepping all bounds of plausibility. A case in point is the attempt by Ernst Benda, then president of the German 'Bundesverfassungsgericht', to derive a prohibition of the technique of cloning right from the 'essence' of humankind. According to

Benda, it is an elementary right of everyone, and an element of his or her dignity as a human being, not to be genetically the exact copy of one of his parents (Benda, 1985, p.224). Characteristically, this kind of 'natural law' argument is presented without any further explanation. No consideration is given to the fact that the existence of identical twins makes it doubtful whether genetic individuality is really part of the 'essence of man' in any descriptive sense. Another case is the reasoning used by the legal commentators of the German 'Embryonenschutzgesetz' (Embryo Protection Act) to justify the legal prohibition of surrogate motherhood (Keller er al., 1992, p.153). These authors suggest that the production of an embryo with a view to surrogate motherhood possibly violates the human dignity of the embryo by virtue of the fact that in this case the embryo is produced for 'foreign ends'.[1] I take this to mean that the production of the embryo is in this case made to serve ends other than its own or its own good. Obviously, either way the argument does not work. On the one hand, the embryo cannot be said to *have* ends, for then it would have to be conscious in some way (which is hard to assume in the case of the early embryo), nor can it be said to *be* an end, since (pace Kant) ends are not human beings but states which human beings want to bring about. If, on the other hand, the production of an embryo is in conformity with human dignity only if it aims at the embryo's *own* good, only a small number of pregnancies would conform to human dignity since it is usually not the good of their future children that people centrally aim at in begetting them. The fact that this argument can at least *appear* to have some plausibility seems largely a matter of psychology. The *technological* aspect of the reproductive process is associatied with *instrumentalising* ways of thinking and acting, whereas in fact the use of technologies is not particularly tied to practices of instrumentalising those to whom it is administered. In medicine, the use of technology is not generally an instrumentalisation of the patient to ends foreign to his own good, but a use of technical instruments exactly for his own good. On the other hand, brutal and morally indefensible ways of instrumentalising people date further back than modern technology. Kant's second formula of the Categorical Imperative reacted to the practice of slavery, bondage and compulsory recruitment rather than to the use of technology.

Arguments for a less-inflated definition of human dignity

There is more than one reason to reject an extensive recourse to the concept of human dignity in bioethics. One reason is that the emphasis and the inherent pathos of the concept often seem to be exploited simply in order to eschew the difficulties of giving rational arguments for moral and legal injunctions against unwelcome practices. One has to admit that these difficulties are sometimes considerable. But the fact that practices like surrogate motherhood and embryo research are rejected, more or less emotionally, by a great majority of the population – and probably also by a majority of intellectuals –, cannot by itself show that these practices are inherently immoral, nor can it by itself justify (at least in a liberal state) the penal sanctions imposed, e.g., by the German 'Embryonenschutzgesetz'. In fact, this remarkable piece of legislation is hardly more than an expressive gesture of public outrage, in the tradition of – as one author (Struck, 1988, p.116) poignantly put it – the practice of public stoning.

Another reason for rejecting an inflated use of the concept of human dignity is its tendency to blur important distinctions. There is a tendency to use the concept of human dignity in a way that makes it coextensive with the principle of sanctity of life as if protection of *life* were the only or the only central concern of the concept, ignoring areas of conflict such as suicide or voluntary euthanasia where the principles have contrary implications. Suicide and voluntary euthanasia (at least its active variants) are clearly ruled out by the principle of sanctity of life, but are clearly compatible with the concept of human dignity. Extracorporal fertilisation is often alleged to be an infringement of the concept of human dignity, but, being a technique of producing life, it is doubtful that it can be thought of as an infringement of the sanctity of life.

The third reason is that an extensive use of the argument of the concept of human dignity tends to weaken the authority and moral emphasis of the concept (Eser 1990, p. 36). This is deplorable because the concept has an important role to play. It would be a pity if by importing subjective and fashionable contents into its meaning the concept loses its normative force and ends up as a piece of empty rhetoric. If Herbert Spiegelberg's dictum is to remain true that 'human dignity seems to be one of the few common values in our world of philosophical pluralism' (Spiegelberg, 1986, p.198) and if the concept is to function – in ethics, law and politics – as a kind of quasi-absolute, its content must as far as possible be free from controversial elements.

This presupposes that the concept does indeed have a role to play and is not, as Schopenhauer argued against Kant, an empty formula both 'insufficent, without proper content and problematical' (Schopenhauer, 1818/1988, p.412). Does the concept of human dignity have a 'proper content'?

I believe that there *is* a content to the concept of human dignity and that this content can be identified both in the ethical and the legal context with a collection of inalienable and unforfeitable *rights*. To respect human dignity means to respect certain *minimal* rights owned by its bearer irrespective of considerations of achievement, merit and quality, and owned even by those who themselves do *not* respect these minimal rights in others. What are these rights?

There are, it seems, four components:

1 provision of the biologically necessary means of existence,
2 freedom from strong and continued suffering,
3 minimal liberty,
4 minimal self-respect.

These four components can be looked upon as minimal 'basic goods' which the principle of human dignity says nobody should be deprived of, where deprivation has to be understood as comprising of both action and omission. Though human dignity is often understood in a purely negative sense, the principle works both as a negative and as a positive right. It sets a minimal standard of acceptibility both to what is done to people and to what people are allowed to suffer. It sets a limit to inhuman treatment (like torture, slavery, capital punishment), but also to inhuman omissions (like letting others starve, or allowing them to be humiliated or persecuted as members of racial, ethnic or religious minorities). This implies that even with the minimality of the rights postulated by human dignity the efforts required by their effective protection may be considerable.

This is especially true, under certain circumstances, of the first component of human dignity, the provision of the necessary means of existence. This component has been widely neglected in the standard explications of the concept, but being a necessary condition of the others, really is its most basic component. The fact that the concept of human dignity is rooted in the essentially liberal tradition of Locke and Kant with its stress on negative rather than positive rights has tended to focus the attention on liberty as the central component of the concept and to blind one to what the effective exercise of liberty requires as its presupposition.

Another component of human dignity is freedom from pain, at least from serious and continued pain. This component is of particular relevance to the German health care system with its scandalous reluctance to provide pain-killing drugs and devices to pain-patients. It is clearly a violation of human dignity to allow a patient to suffer serious and continued pain when the technical means are available or could be made available at reasonable costs.

The two other components, minimal liberty and minimal self-respect, are too widely recognised to need much commentary and are well-established elements of the legal interpretation of the first article of the German 'Grundgesetz'. If there are controversies, they are not about the core content of human dignity in these areas but about where to draw the line between what is minimal and what is more than minimal. Kant's second formula of the Categorical Imperative according to which none must be used by others *only* as a means, does not offer very much help in this respect, not only because this formula does not by itself imply anything about its concrete application apart from Kant's casuistic examples (which are too idiosyncratic to be taken into account nowadays), but because it is too narrow: If the members of a hated minority are lynched by the majority they are not 'used only as means', but they are treated cruelly for their own sakes. If prisoners of war are tortured or starved to death it is not necessarily in the rational pursuit of ends such as gaining secret information, intimidation or deterrence, but it may also be because of strong non-rational interests in retaliation, revenge, and cruelty itself. It is true, historically the concept of human dignity was introduced into the German 'Grundgesetz' mainly in reaction to the characteristic Nazi schizophrenia of irrational (archaic) ends and rational (technological) means. But if intentions, or the rationality of intentions, mattered, the concept of human dignity would paradoxically grant protection only against the technical rationality but not against the arbitrariness and wickedness of tyrants.

The strong, concrete versus the weak, abstract principle of human dignity

There are, thus, good reasons to define the concept of human dignity in a restricted and less-inflated sense, among them the importance of preserving the status of the concept as a moral absolute (or quasi-absolute) and the resultant necessity to keep it out of the common run of ethical value conflicts and political controversies. This, however, is easier said than done, for there are obstacles to such a restriction within the concept itself. The truth is that the inflated use of the concept in recent bioethical debate is foreshadowed in an inner ambiguity of the concept as it is used in informal contexts (Birnbacher 1987). Even in its everyday use human dignity does not only denote a limited sphere of unforfeitable individual minimal rights to be respected irrespective of considerations of merit and quality, but is also used in two extended meanings: one in which it is applied, among others, to the early and the residual stages of human life (human embryos, fetuses, and corpses), and one in which it is applied not to any individuals but to the human species. In Germany, the application of the concept to human embryos was notoriously sanctioned by the 'Bundesverfassungsgericht' in its decision against the liberal abortion law of 1975 when it stated that human dignity 'is a property of human life wherever it exists' (Bundesverfassungsgericht, 1975, p.41), where human life is meant to include the life of the human zygote from conception on, a position echoed in the legal literature (see, e.g., Vitzthum, 1985, p.252). The other extended application – to the human species as such – is exemplified in the common rejection of the production of man-animal-hybrids where the underlying principle is not the consequentialist one that the potential prospects of the beings produced are too uncertain to justify the experiment but the sentiment that such an experiment would destroy the identity of the human species and would overstep boundaries in the order of nature that should somehow be respected.

Both 'abstract' applications of the concept of human dignity cannot be subsumed under its core meaning, that of minimal individual rights. If the concept is invoked to reject (and to prohibit) the production of biological hybrids it is not because of the prospective rights of the individuals produced, but because of an independent principle of species purity. If the concept is invoked to reject (and to prohibit) abortion it is not because of any prospective rights the individuals not carried to term would have if they were carried to term but because of an independent principle that human life as such is endowed with dignity.

Even in its everyday use, then, and most noticeably in its legal use, there is no unitary and homogeneous concept of human dignity, but rather a family of meanings the members of which behave differently not only semantically but also syntactically. While the concept of human dignity in its core meaning needs an individual subject as bearer, this is not necessary with the extended concepts. With them, there need not be a real subject to correspond to the grammatical subject. This is evident where human dignity is applied to the species as such, but it also applies to its use with human zygotes and early embryos, entities which cannot reasonably be assumed to be 'real subjects'. While human dignity in its core meaning postulates minimal individual rights, the concept of human dignity in its extended meaning postulates obligations without corresponding rights since there may be no bearer of rights. With the concept of human dignity in its core meaning the object of respect and protection is the concrete human being. With human dignity in its extended meaning it is humanity, human life, or the identity and dignity of the human species defined by its specific potentialities. This abstractness of the reference of the extended concept, prominent in arguments against germline intervention or against the production of interspecies hybrids (Keller et al., 1992, p.240), is already conspicuous in Kant when he says in a variant of his second formula of the Categorical Imperative that it is not man but *humanity* ('die Menschheit', the human essence) that should never be used only as means (Kant, 1785/1903, p.429).

My thesis is that the distinction between human dignity in its core meaning and in its extended meaning is of considerable importance both in ethics and in law. Its importance lies in the fact that the narrow and the extended concepts carry different moral weight so that conflating them must either lead to an unacceptably weak protection of individual and concrete dignity or to an unacceptably strong protection of generic and abstract dignity.

A concrete concept of human dignity functions as a moral quasi-absolute. Sacrificing the principle for other values or principles is generally held to be acceptable only in exceptional cases. This concept is relevant only to very few of the moral problems specifically associated with modern reproductive techniques. An example would be provided by possible experiments with germline manipulation with a risk of severe suffering in the resulting children or by the potential use of preimplantation diagnosis in a program of compulsory eugenic control. The concept of human dignity which is involved in most of the moral problems specifically associated with modern reproductive techniques is human dignity in the abstract, which is generally thought of as a much weaker principle and does not rule out, as the strong principle does, being given up in favour of other values such as individual autonomy or scientific and medical progress. The respect due to a human embryo or a human corpse is a weak form of respect (Lamb, 1988, p.113), much weaker in any case than that due to a human person with the capacities of consciousness and self-consciousness. The prohibition to sell one's children or one's wife is generally perceived to have a much higher priority than a prohibition to sell living human embryos or live human organs, or a prohibition to sell dead human embryos or parts of human corpses. Whereas the principle of human dignity in its core meaning is generally assigned the highest priority (even higher than that assigned to the principle to protect life), the normative status of its extensions is both lower and more uncertain.

In fact, the difference in normative status is mirrored by a corresponding difference in epistemological status. Whereas for a concrete concept of human dignity a strong justification can be given in terms of the interests and needs of the individual concerned, an abstract concept of human dignity can only be weakly justified, with reference, ultimately, to the sentiments of observers. To justify the minimal rights postulated by individual dignity one does not need more than the weak assumptions of theories of minimal morality such as Bernard Gert's theory of moral rules (Gert 1966), i.e. theories whose essential assumption is the trivial one that people indeed have a strong interest in life, physical integrity, liberty, and self-respect, and a strong interest to live in a society which guarantees at least a minimum of these goods. A justification of the contents of the extended concepts is much more difficult. Whereas the strong principle can be justified via a relatively constant set of basic human needs there is no comparatively elementary justification for the extended concepts. Justifications of these are bound to involve more relative and culture-dependent ideas of value and dignity.

This is evidenced by the fact that roughly the same catalogue of basic human rights is part of nearly all constitutions of the world whereas there is a significant lack of unanimity with reference to, say, the moral status of the human embryo. On this point, opinions diverge widely both between and within national cultures. There is, on the whole, considerable uncertainty about where the ethical truth lies. Personally, I agree with Lamb (1988, p.113) that living human embryos deserve no less, but also no more respect than human corpses or human organs, with the consequence that if the principle of respecting human dignity is applied to them at all, it can have no more moral weight than other principles of piety. But even those who judge differently on this point would not, I presume, go so far as to give the principle of respecting human dignity the same moral weight in this context as in the contexts to which the 'core meaning' of the principle applies.

Note

1 '...dienen menschliche Embryonen, die jemand «herstellt», um sie für eigene oder Drittinteressen zu «benutzen», in geradezu klassischer Weise als Objekt für andere. Deshalb kommt als weiteres geschütztes Rechtsgut (neben dem menschlichen Leben) die Menschenwürde in Betracht.'

References

Benda, E. (1985), 'Erprobung der Menschenwürde am Beispiel der Humangenetik', in Flöhl, R. (ed.), *Genforschung – Fluch oder Segen? Interdisziplinäre Stellungnahmen*, Schweitzer: München, pp. 205-31.

Birnbacher, D. (1987), 'Gefährdet die moderne Reproduktionsmedizin die menschliche Würde?', in Braun, V., Mieth, D. and Steigleder, K. (eds), *Ethische und rechtliche Fragen der Gentechnologie und der Reproduktionsmedizin*, Schweitzer: München, pp. 77-88. Reprinted in Leist, A. (ed.), *Um Leben und Tod. Moralische Probleme bei Abtreibung, künstlicher Befruchtung, Euthanasie und Selbstmord*, Suhrkamp: Frankfurt a.M. 1990, pp. 266-81.

Bundesverfassungsgericht (1975), *Entscheidungen*, Vol. 39, Karlsruhe.

Eser, A. (1990), *Neuartige Bedrohungen ungeborenen Lebens*, C. F. Müller: Karlsruhe.

Gert, B. (1966), *The Moral Rules. A New Rational Foundation for Morality*, Harper & Row: New York.

Kant, I. (1785/1903), *Grundlegung zur Metaphysik der Sitten*, Akademie-Ausgabe, Vol. 4, Reimer: Berlin, pp. 385-464.

Keller, R., Günther, H.-L. and Kaiser, P. (1992), *Embryonenschutzgesetz. Kommentar*, Kohlhammer: Stuttgart.

Lamb, D. (1988), *Down the Slippery Slope. Arguing in Applied Ethics*, Croom Helm: London.

Schopenhauer, A. (1818/1988), *Die Welt als Wille und Vorstellung I, Sämtliche Werke*, ed. Hübscher, 4th Ed., Vol. 2, Brockhaus: Mannheim.

Spiegelberg, H. (1986), *Steppingstones Toward an Ethics for Fellow Existers. Essays 1944-1983*, Reidel: Dordrecht.

Struck, G. (1988),'Die «Würde des Menschen» als Argument und Tabu in der Debatte zur Fertilisations- und Gentechnologie', in Klug, U. and Kriele, M.

(eds), *Menschen- und Bürgerrechte*, Steiner: Stuttgart (*Archiv für Rechts- und Sozialphilosophie*, Suppl. 33), pp. 110-8.
Vitzthum, W. Graf (1985), 'Gentechnologie und Menschenwürde', *Medizinrecht*, Vol. 6, pp. 249-57.

3 Some observations on human dignity and human rights

Deryck Beyleveld

Dieter Birnbacher's contends that there are a number of rights (both negative and positive) that should be treated as absolute or 'quasi-absolute' entitlements of human beings who are 'real subjects', and that the importance of these rights (to 'the provision of the biologically necessary means of existence'; to 'freedom from strong and continued suffering'; to 'minimal liberty', and to 'minimal self-respect' – which he considers to constitute the core values associated with the concept of human dignity) is threatened by 'inflationary' appeals to human dignity that attribute it to 'among others [...] the early and residual stages of human life (human embryos, fetuses, and corpses), and [...] to the human *species.*' While human embryos, etc., do have value, '[t]he respect due to a human embryo or a human corpse is [...] much weaker [...] than that due to a human person with the capacities of consciousness and self-consciousness', being roughly equivalent to the respect due to human organs. To conflate core and extended appeals to human dignity 'must either lead to an unacceptably weak protection of individual and concrete dignity or to an unacceptably strong protection of generic and abstract dignity' (Birnbacher, 1997, pp.328ff).

I have much sympathy with this view. The values that Dieter Birnbacher identifies as constituting the core of human dignity call to mind what Gewirth (1978) identifies as 'basic' rights (rights to 'basic generic needs', the absence of which interferes with, or even precludes, the possibility of action as such). Within the framework of Gewirthian theory, these rights are the most important, and the attribution of such rights to human embryos, human corpses, or the human species *as such* is either wholly untenable or severely restricted. Certainly, none of these rights can be attributed to corpses; at most, it could *perhaps* be argued that fetuses have some right to the provision of the biologically necessary means of existence and to freedom from strong and continued suffering, and that the human embryo has some right to the first of these. Yet, even if such arguments are sound, the protection owed to fetuses or the human embryo will be less than that owed to 'real subjects' or agents. *If* human dignity consists of rights to basic needs, then to conflate protections owed to the human embryo with respect for human dignity will certainly be to weaken the status of basic rights or to unacceptably strengthen the protections owed to the human embryo.

I have, however, three critical observations, which I hope will be constructive.

First, to specify one of the core rights as a right to the provision of the biologically necessary means of 'existence' implies that any living being (or at least human being – in the biological sense) has this right, and produces inconsistencies in Dieter Birnbacher's analysis. Within the general framework of Dieter Birnbacher's thinking, as well as within Gewirthian theory, this right is surely better specified as a right to the provision of the biologically necessary means of *action*. While such a right is, at least in part, a right to life (and the means to it), it is a right to *life-for-action* rather than a right to *life-for-its-own-sake*.

Second, I am not entirely happy with the idea that to possess human dignity is to be owed the basic rights and that to violate human dignity is to violate the basic rights directly. This is mainly because the basic rights include things that are sometimes identified with rights to autonomy, life, integrity, and other values, which are frequently thought to be distinct from the value of human dignity. However, I do not wish to make too much of this, as there is nothing more sterile than a disagreement that boils down to a quibble about how a term is to be used.

This, however, brings me to my third observation. While the important thing is not what we call human dignity, but that we discriminate justifiably between the values of different actions and practices, there is a set of considerations relevant to the use of reproductive technologies that Dieter Birnbacher does not attend to, distinct from respect for the basic rights, that might be said to concern human dignity. What I have in mind is that it might be argued that certain uses of reproductive technologies violate human dignity, not in the way in which they treat the human embryo, but in how they reflect upon the character of those who wish to avail themselves of these technologies. In ordinary usage, persons are characteristically said to act in undignified ways when they display weaknesses that they ought not to display; for example, by failing to display due fortitude in the face of adversity, or by seeking to evade responsibility for their actions. Pursuing this, I can, for example, imagine it being argued that the use of in vitro fertilisation for post-menopausal women is a violation of human dignity (for reasons akin to those that might be used to argue that attempts to prolong life indefinitely by transplantation of organs violate the human dignity of the person attempting to prolong his or her life by these means). I hasten to add that I do not necessarily support such arguments. Any validity they have will need to be assessed on a case by case basis. Furthermore, such arguments might rely on attributions of duties (perfect or imperfect) to oneself, with which I have considerable difficulty – unless these can be derived from perfect duties to others. To my way of thinking, the virtues are predispositions to act in ways that respect the rights of others. Nevertheless, I call attention to this because I believe that appeals to human dignity are not necessarily (unjustifiable) attempts to extend the possession of the basic rights beyond their appropriate bearers, but may be appeals to a different set of considerations altogether. While such considerations are, in my opinion, subordinate to the protection of the basic rights, they still merit careful consideration in the context of reproductive technologies.

References

Birnbacher, D. (1997), 'Do Modern Reproductive Technologies Violate Human Dignity?', this volume, Part Nine.

Gewirth, A. (1978), *Reason and Morality*, University of Chicago Press: Chicago.

4 The 'essentials' of human dignity

Walter Lesch

Dieter Birnbacher's stimulating paper (Birnbacher 1997) leads us to the very centre of our debate on ethical issues in reproductive medicine. The author helps us to clarify the emotional and biased use of moral language and suggests some distinctions which are useful in the discussion about the moral and legal status of the human embryo. Although I agree with the attempt to avoid some of the difficulties caused by the concept of human dignity, I cannot approve of all the critical remarks.

Certainly the idea of human dignity has been developed in a rather special way in recent German bioethics. But it is not an exclusive feature of this particular social, political and historical context. We can find it as well in France or in Italy, in Britain or in the USA. And not only as an old-fashioned 'natural law'-argument maintained by conservative religious groups, but as a normative orientation closely connected to the system of individual human rights. It is undeniable that human dignity is often introduced as a 'conversation stopper'; the same could be said about a lot of other key notions of the current biomedical discourse: autonomy, justice, scientific progress ... There are several ways of defining the 'residual morality' and the 'taboo concepts' of modern societies. Whereas the innovative ideals of medical intervention have the advantage of a dynamic and promising perspective, the advocates of human dignity seem to preach refusal and prohibition because they pretend to possess some kind of metaphysical knowledge about the 'essence' of humankind. Most scientists (and most ethicists) nowadays reject such an inflexible position as fundamentalist.

In spite of the clear rejection of any sort of 'essentialism' in ethical arguments D. Birnbacher defends some *essentials* of human dignity: minimal basic goods and minimal rights which represent a consensus in a world of pluralism. But as he explains himself he cannot escape the necessity of drawing the line between minimal and more than minimal goods. Obviously there is no consensus about a scale of precisely defined *degrees* of basic goods. The distinction finally adopted between a weak, abstract protection of human entities at the beginning and at the end of life and the strong, concrete protection of the agents' individual rights rests arbitrarily. The starting point for ethical embarrassment and ethical reasoning is the intuition that we usually argue in favour of more than just minimal values and rights (for agents and for patients). This constant tension between minimal standards and maximal options exists in scientific research as well as in ethics. Therefore it is unlikely that a moral consensus can be found as a compromise on the lowest level.

Even if we agree that respect of the human embryo is weaker than respect for the person the feeling of piety indicates that there is something special about the beginning and the end of life. Why should we not qualify this characteristic as an aspect of human dignity? Even if it is more the indication of a question than the definitive normative answer. Those who are interested in eliminating all barriers to embryo research might object that such a cautious scepticism with a tendency towards a great respect of the symbolic value of the embryo is not better in its practical consequences than the tough concept of fundamentalism with its quick deduction from nature to normativity. Anyway there is still a lot of work to be done in ethics in order to show that human dignity is not just an ideological article of faith, but a complex and indispensable concept with direct and symbolic implications.

D. Birnbacher focuses on the question whether new reproductive technologies violate the human dignity of the embryo. But we must ask the same question about agents becoming patients when they are undergoing an infertility treatment. Their human dignity has to be protected against all possible attacks by social pressure, discrimination due to problems of unjust allocation, sexism and crude materialism. These would be real cases of physical harm and mental violence. Because of such experiences the controversial notion of human dignity will probably never disappear from our moral language.

Thanks to the open public debate on medical technologies the religion of science has entered the period of enlightenment where the simple reference to the authority of scientists no longer counts as a valid argument if it is not part of a transparent and transdisciplinary procedure. In the project of shaping this process of rational, democratic regulation ethicists and IVF-specialists are in the same boat.

References

Birnbacher, D. (1997), 'Do Modern Reproductive Technologies Violate Human Dignity?', this volume, Part Nine.

5 Moral boundaries of reproductive technology. Some preliminary remarks

Egbert Schroten

The issue of the limits of reproductive technology can be approached from different (e.g. technical, medical, economic) angles. I want to deal with it from a moral point of view. In that case, it will be clear from the outset that it is im possible – or at least very unfruitful – to jump into a discussion, without saying anything about the context and the moral framework within which such a discussion may take place. Before saying something about limiting reproductive technology, then, I want to make some preliminary remarks concerning: plurality in society, the tension between science and technology at one hand and philosophy and ethics at the other, and the possibility of a moral framework, within which the issue can be discussed.

Plural society

It is nearly a truism to say that we live in a plural society. This may be particularly true in view of questions concerning the beginning and the end of life. In this short text, there is no room for an analysis of this complex phenomenon. Only two short remarks: (1) The complexity may be underlined by an ambiguity in public opinion. There is a constant pressure on science and technology to find solutions for problems in the field of human reproduction and of childlessness on one hand, and anxiety about the development of science and technology and the manipulation of the beginning of life on the other. (2) From a moral point of view, however, we should not exaggerate problems as if they were radically new. Even in the so called *corpus christianum*, there has always been discussion in ethics about (the interpretation of) principles and norms and about the priority of some norms over others.

Concerning the plurality of society, three reactions are possible, depending on how we assess it. (1) We could look on plurality, like some 'absolutists' do, as an alibi to avoid entering into a discussion, or (2) we could see it as a thread for our moral and cultural identity and, then, enter into a discussion but in a defensive mood. We could try to stick to our own moral framework and to defend our positions as long as possible. But (3) it is also possible to look on plurality in society as a challenge and try to find a common moral framework in open dialogue with each other. This does not mean that we should betray our own tradition and identity. On the contrary, we should bring them in. But it requires an attitude of openness and respect to other ideas and commitments, and the willingness to walk together and to find common ground and ways to look for solutions for problems we all have to face.

Science and ethics

My second remark is about the tension – sometimes even the gulf – between science and technology and philosophy and ethics. From the Renaissance onwards there has been a 'liberation movement' of various branches of science from theology and philosophy and a development into an independent position of the sciences. Let me, being a theologian, be clear: This has been a healthy and fruitful development. But it had negative consequences as well. Science and ethics are not acquainted any more; hence, they have difficulties understanding each other. They play different language games, to use a Wittgensteinian metaphor, and there are big differences in methodology and in approach. Moreover, in our homo faber culture, science and technology seem to develop rapidly and autonomously, more and more entwined with market economy, whereas philosophy and ethics want to slow down their tempo in order to have the time to ask (moral) questions and to think things over.[1]

This distance and tension are dangerous (at least not fruitful) for society. Science, technology, philosophy and ethics need each other 'to make and to keep human life human' (Paul Lehmann). Besides, ethics has to face the facts, for otherwise it is walking in the clouds. And science and technology need ethics, for otherwise they are rudderless and in danger of getting out of control. In short, science and wisdom need each other. Therefore, in limiting reproductive technology, we need a 'herrschaftsfreie Diskussion' (Habermas) or an 'accompagnement' (Gilbert Hottois) between (reproductive) science and ethics.

A moral framework

In the third place, a 'conscience des limites' needs a moral framework. What I would point out from a moral point of view is that, in spite of the plurality of society and the tension between science and ethics, we do not find ourselves in mere chaos. It seems to be possible to start with an outline of a moral framework, in the light of European cultural tradition. In other words, a common ground may be found, from which a discussion about the limits of reproductive technology could and should start.

In the context of European culture, we could point to the moral tradition of the medical profession, from Hippocrates onwards, with important principles like 'primum non nocere' (non-maleficence) and 'salus aegroti suprema lex' (beneficence). More recently, we could point to the so called 'Georgetown mantra', which adds to these classic principles in medical ethics respect for autonomy and distributive justice. And, finally, we could point to the Convention on Human Rights and Biomedicine (the so called 'Bioethics Convention') of the Council of Europe (1996).

Furthermore, there is, in our society, a broad consensus that children are considered as a blessing, a gift, a joy, a fulfillment of a loving partnership, and that childlessness is a sad thing (although I would emphasise that human life can be fruitful without having children!). Reproductive technology, then, may be assessed positively, insofar as it may contribute to human happiness. There will be a consensus, too, that this technology should meet criteria of safety, carefulness and openness, and that the parents in spe are so well informed that they can take their parental responsibility.

All this is, of course, not meant to deny the problematic side of reproductive technology. We all know that there is a price to be paid, in the form of risks, the loss of human embryos, the medicalisation of pregnancy and the possibility to use this technology for other aims, such as embryo research or sex selection for non-medical reasons. Here the question of limits becomes urgent!

In my personal view, reproductive technology should in principle be limited to reproductive problems. It should therefore in principle be used on medical indication. 'In principle' means that any spin off or alternative use should face a 'no unless', the 'unless' meaning that there should be very good reasons to deviate from the principle. Whether this is the case, should be assessed by a broadly based, independent, multidisciplinary licensing body.

More specifically, I would enter the discussion on the limits of reproductive technology by stating:

- no in vitro fertilisation with the sole aim of creating human embryos for research (cf. Council of Europe, 1996, Art. 18,2);
- no cloning or splitting of embryos for transfer in the womb;
- no genetic modification of sperm, ova or embryos for transfer in the womb;
- no creation of hybrids or chimaeras;
- no sex selection for non-medical reasons.

However, a moral position is as strong or weak as its arguments are, and that must become clear in the course of discussion!

Note

1 There is another tension present in our culture, between 'ars' and 'natura' (the artificial and the natural). Here, I confine myself to referring to the contribution of Hub Zwart (1997).

References

Council of Europe (1996), *Convention on Human Rights and Biomedicine*, Strasbourg.

Zwart, H. (1997), 'Can Nature Serve as a Criterium for the Use of Reproductive Technologies?', this volume, part 9.

6 Nature and Technics. Approaching the underlying concepts in IVF

Barbara Maier

Clarifying the discussion about criteria for a reasonable use of in vitro fertilisation (IVF) means raising awareness of the underlying concepts in reproductive medicine, e.g. of the concept of nature. Reproductive technologies are often critizised for their potential to transform (often called denaturalise) human nature (procreation, parenthood etc.). Seldom is an account given of what is meant by nature.

Our philosophical as well as religious tradition has valued nature as something positive, even of divine origin. Secundum naturam vivere ... as the ancient philosophers told us, should be one of the principles guiding our lives and leading to balance of life. Nature in ancient times was conceptualised as comprising all dimensions of the human being. Managing life according to nature means living in the happy mean, avoiding extreme situations. Mastering nature might provoke strange and alienating developments. In other philosophical as well as religious reflections nature is disqualified, causing pain, illness and at least bringing death. We have to overcome what it brings upon us by mastering it, often by every means disposable to us.

When describing the underlying concept of nature in reproductive medicine we should take the following reflections into consideration: Moral judgements about IVF are prejudiced by the construction of a polarity between natural and artificial. Many misleading conceptions result from this antithetical approach. But what does nature mean? Does the concept of the natural cover the biological, sexual, genetical, also the psychological and mental dimensions, that of the artificial, the planned, controlled, man-made sphere as particularly expressed in and by technology? Where finally could the line between the both dimensions be found?

There is no antithetical, but a dialectical relation between the natural and the artificial. The human being is a cultural being by nature. But does this imply the legitimation of mastering nature, and if, to what an extent? Even when acknowledging the dialectical interwovenness of natural and artificial we have to concentrate on our perceptions of nature and culture. Could we perhaps focus on what might be called 'cultivation of (our) nature' and what it is comprised of? Does it mean (human) 'nature sometimes needs a little help' as it is articulated in an advertising slogan for egg-stimulation substances? And what is the content of that 'little' help? Does this help by so-called artificial means promote (human) nature in all its dimensions, the somatic, psychic, mental etc., or restrict because of resulting negative implications? Measuring technical interventions in our lives often leads to ambivalent judgements. There are fruitful, life-saving technical possibilities, which are performed, for example, in everyday medicine. There are developments which cause anxieties and fears and have no doubt problematic implications in application, not only supportive but really transforming potential for (human) nature – whatever it is, however it has been defined in our cultural traditions.

Kass has entitled one of his excellent papers about reproductive medicine 'The New Biology and the Old Morality' (Kass 1972). What is meant by talking of a new biology against the background of the old (-fashioned) morality? Is the biological base of humankind changeable and, if so, to what extent? How can we cope with the existing changes (in fact, with the possibilities as well as the realities in genetics, reproductive medicine, etc.) morally and ethically? Conditions – even biological conditions – have indeed changed to various degrees. Pregnancies for formerly inescapably childless couples have become a reality. Women aged over fifty years, men with low levels of motile sperm may be rendered fertile; this indicates medicine's success, but is it success only? For whom and at what costs has this success been achieved? Is it really possible to create a 'new biology' in sense of deeply changed human nature in terms of man-made human beings? Is 'old morality' further able to meet the challenges coming from the technical possibilities?

The task of philosophy or ethics should be in demonstrating that 'Technology is much more than technique' (Dyson 1995). Technology has indeed the potential to transform human nature, whatever it is. This potential may materialise according to our concepts of nature. Heidegger (1954) has explained philosophically which consequences creating and applying technology might have. Wherever we use technical means to achieve certain goals a transformation of 'nature' to 'substance' or 'material' is implied, what introduces a series of contingencies through that transformation. This process leads to what Heidegger calls the 'Gestell'. Technical transformation might cover the original way of existence in the world and the nature of things on earth. Unreflected application of technology might imply the loss of all memory of other kinds of being in the world. Nature would be regarded as a 'technicalised' reality hidden and altered in its substance. Whatever its substance is, it might be transformed, cultivated or ruined.

We have to be aware of that transformative potential and reflect upon the resulting implications. Very often man-made, technically produced things (products) would become more perfect, better controlled and therefore regarded superior to so called 'natural' ones. Pursuing this idea in the field of IVF might lead to the following appraisal articulated in an IVF-congress: 'In vitro better than in vivo'. This seems antithetical to the statement mentioned above: 'sometimes nature needs a little help'.

Valuing the natural as superior to the technical does not mean a step further in our discussion. The same is the case for the other reverse. Ambivalent relationship, dialectical interwovenness between nature and technology is the complex situation in which we find ourselves. In using technical means we should think about the desired goals and consequences on the way to achieving them. Technology has changed our world and ourselves. Technologically shaped realities influence in turn our perception and conception of nature. Technology has a persuasiveness which leads us to seek technological fixes. We tend to solve problems technically without thinking about problems which arise in other contexts and demand other problem-solving strategies than technical ones.

So technology might sometimes even be a means to hide problems behind its surface potential. By applying technology we often tend to define problems by reference to the capacities of technologies. The unquestioned adaptation of human acts and passions to the demands of technology, even their subordination, should be a task for philosophical criticism. Accepting and applying technology means creating new realities; our lives become more or less, consciously or subconsciously, modified. Reproductive medicine enables us to produce and control at will within a very intimate sphere, thus often not increasing but decreasing personal autonomy. The ethical assessment of technology, according to Henk ten Have (1995), is not another technical problem-solving strategy, but a critisism from a philosophical point of view, discussing our concepts of nature, culture, etc.

The increasing nature-mastering potential of our modern technology seems to open a wide, almost unlimited range of options for the individual, but creates at the same time dependency on technology and on the consequences of its application. In getting rid of restrictions given by nature we often get entangled in the implications of our options.

References

Dyson, A. (1995), *The Ethics of IVF*, Mowbray: London.

Kass, L.R. (1972), '«Making Babies» – The New Biology and the Old Morality', *The Public Interest*, Washington, pp. 18-56.
Heidegger, M. (1954), 'Die Frage nach der Technik', *Jahrbuch der Bayerischen Akademie der Schönen Künste*, Vol. 3, R. Oldenburg: München, p. 70 ff.
ten Have, H. (1995), 'Medical Technology Assessment and Ethics: Ambivalent Relations', *Hastings Center Report*, Vol. 25, No. 5, pp. 13-9.

7 Can nature serve as a criterium for the use of reproductive technologies?

Hub Zwart

Introduction

Contemporary ethical discourse is faced with a remarkable ambiguity. On the one hand, we find the human subject thoroughly de-naturalised. Self-determination is regarded as the starting-point for moral decision-making, human nature is reduced to being free and reasonable, and the idea that nature might serve as a criterium for moral behaviour or as a standard for moral guidance seems to have lost all credibility. On the other hand, however, we are faced with the opposite effort as well, namely to *naturalise* human beings, considering them solely in biological terms and reducing them to one particular species among others, displaying a life-pattern that can be described in purely instinctual terms.

A philosophical tradition of long standing, which apparently has fallen into oblivion (at least as far as medical ethics is concerned), tried to avoid both forms of one-sidedness by considering moral life in rational as well as in natural terms. It pointed out that to be rational basically means to organise one's life in accordance with nature. Human beings are not animals because they have the ability to shape their lives in an active, self-conscious and rational manner. Yet, their basic moral goals and objectives, the basic constituents of a full human life, must still be regarded as natural.

Several debates in contemporary ethics have been affected by the fundamental ambiguity described above. One of them is the debate which arose in 1993 when it was made public that in Italy, two elderly women who had passed the menopause (one of whom was fifty-nine and the other sixty-two) successfully applied for in vitro fertilisation (IVF) (Zwart 1994). Some participants in the ensuing debate claimed that menopausal IVF posed a threat to the physical well-being of the mother herself, who perhaps might not be able to physically cope with the burdens of pregnancy and delivery. Others claimed that having an elderly mother might (for several reasons) harm the psychological well-being of the off-spring. And finally, it was considered objectionable because menopausal pregnancy is against nature. The latter objection, however, which is the subject of my paper, entails a great number of difficult conceptual problems. What do we mean by nature? Is it not the basic goal of medicine to liberate us from the physical harms and restrictions caused by nature?

As a rule, the appeal to nature is not regarded as a convincing argument in contemporary bioethics. Rather, it is claimed that everything medicine does must be considered unnatural, that human self-determination ought to prevail over natural restrictions, and that mere biological facts can never be regarded as plausible arguments in a secular ethical debate. At times, it is even demanded that the concept of nature be excluded from the vocabulary of ethics. I agree that the debate triggered by the claim that menopausal IVF must be regarded as unnatural, was confused and unsatisfactory from the outset, due to conceptual obscurities surrounding the moral significance of nature. We no longer seem to know what nature is. Still, I am convinced that the exclusion of nature as a concept from our moral vocabulary would entail a deplorable impoverishment of moral language, thereby reducing our ability to articulate important aspects of moral experience. In order to become employable, the concept of nature is in need of thorough philosophical reconsideration. Most notably, we must be aware of the fact that in the course of history several incompatible *models of understanding nature*, several incompatible *possibilities of experiencing nature* have emerged. These models have profoundly influenced moral reflection on the relationship between medicine and nature up to the present. They are bound to interpret arguments concerning nature in heterogeneous and divergent ways. In my paper, two models will be introduced, an ancient and a modern one. Moreover, the present ignorance of nature with regard to assisted procreation will be compared to a rather similar experience in the nineteenth century. Finally, I will argue that, rather than unequivocally enhancing human liberation, the on-going eclipse of nature will produce unprecedented *forms* of dependence and restriction of its own.

Nature and medicine: an ancient perspective

In the first book of his *Politics*, Aristotle (1982) claims that man and wife, unable to exist without one another, are bound to seek each other's company, for the sake of the continuance of the species, out of a natural drive humans share with other animals. Likewise, in a famous passage of his *Summa Theologica*, Thomas Aquinas (1922, I-II 94,2) acknowledges that the natural inclination to secure the future existence of the human race and to care for one's off-spring must be regarded as one of the basic moral objectives of humankind. Yet, both Aristotle and Thomas emphasise that this inclination, although similar to the instinct of procreation encountered in the animal world, is to be moulded and cultivated in a human way. In the *Nicomachean Ethics*, for example, Aristotle points out that (unlike animals) humankind does not display natural behavioural patterns automatically. Although we are naturally *inclined* to realise our natural moral goals (such as procreation), we have to resort to education and culture in order to do so in a truly human – that is: virtuous – manner. This does not imply, however, that procreation thereby becomes unnatural.

In short, nature counted as a basic principle in ancient ethical discourse. The basic attitude of respect towards nature, the basic willingness to comply with nature also emerged in ancient moral discourse on medicine. According to Hippocrates, medicine aims at serving rather than at mastering nature and in the second book of his *Physics*, Aristotle (1980, B 1) uses medicine to explain the difference between the natural and the technical (cf. Heidegger 1967). According to Aristotle, nature is the basic principle of health. If a physician successfully treats a patient, the patient's health has two causes: a natural and a technical one. Yet, the technical cause (medical treatment) would be of no avail if it did not comply with and rely on the natural tendency of the body itself to restore its health. The art of medicine is in support of and complimentary to nature, and nature remains the basic standard for medical practice. Medicine basically aims at restoring the body's natural condition – health. If, to take a more or less modern example, a patient suffers from a complicated fracture of the leg that will not allow for spontaneous recovery, the act of hammering a metal pin into the patient's limb must not be regarded as unnatural. Rather, the intervention will allow nature to resume its salutary work, and the whole process of healing and recovery basically remains a natural one.

What does such a view imply when it comes to assessing IVF? As we have seen, the Aristotelian-Thomistic view acknowledges a limited range of natural human pursuits, directed at achieving certain natural moral objectives, with the implication that the basic conditions of life are similar for all of us. Human life displays a common moral pattern. In the case of medicine, an intervention is justified if the effort to realise these basic human goals or goods will be enhanced by it, if human flourishing will be supported by it. In principle, therefore, an Aristotelian-Thomistic view will be in support of IVF because it intends to enable the woman involved to realise a basic moral goal of life. Moreover, one could argue that the medical intervention does not render the pregnancy as such unnatural, but will rather allow nature to resume its course and sway once the woman in question has become artificially impregnated. Although highly technological in itself, the intervention is still in service of and in compliance with nature.

Yet, to all the goals of life, there is a season. The idea of human flourishing, of a full human life, entails the idea of human finitude. Those who allowed the natural opportunity to realise one of their basic moral goal to pass, should not turn to medicine with the intention of violating the natural patterns and cycles of bodily life. If an elderly woman who has reached the menopause at a normal age applies for IVF in order to fulfil her wish to bear a child, such an intervention will be considered as unnatural in view of the fact that infertility due to having reached the menopause cannot be regarded as pathological or premature ('praecox'). Menopausal IVF would imply mastery of, rather than compliance with nature. It is not the intervention in itself which is regarded as unnatural, but rather the manner in which it is used, the objective supported by it, the stance towards nature implied in it.

In other words, the ancient perspective entails a distinction between two basic attitudes towards bodily life, which can be referred to as *management* and *mastery*. In the one case ('management'), we use medicine to shape our physical existence in compliance with the natural patterns and cycles of bodily life. In the latter ('mastery'), however, these patterns and cycles are overruled and regarded as morally insignificant, they are subordinated to human self-determination. Rather than allowing nature to take its course, the technical takes precedence over the natural and our dependence on medical technology and expertise takes precedence over our dependence on nature.

Nature and medicine: a modern perspective

The model described above excels in respect for and reliance on nature. There is another model, however, another basic possibility of experiencing nature which discerns that, rather than being the principal cause of health, nature is what causes the disease. And rather than trying to comply with nature, nature has to be mastered in order for human life to flourish. Allow me to exemplify this model by means of an example.

In his poem *The Anatomy of the World* John Donne (1572-1631) makes a crushing diagnosis regarding the physical condition of nature. Our natural world, he claims, is thoroughly corrupted and putrefied. Both nature at large and the bodily life of man suffer from a 'sicknesse without remedie'. Whoever is born into this world, will find himself intrinsically damaged. The best we can hope to achieve is absence of disease, but we will never enjoy true health:

> There is no health; Physitians say that wee,
> At best, enjoy but a neutralitie.
> And can there be worse sicknesse, then to know
> That we are never well, nor can be so? (91-94)

In one of his sermons he provides a commentary to these lines: '*Non sanitas*, there is no health in *any*, so universall is sickness; nor at *any time* in any so universall; and so universall too, as that *not in any part* of any man, at any time' (Allen 1975, p.96). Further on in the *Anatomy of the World*, Donne claims that every part of our natural frame is maimed:

> Then, as mankinde, so is the worlds whole frame
> Quite out of joynt, almost created lame...
> The world did in her cradle take a fall,
> and turn her braines, and took a generall maime,
> Wronging each joynt of th'universall frame... (191-198)

Whereas the general physical condition of humankind is deplorable, the worst intrinsic deficiency is the brevity of life:

> Alas, we scarce live long enough to try
> Whether a true made clocke run right, or lie...
> So short is life, that every peasant strives,
> In a torn house, or field, to have three lives. (129-134)

The traditional (Hippocratic) methods to regain one's health by restoring the body's natural condition of balance ('health') are to be considered futile, for the harm is not caused by any specific form of lack or excess, but by the miserable, congenital condition of the body as a whole:

> [This] worlds generall sicknesse doth not lie
> In any humour, or one certain part;
> But as thou sawest it rotten at the heart,
> Thou seest a Hectique feaver hath got hold
> Of the whole substance, not to be contrould. (240-244)

Measure and balance are absent – *proportion is dead*. In other words, whereas the sixteenth century still to a considerable extent relied on Hippocratic medicine, and Donne himself was fairly aquainted with Renaissance medical philosophy (most notably with Paracelsus, cf. Allen 1975), he appears to us very much as someone belonging to the era of the dawn of modern science. His poetry is modern to the extent that the time-old Christian theorem about the decay of the world and the corruption of nature, due to man's original sin, no longer seems to be moderated or toned down by a more positive, medieval, Aristotelian-Thomistic counter-point. The idea *as such* of the depravity of nature, is of course Biblical – cf. Ps. 38,3: 'There is no soundness in my flesh', 'Non est sanitas in carne mea' (Milgate, 1978, p.133). What is new in Donne's poem is the radical, one-sided way the frailty and evil of the natural world and body is being exposed. The attitude articulated in his poem, derived from a Christian origin but reformulated and reinforced in the seventeenth century, encouraged a new way of perceiving the body, and eventually encouraged the emergence of a new science of medicine.

Donne was very much concerned with health, both personally and in general. Allen (1975) stresses that he was more interested in 'the intrinsic agonies of his own viscera' than in anything else:

> Were all biographical evidence wanting and the corpus of Donne's work reduced to just the poetry and sermons, we should not hesitate to label him as a valetudinarian. Medical data, anatomical terminology, physiological theory, apothecary's 'drug tongue', and physician's jargon elbow from the pages... [in the sermons] he unwinds his medical knowledge to the delight of the hypochondriacs of his parish... The *Devotions Upon Emergent Occasions* is a fine clinical account of the progress of an illness; the *Letters to Severall Persons of Honour* contain many reports of Donne's maladies. (p. 93)

His trust in medicine, however, was still rather limited and he considered 'ignorant, and torturing Physitians' as one of the scourges sent to us by God. One of his poems, the *Devotions*, is referred to by Allen as a 'treatise on the futility of medicine'.

It is obvious that the basic experience of nature articulated in Donne's poem is out of tune with the ancient one previously described. Health and well-being are no longer regarded as part of our natural condition. Rather, nature is sickening. In order to improve our physical condition, Donne urges us to rely on God. Only God can save us and the prospects for medicine are rather bad. Due to the growth of medical knowledge, however, the expectation that nature's sickening sway *can* be diminished by relying on the benefits of medicine, has gained much ground since then. In other words, the model articulated in a cheerless tone of voice by Donne, suffered a secular, anthropocentric and rather optimistic turn, but its assessment of nature remained similar to the one developed within its original, theocentric and much more pessimistic version.

In view of the subject matter of this paper it is interesting to note that at a certain point, Donne utters the claim that, ever since the fall, the seasons of our world deteriorated and became like the sons 'of women after fifty':

> So did the world from the first houre decay,
> That evening was beginning of the day,
> And now the Springs and Summers which we see,
> Like sonnes of women after fifty bee. (201-204)

Whereas Donne's complaint about the deterioration of the seasons goes back to the Church Father St Cyprian, it was Pliny who said that a woman does not bear children after the year of fifty (Milgate, 1978, p.140). Menopausal IVF not only aims at providing women after fifty with the possibility of bearing children (a possibility denied to them by nature), but also at foregoing the natural deterioration of the healthiness of an elderly woman's off-spring, hinted at by Donne.

In the current debate on IVF in elderly woman, as well as in other debates concerning IVF (or other forms of assisted procreation), a Donne-like understanding of nature still appears to be at work. Nature is regarded as the cause of human illness and fragility, as the source of our physical malaise, and as the origin of severe restrictions on human flourishing and self-determination. Medicine has to explore nature in order to conquer it, control it, so that human freedom and happiness become attainable. Nature is the cause of human infertility problems, most notably of the fact that humans as a species are remarkably infertile as compared to other species. Indeed, during this very conference, several contributions seemed to concur with the understanding of nature in terms of deficiency, restriction, deterioration and malaise. For example, at a certain point during the discussion, our colleague Farhan Yazdani from Annecy stated that 'as human beings we are prisoners of nature; someone who has an infertility problem is a prisoner of nature'.

Although it was John Donne's sincere conviction that only God can save us, I already pointed out that subsequent generations increasingly relied on science and reason. During recent decades, complete mastery of nature became medicine's ultimate objective. And rather than relying on nature as a moral argument, self-determination became the principal standard of ethics. Medicine has the fundamental right to restore the intrinsic harms of nature. And since the intrinsic finitude of life is regarded as harmful, the elderly woman has a right to demand a second life (the principle of self-determination). Although certain restrictions can and must be imposed on the principle of self-determination, these restrictions cannot be derived from the natural patterns and cycles of bodily life. Rather, they have to be formulated in terms of harm (to self or others) and scarcity. Only if harmful consequences, either for herself or for the child, would undeniably result from her decision (the harm principle), or if other human beings, whose health care needs are regarded by society as more urgent and pressing, would be put at a disadvantage by it (the distributive justice principle), the right to exercise her freedom by applying for IVF could be denied to her. In short, the right to self-determination entails the right to counter the intrinsic harms of nature, such as the natural limits to fertility. Nature, being deficient in itself, cannot provide medicine with a moral standard, nor can it offer moral guidance.

The Donne poem reveals that the apparent optimism of modern medicine is grounded in a basic attitude of pessimism and distrust, and that the utopian prospects fostered by modern medicine, originate from a rather negative assessment of the quality of a more natural kind of life. Due to nature, the success rate of natural human intercourse is deplorable when compared to those of other animals, and human beings are among the least fertile of all mammals. Nature is the cause of the problem, technology the solution. Nature is the origin of disease, technology is the cause of health and we have to rely on medicine in order to counter the threats and harms inherent in nature. The principal form of natural malaise is our inability to pursue certain basic goals of life (such as the reproduction of an off-spring of one's own), either due to our infertility problems, or to the brevity of human life (in combination with the exactingness of other life goals, most notably the will to excel in one's professional career). The freedom to pursue these goals, denied to us by nature, is restored by medicine; for example by allowing us to become pregnant at a time when, having successfully lived through the decisive years of our professional career, we are finally in the position to broaden the scope of our life goals. To a certain extent, this possibility of experiencing nature, either in its original, pessimistic version or in its more modern, optimistic version, will strike us as plausible and convincing. Yet, we also remain aware of the fact that it cannot be the whole story. A sense of unease is bound to emerge if nature is ignored or eclipsed completely.

The eclipse of nature

To every thing, there is a season. In the sixties, this phrase from the Scriptures (Eccl. 3,1-2), quite in tune with the traditional stance towards nature described above, became the opening line of a very famous song. It seems to convey a cyclical, natural way of experiencing time and human existence, one intimately connected with traditional forms of agriculture and social or family life. To everything, there is a season; a time to sow, a time to reap – a time to procreate. Menopausal IVF seems to be quite at odds with this traditional possibility of experiencing nature. Nowadays we ask ourselves why a medical treatment, readily offered to a woman of thirty-five, should be denied to a woman who is twenty years her senior?

This attitude of ignoring nature is the outcome of a long, historical development. In the previous section, one chapter of this history was briefly summarised. During the first half of the nineteenth century, however, the negative assessment of nature expressed by Donne came to be reinforced in a decisive manner. In those days, a remarkable perplexity concerning the significance of nature occurred in the field of labour, a perplexity rather similar to the one we now experience with regard to IVF – and I cannot refrain from briefly referring to this historical episode.

Due to the Industrial Revolution, the natural distinction between day and night, between childhood and adulthood was rendered obsolete and had to be replaced by an exact definition of what constitutes a working day, by an exact demarcation between productive and reproductive time.[1] In chapter 8 of his book *The Capital* Karl Marx (1962) described the fierce political struggles which evolved over the definition of a 'natural' working day. Initially, a natural working day was said to contain twelve hours. Subsequently, factory owners managed to extend it to sixteen hours. The labour movement, however, protested against such a bold and violent transgression of 'natural' restrictions on the exploitation of bodily resources. Gradually, it managed to reduce it to eight hours. Yet, the awareness that all limits are arbitrary and open to negotiation, had become almost self-evident by then.

A similar struggle occurred with regard to the natural age at which someone could be regarded as fit for work. As Marx cynically points out, nineteenth-century capitalism refrained from 'discrimination on the ground of age' (p.269). All individuals, including children, were granted the 'liberty' to enter the labour market. Indeed, the factory owners managed to have it established as a standard that the natural transition from childhood to adulthood occurred at the age of twelve. Gradually, the labour movement succeeded in postponing it to the age of sixteen. Still, all traditional natural restrictions on productive time, all natural distinctions between day and night, childhood and adulthood became useless and meaningless. They had to be determined in an exact and arbitrary manner, they became the temporary outcome of a process of political struggle and negotiation.

In the course of the nineteenth century, as the living conditions of the labour population, extremely deplorable at first, gradually ameliorated, another question had to be raised: should there be a natural age limit to productive labour? In Germany, Bismarck was the first to establish such a limit. At the age of sixty-five, the labour population, instead of being expected to work, was afforded with a pension. The reason for setting the limit at this particular age was that in those days, only twenty per cent of the working population was expected to reach the age of sixty-five. By that time, the risk of having to provide a former labourer with a pension had become acceptably low.

Why do I commemorate all this? To begin with, it seems that underneath the socio-economical development called the Industrial Revolution, a conceptual transition occurred among the popular masses of Europe from a more or less traditional understanding of nature, intimately connected with traditional forms of agriculture, to an unprecedented one, an understanding of nature (and this includes the human body) in terms of resources, open to technological exploitation. An understanding which was aimed at exhausting natural or bodily possibilities to the full, ignoring any inherent restrictions to industrial expenditure whatsoever. The kind of society which emerged in the course of the nineteenth century throughout Europe, entailed a basic understanding of, a basic stance or attitude towards nature, a basic possibility of experiencing nature. Nature and natural bodies were transformed into a huge collection of natural resources deprived of intrinsic value.

The second reason for drawing attention to the historical debate just mentioned is that nowadays we seem to be faced with a somewhat similar debate. In the Netherlands, the commission for medical ethics of the Royal Dutch Society of Medicine (KNMG) recently tried to establish an age limit to IVF and concluded that, notwithstanding a certain unease with regard to menopausal IVF (due to the impression that natural limits are being ignored), all efforts to determine a natural age limit for the use of IVF must be regarded as futile, because all age limits are ultimately arbitrary (KNMG 1996, Zwart 1996). Rather than being derived from a profound understanding of what nature is, age limits must be based on the opinions of medical, ethical and other experts with regard to the potential harms inflicted, either on the woman herself, the child, or society at large. Nature can no longer serve as a standard for decision-making in medical practice. Instead, we become dependent on the (ultimately arbitrary) judgements of expert committees.

Discussion

Whenever nature emerges as an argument in contemporary bioethics, we have to be conscious of the fact that incompatible models for moral assessment are involved. Those who feel more are at home in the one, will never be completely convinced by arguments derived from the other, and vice versa. If the incompatibility of both models or attitudes is being neglected, the debate becomes confused and unsatisfactory. Awareness of their incompatibility, therefore, and of the original profoundness of both, although it will not allow us to solve the problem, will at least allow us to improve the quality of the debate. Whenever the nature-argument arises, the question is: whose nature, which nature? Incompatible understandings are at stake. I suspect no one will be completely engrossed in the one and completely indifferent to the other. Rather, both attitudes, both possibilities of experience are present in all of us.

Although this kind of analysis cannot answer the question whether postmenopausal IVF is illicit or unreasonable, it helps us to formulate another question, namely whether (from an ethical point of view) postmenopausal IVF constitutes a *different kind* of intervention as compared to other forms of medical practice (such as IVF in younger women). It provides us with a conceptual distinction between management and mastery of nature that will be considered viable by protagonists of the one model of assessment, and irrelevant by proponents of the other. Several answers to the question what nature is – a standard for moral behaviour, a sickening environment, or a resource for exploitation – are possible, and menopausal IVF is in agreement with some answers rather than with others. It unequivocally implies a mastery-stance towards nature. But this is not the only possibility of experiencing nature. Indeed, it is my contention that, in a comprehensive view of nature, the understanding of nature as that which provides us with basic possibilities of human existence (such as procreation) ought to take precedence over the understanding of nature as the cause of our restrictions and malaise. More important still, a philosophical analysis reveals that the modern model, rather than liberating us from all limits, confronts us with new forms of limit and restriction, imposed by human judgement. The modern experience of nature has made us increasingly dependent on scientific, technological and ethical expertise.

Therefore, the opposition between ancient and modern possibilities of experiencing nature must not be identified with the opposition between restriction and freedom. Rather, the modern stance towards nature (either as a sickening environment or as a natural resource for exploitation) introduces new *forms* of restriction of its own. Forms of restriction, moreover, which might eventually turn out to be more compelling that the ancient ones. In the case of IVF in elderly woman, medical, psychological, juridical, economical and ethical experts, assembled in hospital or government committees, will set new limits. They will determine what needs and preferences can be regarded as reasonable. Human decisions, that is, will impose new and artificial boundaries and restrictions. Moreover, menopausal IVF might perhaps make it more difficult for individuals to accept the fact that they will have no children, or to resist the increasing demand to keep their bodies completely available for participation in professional life when they are in their thirties or forties. This does not imply, of course, that IVF ought to be banned completely, or something like that. Rather, a philosophical reconsideration might trigger our responsiveness to important aspects of the case which tend to be neglected by 'normal' bioethical discourse.

Notes

1 'Nachdem das Kapital Jahrhunderte gebraucht, um den Arbeitstag bis zu seinem normalen Maximalgrenzen und dann über diese hinaus, bis zu den Grenzen des natürlichen Tags von 12 Stunden zu verlängern, erfolgte nun, seit der Geburt der großen Industrie im letzten Drittel das 18. Jahrhunderts, eine lawinenartig gewaltsame und maßlose Überstürzung. Jede Schranke von Sitte und Natur, Alter und Geschlecht, Tag und Nacht, wurde zertrümmert. Selbst die Begriffe von Tag und Nacht, bäuerlich einfach in den alten Statuten, verschwammen so sehr, daß ein englischer Richter noch

1860 wahrhaft talmudistischen Scharfsinn aufbieten mußte, um «urteilskräftig» zu erklären, was Tag und Nacht sei' (Marx, 1962, p.294).

References

Allen, D.C. (1975), 'John Donne's Knowledge of Renaissance Medicine', in Roberts, J. (ed.), *Essential Articles for the Study of John Donne's Poetry*, The Harvester Press: Columbia, pp. 93-106.

Aquinas, T. (1922), *Summa Theologica* (6 volumes), Marietti: Taurini.

Aristoteles (1980), *Physics 1-4*, The Loeb Classical Library 4, Harvard University Press: Cambridge / Heinemann: London.

Aristoteles (1982), *Politics 1-8*, The Loeb Classical Library 21, Harvard University Press: Cambridge / Heinemann: London.

Donne, J. (1912/1953), 'An Anatomie of the World. Wherein, by the Occasion of the Untimely Death of Mistris Elisabeth Drury, the Frailty and the Decay of This Whole World is Represented (The First Anniversary)', in Grierson, H. (ed.), *The Poems of John Donne, Vol. 1*, Oxford University Press: Oxford; Cumberlege: London, pp. 229-45.

Heidegger, M. (1967), 'Vom Wesen und Begriff der *Physis*. Aristoteles' Physik B, 1', in *Wegmarken*, Klostermann: Frankfurt am Main.

KNMG (1996), 'IVF op latere leeftijd', *Medisch Contact*, Vol. 51, No. 18, pp. 620-7.

Marx, K. (1962), *Das Kapital 1* (MEW), Dietz Verlag: Berlin.

Milgate, W. (1978), *John Donne. The Epithalamions, Anniversaries and Epicedes. Edited with Introduction and Commentary*, Clarendon Press: Oxford.

Zwart, H. (1994), 'De morele betekenis van onze biologische natuur: ethische aspecten van postmenopauzaal moederschap', *Tijdschrift voor Geneeskunde en Ethiek*, Vol. 4, No. 2, pp. 39-42.

Zwart, H. (1996), 'De natuur heeft zich van ons afgekeerd. Over het standpunt van de Commissie Medische Ethiek van de KNMG inzake postmenopauzale IVF', *Tijdschrift voor Gerontologie en Geriatrie*, Vol. 27, No. 3, pp. 94-6.

Index